Breast Cancer Nursing Care and Management

Second Edition

Edited by

Victoria Harmer

RN, BSc (Hons), Diploma (Breast Care), MBA, AKC
Clinical Nurse Specialist
Breast Care Unit
Imperial College Healthcare NHS Trust
London, UK

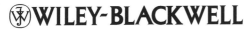
A John Wiley & Sons, Ltd., Publication

Library of Congress Cataloging-in-Publication Data
Breast Cancer Nursing Care and Management / edited by Victoria Harmer. – 2nd ed.
     p. ; cm.
   Includes bibliographical references and index.
   ISBN 978-1-4051-9866-0 (pbk. : alk. paper)   1. Breast–Cancer.   2. Breast–Diseases–Nursing.
3. Cancer–Nursing.   I. Harmer, Victoria.
   [DNLM: 1. Breast Neoplasms–nursing.   2. Breast Neoplasms–therapy.   3. Oncologic Nursing–methods.
WP 870]
RC280.B8B6728   2011
616.99′449–dc22

                                                                                                    2010031133

A catalogue record for this book is available from the British Library.

Set in 10/12 pt Times by Aptara® Inc., New Delhi, India

1   2011

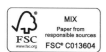

Contents

Colour plate section follows page 114

Preface

Although there is much literature available for people with breast cancer, there are very few books for nurses and other health-care professionals.

Breast cancer is increasing in prevalence as the population ages. One in six women has a first-degree relative with breast cancer. This book aims to provide a well-balanced approach to all aspects of management of this malignancy. Generalities are not enough. Expert nurses in these topics deal with the specific details of special care. However, the importance of writing from a complete nursing perspective is underlined so that the essence of support and bedside care is not missed.

This book teaches us about breast cancer treatments, and how to manage, nurse and empower patients through each modality, as well as how to give sound, evidence-based information on possible side effects and how to combat them.

Nurses need to have the necessary information to enable seamless, individualised treatment for the patient. This book is applicable to any stage of the cancer journey, from the biological aspects of care to the psychological issues for people facing this potentially life-threatening disease.

This comprehensive handbook has been updated to act as a resource for any nurse or health-care professional caring for a person with breast cancer.

Victoria Harmer

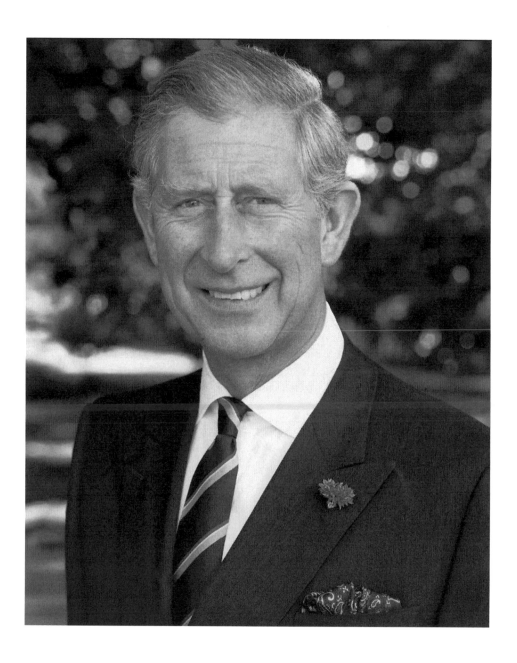

It is of immense concern to us all that nearly 46,000 women are diagnosed with breast cancer in the UK every year. While the statistics speak volumes, there is nothing like first-hand experience to bring home the truly devastating effects of the disease – at some stage in our lives most of us will meet or know someone who has been diagnosed with cancer.

As Patron of Breakthrough Breast Cancer, and through witnessing the work of the many Hospices with which I am closely involved, I have seen the terrible toll that breast cancer has taken.

Expert nursing care at this time is fundamental to treatment and recovery. Only with a thorough understanding of the disease and the treatments available, including appropriate complementary therapies, can nurses ensure that each patient receives the best individualized care at this distressing and difficult time.

I am delighted that Victoria Harmer and her team of contributors have produced a book that will help nurses to understand thoroughly not only the physical aspects of the disease and its treatment, but also the emotional stresses faced by people with breast cancer, and so be able to offer relief, practical help and comfort. I am sure this inspiring book could become a handbook for every breast cancer nurse in the UK.

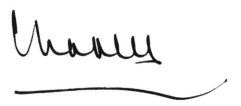

Words of Encouragement for Nurses

If it wasn't for your commitment to helping the needy, the world would certainly be a far crueller place. Your role in the fight against breast cancer starts from day one. You have the power to save a person from giving into the disease. It is your encouragement, patience and support which is invaluable . . . thank you.

Warm regards

Stella
Stella McCartney

Contributors

Chapter 1 An Overview of the Breast and Breast Cancer
Elisabeth Grimsey RN, MSc, Macmillan Consultant Nurse – Breast Care, East Sussex Hospitals NHS Trust

Chapter 2 The Histopathology of Breast Cancer
Helen E. Froyd RGN, BSc (Hons), Dip (Onc), MSc, Advanced Nurse Practitioner – Breast Care, Guy's and St. Thomas' NHS Foundation Trust, London

Victoria Harmer RN, BSc (Hons), Dip (Br Ca), MBA, AKC, Clinical Nurse Specialist – Breast Care, Imperial College Healthcare NHS Trust, London

Chapter 3 Genetic Factors in Breast Cancer
Audrey Ardern-Jones RGN, MSc, Dip (N), Genetics Cert, Nurse Specialist in Cancer, Genetics/Associate Lecturer in Cancer Genetics, The Royal Marsden NHS Foundation Trust, Sutton

Chapter 4 Breast Screening
Ann-Marie Fretwell BHSC, PgA, Lead Mammography Educator, Nottingham Breast Institute, Nottingham

(previous contribution by) Linda Lee DCR Med, Radiographic Services Manager, Breast Directorate, Nottingham City Hospital NHS Trust

Chapter 5 Surgery for Breast Cancer
Victoria Harmer RN, BSc (Hons), Dip (Br Ca), MBA, AKC, Clinical Nurse Specialist – Breast Care, Imperial College Healthcare NHS Trust, London

Chapter 6 Physiotherapy for Patients with Breast Cancer
Helen Macleod MCSP SRP, Senior Physiotherapist, The Royal Marsden NHS Foundation Trust, Sutton

Pauline Koelling MCSP SRP, Formerly Senior Physiotherapist, The Royal Marsden NHS Foundation Trust, London

Chapter 7 Breast Reconstruction
Nicola West RGN, BN, PGFETC(cert ed), MA, Consultant Nurse/Lecturer Practitioner, Cardiff and Vale University Health Board, Wales

Chapter 8 Chemotherapy as a Treatment for Breast Cancer
Dr Elaine Lennan D ClinP RGN Onc Cert BN, MSc, Consultant Nurse, Southampton University Hospitals Trust, Southampton

(previous contribution by) Joan Klein née McCoy RGN Onc Cert, BSc (Hons), PgDip, Consultant Nurse, Imperial College Healthcare NHS Trust, London

Chapter 9 Radiotherapy as a Treatment for Breast Cancer
Karen Burnet MSc, BSc, RGN, CRUK Senior Research Nurse, Cambridge University Hospitals Trust, Cambridge

Chapter 10 Endocrine Treatment for Breast Cancer
Dr Deborah Fenlon RGN, Senior Research Fellow, Macmillan Survivorship Research Group, School of Health Sciences, University of Southampton, Southampton

Kay Townsend RCN, BSc (hons), Lecturer, School of Health Sciences, University of Southampton, Southampton

Chapter 11 Lymphoedema and Breast Cancer
Mary Woods BSc (Hons), MSc, RGN Onc Cert, Clinical Nurse Specialist – Head of Lymphoedema Services, The Royal Marsden NHS Foundation Trust, Sutton

Chapter 12 Fungating Wounds
Victoria Harmer RN, BSc (Hons), Dip (Br Ca), MBA, AKC, Clinical Nurse Specialist – Breast Care, Imperial College Healthcare NHS Trust, London

(previous contribution by) Rachael King RN, BSc (Hons), Formerly Clinical Nurse Specialist – Tissue Viability, St Mary's Hospital NHS Trust, London

Chapter 13 Advanced Disease
Elizabeth Sumner RN, BA (Hons), Dip (N), Clinical Nurse Specialist – Palliative Care, Watford General Hospital, Watford

Chapter 14 Complementary and Alternative Therapies
Rosemary Lucey RGN, RMN, Head of Centre, Lynda Jackson Macmillan Centre, Mount Vernon Hospital, Middlesex

Chapter 15 Psychological Issues for the Patient with Breast Cancer
Jane Rogers SEN, RN Dip (Onc), MSc, Specialist Breast Care Nurse, Lancashire Teaching Hospitals NHS, Foundation Trust, Lancashire

Dr Mary Turner RGN, BA (Hons), Research Fellow, International Observatory on End of Life Care, Lancaster University, Lancaster

Chapter 16 Survivorship Issues
Dr Carmel Sheppard RGN, BSc (Hons), MSc, Dip (Counselling), DBMS, Consultant Nurse – Breast Care, Portsmouth Hospitals NHS, Trust/University of Southampton

Chapter 17 Specialist Nursing Roles: What Are the Challenges?
Dr Emma Pennery RGN, MSc, Clinical Director, Breast Cancer Care

Acknowledgements

I have been lucky with the calibre of the contributors and would like to thank them for agreeing to be part of this second edition. This book would not be possible without them; they are the prominent names in breast care nursing, and it is their expertise and reputation that makes this book so robust.

I am also grateful for the continued support of His Royal Highness The Prince of Wales and Stella McCartney.

A special mention should go to Mr D.J. Hadjiminas and my colleagues in the breast unit at Imperial College Healthcare NHS Trust, and thanks to my family – my parents, Lola and Rex.

This book is a tribute to the wonderful patients that it has been my privilege to meet.

1 An Overview of the Breast and Breast Cancer

Elisabeth Grimsey

INTRODUCTION

Breast Cancer is the most common cancer in women in the UK, with a lifetime risk of 1 in 9 (Cancer Research UK, 2009). Approximately 44 000 women are diagnosed annually in the UK. It is therefore very likely that most nurses will find that they will care for women with breast cancer at some point in their career or will have a personal connection with someone who has breast cancer.

Worldwide, breast cancer has a high media and political profile. October is breast cancer awareness month, which is hard to escape anyone's attention. Magazines, broadsheets and tabloids alike will have articles about breast cancer, people come to work dressed in pink for 'Wear it Pink' day, and the shops are adorned with pink ribbons and pink products. With women forming a large proportion of the voting public, breast cancer and breast cancer screening is high on the political agenda.

Women are increasingly well informed about breast cancer and its treatments. Therefore, to nurse these women with care and understanding, it is vital to have a good theoretical and practical working knowledge regarding the breast, breast cancer and treatments.

This chapter will look at the anatomy and physiology of the normal breast, the incidence and aetiology of breast cancer, the risk factors of developing breast cancer, the diagnostic pathway, certain characteristics of breast cancer and the staging of breast cancer.

ANATOMY AND PHYSIOLOGY OF THE BREAST

Breast development

The breasts, also known as the mammary glands, exist in both males and females but are only usually enlarged in the woman. The breasts begin to develop in the foetus at around the seventh week of gestation and progress to the budding stage at the twelfth week. They are formed from the ectodermal mammary ridge that runs from the axilla to the groin, often referred to as the nipple line. Between weeks 13 and 20, the epithelial bud branches and canalises to form the 16–20 major ducts found in the adult breast.

Occasionally at birth, a baby may produce a small amount of milk. This is due to high levels of luteal and placental hormones crossing the placenta and entering the foetal

Breast Cancer Nursing Care and Management, Second Edition, Edited by Victoria Harmer
© 2011 by Blackwell Publishing Ltd.

circulation during the late stage of pregnancy thus stimulating the foetal breast. At birth, the foetal and maternal circulatory systems are separated, resulting in the rapid fall of sex steroids in the baby's blood, whereas the baby's pituitary gland continues to secrete prolactin. The baby's prolactin level then declines and the secretions dry up. This is classed as a normal physiological event. Accessory nipples may also be found along the ectodermal ridge, most commonly below the normal breast. These are harmless and only need to be removed if they cause distress to the individual.

Changes at puberty

The female breast starts to change at the time of puberty. The pituitary gland begins to produce the gonadotrophins, follicle stimulating hormone (FSH) and luteinising hormone (LH). As the levels of these hormones rise, the egg follicles within the ovary start to produce oestrogen, which is responsible for the first stages of breast development. At around the age of 10 years old, the mammary tissue behind the nipple enlarges, producing the characteristic swelling referred to as a breast bud that may often be asymmetrical. Oestrogen also induces the connective tissue and vascular growth that is required to support the ductal system. The connective tissue in turn stimulates fat deposition. Once the ovulation cycles begin, the increased output of progesterone balances the oestrogen output and results in the maturation of the glandular tissue (Hughes *et al.*, 2000).

Anatomy of the adult breast

Gross structure

The breasts are situated on either side of the sternum between the second and sixth rib, overlying the pectoralis major muscle. The shape of the breast is hemispherical with a tail of tissue extending into the axilla, known as the tail of Spence. They are stabilised by a suspensory ligament known as Cooper's ligament, named after Sir Astley Cooper. The size of the breast will vary with the stage of development and age and will also vary between individuals. It is common to have one breast slightly larger than the other.

Centrally on each breast lies the nipple–areola complex. The areola is the pigmented circular area, measuring approximately 2.5 cm in diameter. The colour varies from pale pink in fair-skinned women to dark brown in dark-skinned women and will darken during pregnancy. On the surface of the areola are a number of small protuberances known as Montgomery's tubercles, which are modified sebaceous glands whose purpose is to lubricate the nipple during lactation. The nipple lies in the centre of the areola and is approximately 6 mm in length. The surface of the nipple is perforated by the openings of the lactiferous ducts. The nipple–areola complex is rich in smooth muscle fibres, which are responsible for nipple erection.

Microscopic structure

The breast is composed of fibrous, glandular and fatty tissue and is covered by the skin.

Fibrous bands divide the glandular tissue into approximately 16–20 lobes. Clinical findings, however, find the number to be more in the region of 7–8 lobes (Hughes *et al.*, 2000). Within each lobe is the milk-producing system. The lobe contains up to 40 lobules that contain 10–100 alveoli (or acini) which are the milk-secreting cells. The alveloi are

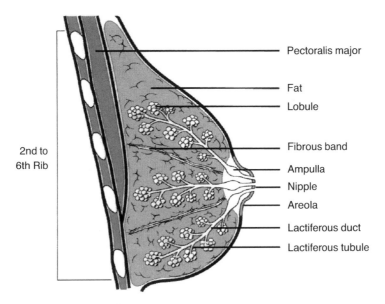

Fig. 1.1   Microscopic structure of the breast.

connected to lactiferous tubules, which in turn connect to the lactiferous duct, which is lined with epithelial cells. The lactiferous duct runs up towards the nipple and, when approaching the nipple, widens to form the ampulla, which acts as a reservoir for the milk to be stored. The lactiferous duct than continues on from the ampulla to open out onto the surface of the nipple (Fig. 1.1).

The glandular tissue of the breast is surrounded by fat. If weight is lost or gained, the breast will vary in size.

Blood supply

The blood supply is from the axillary artery and the internal mammary artery. The venous drainage is through the corresponding vessels into the internal mammary and axillary veins.

Nerve supply

The nerve supply to the breast is mainly from the somatic sensory nerves and the autonomic nerves accompanying the blood vessels. The most sensitive part of the breast is the nipple–areola complex, which is supplied by the somatic sensory nerves. The rest of the breast is supplied by the autonomic supply.

The somatic sensory supply is served via the supra-clavicular nerves (C3, C4) superiorly and laterally from the lateral branches of the thoracic intercostal nerve (3rd and 4th). The medial aspects of the breast receive supply from the anterior branches of the thoracic intercostal nerves, which penetrate the pectoralis major to reach the skin. The nerve supply to the upper outer quadrant of the breast is provided by the intercostobrachial nerve (C8, T1) (Hughes *et al.*, 2000).

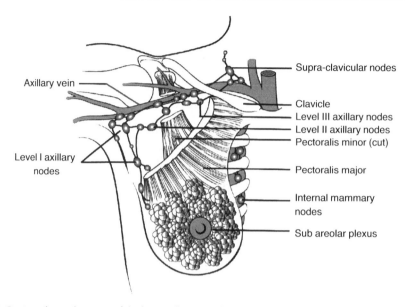

Fig. 1.2 Lymphatic drainage of the breast illustrating levels of axillary nodes.

Lymphatic system

The lymph fluid from the outer quadrants of each breast flows into the ipsilateral axillary lymph nodes along a chain which begins at the anterior axillary nodes and continues into the central and apical node groups. Lymph fluid from the medial quadrants drains towards the sternum via the inframammary nodes.

The major lymphatic drainage of the breast is to the axilla, and the axillary nodes are the first place a breast cancer will spread to. The axillary nodes are divided into three levels (Fig. 1.2).

- Level I – the nodes lie lateral to the lateral border of the pectoralis minor muscle.
- Level II – the nodes lie behind the pectoralis minor muscle.
- Level III – the nodes are located medial to the medial border of the pectoralis minor muscle.

Cyclical changes

During the menstrual cycle, the breasts undergo cyclical changes due to the changing levels of the hormone prolactin, which controls the secretion of the ovarian hormones, oestrogen and progesterone. These hormones cause the breast tissue and ducts to enlarge. The breast may change in size and consistency and become tender and nodular, usually 10–14 days prior to menstruation. These symptoms tend to resolve once menstruation occurs.

Changes during pregnancy

Changes in the breast are often the first symptoms of pregnancy. The woman may complain of fullness, tenderness and an increase in size. Veins become more prominent as the blood supply is increased and the areolar and nipple darken.

These changes are due to firstly oestrogen and progesterone and then to hormones produced by the placenta. Oestrogen stimulates the nipple–arcolar complex, causing it to darken; progesterone causes proliferation of the alveoli in preparation for milk production. As the placenta enlarges, it secretes human placental lactogen, which works alongside oestrogen and progesterone to stimulate the hypothalamus to secrete prolactin-releasing hormone (PRH). This hormone stimulates the anterior pituitary gland to secrete more prolactin, and this is responsible for milk production. After 12 weeks, a clear watery fluid known as colostrum is secreted by the breasts and expressed from the nipple. Its main function is to clear the lactiferous ducts and tubules of dead epithelial cells to make way for the free flow of milk.

After birth and the expulsion of the placenta, an alteration in the levels of the hormones oestrogen and progesterone occurs, resulting in the release of prolactin from the anterior pituitary gland. Oestrogen suppresses the action of prolactin, so it is not until about 3 days that the milk 'comes in'. In the meantime, the baby feeds off the colustrum, which is low in fat and contains vitamin A, protein and minerals.

Post-menopausal changes

When ovarian activity ceases at the menopause, causing the fall of oestrogen and progesterone, the glandular tissue in the breast starts to involute and atrophy, and is replaced by fat. The breasts tend to feel softer and become more pendulous. If hormone replacement therapy (HRT) is prescribed, the breasts may become fuller and can be tender.

INCIDENCE AND AETIOLOGY OF BREAST CANCER

Cancer is a common disease with a lifetime risk of more than one in three. Of all the cancers diagnosed in the UK, breast cancer is the most common female cancer, accounting for 31% of all new cases. Approximately 46 000 women are diagnosed in the UK annually. The estimated lifetime risk is now quoted to be one in nine (Cancer Research UK, 2009). Breast cancer in men is rare, with approximately 300 new cases annually (Cancer Research UK, 2009).

Although the incidence of breast cancer is seen to be rising, the mortality rate is fortunately on the decrease. In the UK in 2006, 12 319 women died from breast cancer compared to 15 625 in 1989. This reduction is thought to be due to earlier detection and improvement in treatment (Cancer Research UK, 2006). The 5-year relative survival rate for women with breast cancer is now estimated to be 82% (Office for National Statistics, 2005) compared to 50% for women diagnosed in 1971–1975.

Risk factors

The cause of breast cancer is not yet fully understood; however some risk factors have been identified. The risk factors can be divided into two: definite risks and potential risks.

Definite risks

Definite risks are the known risks that have been shown by research to increase the risk of developing breast cancer.

Gender

Being female increases the risk of breast cancer. As stated earlier, males do get breast cancer but it is rare.

Age

As we get older, our chance of getting breast cancer increases. Breast cancer is rare in women under the age of 35 years; however, after that age, the incidence starts to rise. More than 80% of cases occur in women over 50 years of age (Cancer Research UK, 2005)

Strong family history

Having a strong family history of breast cancer increases the risk of developing breast cancer. Much research is being undertaken to identify faulty genes that are associated with the increased risk. Two such genes have been identified so far: *BRCA1* and *BRCA2*, and these will be discussed in depth in Chapter 3.

Not everyone who has a family history of breast cancer will be at a higher risk of developing breast cancer than the average population.

A family history may be described as significant in the following situations (NICE, 2006).

- One first-degree relative and one second-degree relative diagnosed with breast cancer before the average age of 50 years;
- Two first-degree relatives diagnosed before the average age of 50 years;
- Three or more first- or second-degree relatives diagnosed at any age;
- One first-degree male relative diagnosed with breast cancer at any age;
- One first-degree relative with bilateral breast cancer where the first primary was diagnosed before the age of 50 years;
- One first- or second-degree relative with ovarian cancer at any age and one first- or second-degree relative with breast cancer at any age (one should be a first-degree relative).

Those who fit the above criteria should be offered a referral to a Family History clinic, where they can have their risk assessed and have regular screening, where appropriate. Referral to a Regional Genetic Unit may be appropriate following assessment.

Exposure to hormones

The number of menstrual cycles a woman undergoes is a powerful determinant of breast cancer risk. A woman who has an early menarche and late menopause has an increased risk of developing breast cancer. It has been shown that women who undergo a bilateral oophrectomy under the age of 50 years have a 50% reduction in breast cancer for up to 9 years post-surgery (Fentiman, 2001). A woman who has had her first baby after the age of 35 years, or is nulliparous, also carries a higher risk of developing breast cancer.

These findings suggest that the unopposed circulating oestrogen increases the breast tissue's susceptibility to other risk factors for breast cancer (MacPherson *et al.*, 2000).

Benign breast disease

Several studies have looked at the correlation between breast cancer and benign breast disease (Fentiman, 2001). A consensus paper published by the American College of Pathologists (Winchester, 1985), based on the work of Dupont and Page (1985), uses three classifications: no risk, slight risk and moderate risk. Those in the slight-risk group (1.5–2 times) include: moderate or florid hyperplasia with no atypia, intraduct papillomas. Those in the moderate-risk group (5 times) include: atypical lobular or ductal hyperplasia. More recently, a group in the USA studied a large cohort of women with benign breast disease and made similar findings (Hartmann *et al.*, 2005). The relative risk associated with atypia was 4.24, compared with a relative risk of 1.88 with proliferative changes without atypia and 1.27 with non-proliferative lesions.

Ionising radiation

Exposure to ionising radiation is known to increase the risk of breast cancer, as was found in studies in the use of radiation to treat benign conditions such as ringworm and enlarged thymus (Modan *et al.*, 1989; Hildreth *et al.*, 1989; Preston *et al.*, 2002).

  Women who have had radiotherapy to their chest for Hodgkin's lymphoma before their early thirties are at an increased risk of breast cancer and should be referred for early breast screening (Travis *et al.*, 2005).

  It must be stressed that the amount of radiation delivered by a screening mammogram is very small, and the potential benefits obtained outweigh the small risk.

Oral Contraceptive pill

The Collaborative Group on Hormonal Factors in Breast Cancer (CGHFBC, 1996) carried out a meta-analysis of results of 54 studies which included 53 297 breast cancer cases and 100 239 controls. It found that those who had used oral contraceptives (both combined or progesterone only) has a small but statistically significant risk that disappeared 10 years after cessation. However, it is important to remember that these studies were using the older-style contraceptive pills, which tended to have a higher dose of oestrogen. It is not clear whether the modern, low-dose preparations of the combined pill are associated with the same breast cancer risk as the older higher-dose preparations. One population-base case-control study in the USA suggested that the new lower-dose pills may impart a lower risk of breast cancer than the older higher-dose preparations (Althius *et al.*, 2003).

  It is important to remember that breast cancer is uncommon in young women (the age group more likely to use oral contraception) so this only leads to a few extra cases per year. The combined pill also reduces the risk of ovarian cancer (Hannaford *et al.*, 2007).

Hormone Replacement Therapy

Several studies have looked at HRT and its affect on breast cancer risk. In 2003, the results of the Million Women Study were published which showed that if you took a combined HRT you had a relative risk of 2.00 compared to 1.30 if you took an oestrogen only preparation. This risk returns to the same level as in women who have never taken HRT, 5 years after stopping it. In real terms, this means that 10 years of use of a combined HRT will contribute to an extra 19 cases per 1000 users and to five extra cases per 1000 users if oestrogen-only HRT is taken (Million Women Study Collaborators, 2003).

Obesity

Most studies have shown that obesity is a protective factor in pre-menopausal women but increases the risk in post-menopausal women (Van den Brandt *et al.*, 2000). This is because in post-menopausal women the major source of oestrogen comes from peripheral aromatisation of adrenal adrogens in fat. Therefore obesity increases the risk of breast cancer (Ziegler *et al.*, 1996, Sellers *et al.*, 1992, Van den Brandt, 2000).

Alcohol intake

In a pooled analysis of cohort studies looking at the effect of alcohol consumption on the risk of breast cancer, Smith-Warner *et al.* (1998) found that it is associated with an increased risk. The type of alcohol consumed did not strongly influence risk estimates.

Potential risks

Potential risks are those that have not been proven but have led scientists to research further.

Diet

As yet there is no scientific evidence to link breast cancer with diet (McPherson *et al.*, 2000). The intake of fat in the diet has been studied showing no significant risk. Hunter *et al.* (1996) pooled the results from eight major cohort studies and showed no effect of fat intake on the risk of breast cancer. It showed that women whose intake of fat comprised of less than 20% of their calorie intake did not have any reduction in risk. Therefore, if western women reduce their fat intake, it is unlikely to lead to any significant reduction in breast cancer risk reduction.

There has been no conclusive evidence to suggest that a diet high in fruit and vegetables reduced the risk of breast cancer (Smith-Warner *et al.*, 2001).

Height

There has been inconsistency regarding the research findings regarding the influence of height on breast cancer risk. In studies where height was self-recorded there was no increased risk identified but in studies where the participants were formerly measured there was found to be a positive association between increased height and breast cancer risk (Fentiman, 2001).There is no strong evidence to suggest why height has a part to play in breast cancer risk. It is hypothesised that childhood diet, affluence and physical activity during puberty may have an influence (Van den Brandt *et al.*, 2000).

The diagnostic pathway

There are two main diagnostic pathways: screening and symptomatic. Breast screening is extensively covered in Chapter 4 so this chapter will focus on the symptomatic diagnostic pathway.

Patients should be referred to a specialist breast unit by their General Practitioner (GP). In 2005, the National Institute for Health and Clinical Excellence (NICE, 2005) produced guidelines for referral for suspected breast cancer. By December 2009, all breast referrals should be seen within 2 weeks of referral (Department of Health, 2007).

Specialist breast units offer triple assessment which involves clinical examination, radiological assessment and pathological assessment. Many specialist units offer a 'one-stop' service, where the patients get the results on the same day. This is especially advantageous for those who have benign disease. It can however be difficult for a patient who is diagnosed with breast cancer, who has not been prepared for the news. It is therefore important that the GP informs the patient of the process and warns them of any suspicions. With the increasing use of core biopsy, in the diagnosis of breast cancer, a 'two-stop' service is also common.

Methods of assessment

History taking

Before examining the patient, a detailed history should be taken. It is useful in helping make the diagnosis and identifying risk factors.

The details obtained should include the following:

- Patient's age;
- Past medical history;
- Family history of breast and ovarian cancer;
- Age at menarche/age at menopause;
- Date of the last menstrual period (LMP);
- Use of the combined oral contraceptive pill and hormone replacement therapy;
- Number of pregnancies;
- Age at first pregnancy;
- Whether the patient breast-fed her babies;
- Nature of the presenting symptom and its duration.

Clinical examination

It is important to ensure the environment is as pleasant as possible. A gown should be provided, curtains surrounding the examination couch drawn and the door closed to ensure privacy. A chaperone may be present, depending on individual hospital policy.

The clinical examination is divided into two parts:

1 Palpation;
2 Inspection.

Palpation

The patient is first examined lying supine on the couch with the arms above the head. This flattens out the breast tissue making it easier to examine. The clinician, having washed and warmed their hands, should use the flats of the fingers to palpate the whole of the breast using a steady medium pressure. Any abnormality found is then examined with the fingertips to assess for mobility and fixation. It is important to examine both breasts for comparison and ideally the 'normal' breast should be examined first. The breasts should also be examined in the sitting position.

The axillary nodes should also be palpated either in the supine position or sitting up. The arm should be supported to ensure the muscle is relaxed. It is easy to miss nodes in a fatty axilla and it has been found that correlation between clinical examination and pathology is poor (Dixon and Sainsbury, 1998). The use of ultrasound is increasing used in staging the axilla.

When the patient is sitting the supraclavicular nodes should be palpated and the examiner should sweep their hands down the chest wall feeling for any enlarged inframammary nodes.

The Royal College of Nursing (2002) and The Department of Health (1998) have recommended that nurses do not undertake the practice of breast palpation. It does however acknowledge that a small number of nurses with specialist training and who work within a specialist breast unit can practice breast examination.

Inspection

The patient should be in a sitting position. There are three different positions to inspect the breast:

1 Hands relaxed by the side;
2 Hands in the air;
3 Hands on the hips pushing in, contracting the pectoralis major muscle.

The signs to look for are:

• Size and contour of the breasts – is one breast larger than the other, has it always been? Is there any change in shape?
• Skin changes such as dimpling, increased vascularity and skin lesions.
• Nipple changes such as eczematous changes, discharge, crusting and a recent inversion.

Investigations

Following examination and inspection the clinician may organise further investigations. The following investigations are commonplace:

Mammography

A mammogram is a low-dose X-ray of the breast tissue. The dose of radiation is less than 1 Gy. Mammograms are generally not performed on women under 35 as the breast tissue in young women is relatively radio dense. Mammography is discussed in more depth in Chapter 4.

Ultrasound

Ultrasound is a painless procedure that uses high-frequency sound waves. It is a useful in women under 35, as an aid to mammography, measuring lesions and differentiating between a cystic or solid mass.

Magnetic Resonance Imaging

Breast magnetic resonance imaging (MRI) is increasing used in breast assessment although it not routinely used. It is used as an addition to mammograms and ultrasound in complex cases. MRI of the breast is the best technique for imaging implants and the post-surgical breast where local recurrence needs to be excluded. It is also beneficial in assessing the extent of lobular carcinoma in the breast or for multifocal disease. Breast MRI is now recommended for screening high-risk family history patients and those with known gene mutations (NICE, 2006).

To image the breast, the patient has to lie prone and an intravenous contrast is required.

Fine-needle aspiration cytology

Fine-needle aspiration cytology (FNAC) can be performed freehand by the clinician in the outpatient department or under ultrasound guidance. Usually a 10-ml syringe with a 21Gor 23G needle is used. The skin is cleaned and the needle is inserted into the lump. Suction is applied whilst several passes are made into the lump in different directions. The material obtained is spread thinly on a slide and is left to air dry. The slides are then reported by the cytologist (Button *et al.*, 2004). The results are graded using a numerical system: C1 = inadequate, C2 = benign, C3 = indeterminate probably benign, C4 = indeterminate, probably malignant and C5 = malignant.

Core Biopsy

If the FNAC results are not conclusive, or histology is required, a core biopsy can be taken. Increasingly the use of core biopsy is replacing FNAC.

Core biopsies can be taken free hand or under image guidance. Local anaesthetic is injected into the breast, a small incision is made with a scalpel and a trocar/biopsy needle is inserted until the tip touches the lump. The biopsy gun is fired which takes a small core of tissue. Several passes are taken to gain a representative sample. The cores are then sent to histology. Pressure should be applied to prevent bruising. Caution should be taken with patients on warfarin, as they should have their INR taken first.

Core biopsies are graded the same way as cytology results but with a preceding 'B', e.g. B1, B2.

Staging investigations

If breast cancer is diagnosed staging investigations may be undertaken to assess for metastatic disease. Depending on need and individual hospital policy, blood tests (full blood count, urea and electrolytes, liver function and bone profile), a chest X-ray, a bone scan, abdominal ultrasound, computed tomography (CT) or MRI can be requested.

Psychological support

Being given a diagnosis of breast cancer is a very difficult time for women. For women who are diagnosed via the screening programme it can come as a complete shock as they were asymptomatic, whilst women who present with a symptom may have undoubtedly questioned in their minds whether they have cancer. It is therefore important that the Breast

Care Nurses are available to give support and advice throughout the diagnostic pathway. Psychological support will be dealt with in more depth in Chapter 15.

Staging breast cancer

The pathologist is responsible for reporting the histological findings. The results should be discussed at a multidisciplinary team meeting. The core members of this team should include a consultant histopathologist, consultant cytologist, consultant radiologist, consultant surgeon, consultant medical oncologist, consultant clinical oncologist and breast care nurse. Other members include a plastic surgeon, radiographer, trials coordinator, clinical psychologist, a geneticist and administration staff. The histological factors will help to determine the appropriate treatment for the patient.

The pathologist will report of different characteristics of the tumour including:

Size

The size of the tumour is one of the most significant prognostic indicators. The smaller the cancer is, the better the prognosis.

Grade

The tumour is graded according to the cellular differentiation i.e. the degree to which the cancer cells resemble their tissue of origin (King, 1996). A commonly used grading system is the modified Bloom and Richardson system (Elston and Ellis, 1998). It uses three grades: Grade I, Grade II and Grade III.Grade I is the slowest growing cancer; a well-differentiated tumour with the cells closely resembling their tissue of origin. Grade II is a moderately differentiated tumour where the cells are less like their tissue of origin and Grade III is a poorly differentiated tumour where the cells look very unlike their tissue of origin, it is the most aggressive grade of breast cancer.

Grade alone is an important prognostic indicator. It is known that 85% of patients with a grade I tumour are alive and well at 5 years as opposed to 45% of those with a grade III tumour (Ellis *et al.*, 1992).

Vascular and lymphatic invasion

If the tumour has invaded the blood or lymphatic vessels this is a poor prognostic feature.

Lymph node status

The number of lymph nodes involved with cancer cells determines the chance of survival for that individual and is one of the most important prognostic indicators. If positive nodes are identified it will impact on the type of treatment offered.

Hormone Receptor status

The tumour is analysed to test for the presence of the steroid hormone receptors, oestrogen (ER) and progesterone (PR). The presence of such receptors will determine the effectiveness of endocrine therapy such as tamoxifen and the aromatase inhibitors. It has been shown that those with an oestrogen receptor positive tumour have a better outcome.

For over 30 years tamoxifen has been the gold standard endocrine therapy used for oestrogen receptor positive breast cancers, and still is for pre-menopausal women. The Early Breast Cancer Trialists' Collaborative Group (1998) produced a meta-analysis which showed that if tamoxifen was taken for 5 years, it reduced the recurrence rate by 50%. However, tamoxifen is known to increase the risk of thromboembolic events and endometrial cancer.

Since 2005, the use of aromatase inhibitors has increased following the publication of several studies (Howell *et al.*, 2005; Goss *et al.*, 2003; Coombes *et al.*, 2004). The three most commonly used aromatase inhibitors are anastrozole (Arimidex), exemestane (Aromasin) and letrozole (Femara). They can be given as an upfront treatment, switching therapy after 2–3 years of tamoxifen or as extended therapy after 5 years of tamoxifen. It is important to note they are only suitable for post-menopausal women.

Endocrine therapy will be discussed in more depth in Chapter 10.

Oncogenes

Changes to the genes in a normal cell can result in cell proliferation and malignant proliferation. Proto-oncogenes are involved in stimulating the cell through the normal cell cycle resulting in proliferation, while tumour suppressor genes inhibit excessive cell proliferation. However, either mutation or amplification of proto-oncogenes, and inactivation or loss of tumour suppressor genes can result in uncontrolled cell proliferation and cancer formation (Cooke *et al.*, 1999).

Many proto-oncogenes encode for epidermal growth factor receptors, and the two most important growth factors that have been discovered so far are the human epidermal growth factor receptor – 1 (HER1) and the human epidermal growth factor – 2 (HER2). These are sometimes referred to as c-*erb1* and c-*erb2*, respectively, and are located on Chromosome 17.

HER2 has been shown to be over-expressed in 25–30% of all human breast cancers, and women whose tumours over-expresses HER2 have a shorter disease-free survival and worse overall survival (Slamon *et al.*, 1987; Slamon *et al.*, 1989).

In 2005, results of the HERA trial (Trastuzumab after Adjuvant Chemotherapy in HER2-positive Breast Cancer) were published showing a significant improvement in disease-free survival among women with HER2-positive breast cancer (Piccart-Gebhart *et al.*, 2005). It was shown that if trastuzumab was given, for 1 year, to HER2-positive patients who had completed adjuvant chemotherapy, it reduced the rate of recurrence, particularly distant recurrence by approximately 50%.

Therefore, if a patient's tumour over-expresses HER2, they will be deemed HER2-positive and will be eligible for trastuzumab (Herceptin). This will be discussed in more depth in Chapter 8.

New drugs are being developed to target epidermal growth factor receptors; for example, lapatinib (Tykerb) – a dual tyrosine kinase inhibitor – targets both HER1 and HER2. Ongoing trials are assessing effectiveness and safety (Petrelli *et al.*, 2008).

Targeted therapies are a new and exciting development in the treatment of breast cancer, and future research may result in the development of additional targeted therapies.

Classification of stage

Staging refers to the grouping of patients according to the extent of their disease. The purpose of this grouping is as follows (Sobin and Wittekind, 2002).

- To aid the clinician in the planning of treatment;
- To give some indication of prognosis;
- To assist in the evaluation of the results of treatment;
- To facilitate the exchange of information between treatment centres;
- To contribute to the continuing investigation of human cancer.

Several classification systems are in use, most commonly the UICC (International Union Against Cancer) TNM system and the Nottingham Prognostic Indicator.

The TNM system

The TNM system was developed in France between 1943 and 1952 and is used for all tumour types, not solely breast. The TNM system is based on three main components:

1 **T** – the extent of the primary tumour;
2 **N** – the absence or presence and extent of regional lymph node metastasis;
3 **M** – the absence or presence of distant metastasis.

The TNM system is summarised in Table 1.1. The TNM classification categories can be relatively complex and, for convenience, they can be condensed to make a more manageable stage group that gives an indication for survival. There are five stages, as shown in Table 1.2.

To put this in practice, a woman who presents with a 3-cm tumour with a moveable node in her ipsilateral (same side) axilla, but has no evidence of metastatic disease, is said to have a T2 N1 M0 invasive breast cancer, which is stage IIB. The lower the stage, the better is the prognosis.

Nottingham Prognostic Indicator

The Nottingham Prognostic Indicator (NPI) is an integrated prognostic index that combines tumour size, lymph node status and grade. The index is calculated by $0.2 \times$ the tumour size (cm) + grade (1–3) + lymph node status (1 = no nodes; 2 = 1–3 nodes; 3 = 3 or more nodes are involved). This separates patients into three prognostic groups: good (score <3.40), moderate (score 3.4–5.4) and poor (score >5).

Adjuvant! Online

Adjuvant! Online is a website that is aimed to help health professionals and patients discuss the risks and benefits of adjuvant treatment for early breast cancer (chemotherapy and endocrine therapy). Information is entered about the patients and their tumours (for example: age of patient, tumour size, grade, nodal involvement, etc.). A printout from the website illustrates the estimated risk of cancer-related mortality or relapse without

Table 1.1   TNM classification

Stage	Characteristics
T-primary tumour	
TX	Primary tumour cannot be assessed
T0	No evidence of primary tumour
Tis	Carcinoma in situ: Tis (DCIS): Ductal carcinoma in situ Tis (LCIS): Lobular carcinoma in situ Tis (Paget): Paget's disease of the nipple, no tumour
T1	Tumour 2.0 cm or less in greatest dimension T1mic: Microinvasion 0.1 cm or less in greatest dimension T1a: More than 0.1 cm, but not more than 0.5 cm in greatest dimension T1b: More than 0.5 cm, but not more than 1 cm in greatest dimension T1c: More than 1 cm, but not more than 2 cm in greatest dimension
T2	Tumour more than 2 cm, but not more than 5 cm in greatest dimension
T3	Tumour more than 5 cm in greatest dimension
	Tumour of any size, with direct extension to chest wall or skin
T4	T4a: Extension to chest wall T4b: Oedema (including peau d'orange), or ulceration of the skin of the breast, or satellite skin nodules confined to the same breast T4c: Both 4a and 4b, as above T4d: Inflammatory cancer
N-nodal status	
NX	Regional lymph nodes cannot be assessed (e.g. previously removed)
N0	No regional lymph node metastasis
N1	Metastasis in moveable ipsilateral axillary node(s)
N2	Metastasis in fixed ipsilateral axillary node(s) N2a: Metastasis in axillary lymph nodes fixed to one another or to other structures N2b: Metastasis in only clinically apparent internal mammary lymph node(s) and in the absence of clinically evident axillary lymph node metastasis
N3	Metastasis to ipsilateral internal mammary lymph node(s) N3a: Infra-clavicular N3b: Internal mammary and axillary N3c: Supra-clavicular
M-distant metastasis	
MX	Presence of distant metastasis cannot be assessed
M0	No distant metastasis
M1	Distant metastasis present

systematic adjuvant therapy and with systemic therapy. The website is available to view on http://www.adjuvantonline.com.

CONCLUSION

Chapter 1 has given an overview of breast cancer, including the anatomy and physiology of the breast, and has also looked at the symptomatic diagnostic pathway. This overview will

Table 1.2   Five stages of the TNM classification.

	T	N	M
Stage 0	Tis	N0	M0
Stage I	T1	N0	M0
Stage IIA	T0	N1	M0
	T1	N1	M0
	T2	N0	M0
Stage IIB	T2	N1	M0
	T3	N0	M0
Stage IIIA	T0	N2	M0
	T1	N2	M0
	T2	N2	M0
	T3	N1, N2	M0
Stage IIIB	T4	N0, N1, N2	M0
Stage IIIC	Any T	N3	M0
Stage IV	Any T	Any N	M1

hopefully provide a good knowledge base for healthcare professionals caring for women with breast cancer.

REFERENCES

Althius MD, Brogen DR, Coates RJ *et al.* (2003) Hormonal content and potency of oral contraceptives and breast cancer risk in young women. *British Journal of Cancer* 88, 50–57.

Button F, Kirkham B and Pennery E (2004) Breast aspiration and seroma drainage. In: Doherty L and Lister S (Eds) *The Royal Marsden Manual of Clinical Procedure.* Oxford: Blackwell.

Cancer Research UK (2005) *Cancer Statistics.* Online. Available http://www.cancerresearchuk.org/cancerstats.

Cancer Research UK (2006) *Cancer Statistics.* Online. Available http://www.cancerresearchuk.org/cancerstats.

Cancer Research UK (2009) *Statistical Information Team.* Online. Available http://info.cancerresearchuk.org/cancerstats/types/breast/incidence/#Lifetime.

Collaborative Group on Hormonal Factors in Breast Cancer (1996) Breast cancer and oral contraceptives. *The Lancet* 347: 1713–1727.

Cooke T, Rovelon P, Slamon D and Bohme C (1999) I am HER2-positive – what does this mean? Providing answers to patient concerns. *Program and Abstracts of European Cancer Conference*: Sept. 12–16, Vienna, Austria. EONS Symposium.

Coombes RC, Hall E, Gibson LG *et al.* (2004) A randomised trial for exemestane after two to three years of tamoxifen therapy in postmenopausal with primary breast cancer. *New England Journal of Medicine* 154: 1081–1092.

Department of Health (1998) *Clinical Examination of the Breast.* London: HMSO. Online. Available http://www.dh.gov.uk.

Department of Health (2007) *Cancer Reform Strategy.* London: HMSO. Online. Available http://www.dh.gov.uk.

Dixon JM and Sainsbury R (1998) *Diseases of the Breast* (2nd edn.). London: Churchill Livingstone.

Dupont WD and Page DL (1985). Risk factors for breast cancer in women with proliferative breast disease. *New England Journal of Medicine* 312: 146–151.

Early breast Cancer Trialists' Collaborative Group (1998) Tamoxifen for early breast cancer: an overview of randomised trials. *The Lancet* 351: 1451–1467.

Ellis IO, Galea M, Broughton N, Locker A, Blamey RW and Elston CW (1992) pathological prognostic factors in breast cancer – relationship with survival in a large study with long-term follow-up. *Histopathology* 27: 479–489.

Elston CW and Ellis IO (1998) *The Breast*. Edinburgh: Churchill Livingstone.

Fentiman IS (2001) Fixed and modified risk factors for breast cancer. *International Journal of Clinical Practice* 55(8): 527–530.

Goss PE, Ingel JN, Palmer MJ *et al.* (2003) A randomized trial of letrozole in postmenopausal women after five years of tamoxifen for early-stage breast cancer. *New England Journal of Medicine* 349: 1793–1802.

Hannaford PC, Selvasbramaniam S, Elliot AM, Angus V, Iversen L and Lee A (2007) Cancer risk among users of oral contraceptives: cohort data from the Royal College of General Practitioner's Oral Contraceptive Study. *British Medical Journal* 335: 651.

Hartman LC, Sellers TA, Frost MH *et al.* (2005) Benign breast disease and the risk of breast cancer. *New England Journal of Medicine* 353: 229–237.

Hildreth NG, Shore RE and Dvoretsky P (1989) The risk of breast cancer after radiation for the thymus in infancy. *New England Journal of Medicine* 321: 1281–1284.

Howell A, Cuzich J, Baum M *et al.* (2005) ATAC Trialists' Group. Results of the ATAC (arimidex, tamoxifen, alone or in combination) trial after completion of 5 years' adjuvant treatment for breast cancer. *The Lancet* 365: 60–62.

Hughes LE, Mansel RE and Webster DJT (2000) *Benign Disorders and Disease of the Breast: Concepts and Clinical Management*. London: W.B. Saunders.

Hunter DJ, Spiegelman D, Adami H-O *et al.* (1996) Cohort studies of fat intake and the risk of breast cancer – a pooled analysis. *New England Journal of Medicine* 334: 6, 334–361.

King RJB (1996) *Cancer Biology*. Harlow: Longman.

MacPherson K, Steel CM and Dixon JM (2000) Breast cancer: epidemiology, risk factors and genetics. In: Dixon JM (Ed.) *ABC of Breast Diseases*. London: BMJ Publishing.

Million Women Study Collaborators (2003) Breast cancer and hormone replacement therapy in the Million Women's Study. *The Lancet* 362: 419–427.

Modan B, Chetrit A and Alfanary E (1989) Increased risk of breast cancer after low-dose radiation. *The Lancet* ii: 629–631.

National Institute for Health and Clinical Excellence (2006) *Familial Breast Cancer – The Classification and Care of Women at Risk of Familial Breast Cancer in Primary, Secondary and Tertiary Care. Clinical Guidance 14*. Online. Available http://www.nice.org.uk/Guidance.

National Institute for Health and Clinical Excellence (2005) *Referral Guidelines for Suspected Cancer*. Online. Available http://www.nice.org/Guidance.

Office for National Statistics (2005) *Long term Breast cancer Survival, England and Wales, up to 2003*. Online. Available http://www.statistics.gov.uk/statbase/Product.asp?vlnk=14172&More=Y.

Petrelli F, Cabiddu M, Cazzaniga M, Cremomesi M and Barni S (2008) Targeted therapies for the treatment of breast cancer in the post-trastuzumab era. *The Oncologist* 13: 373–381.

Piccart-Gebhart MJ, Procter M, Leyland-Jones B *et al.* (2005) Trastuzumab after adjuvant chemotherapy in HER2-positive breast cancer. *New England Journal of Medicine* 353(16): 1659–1672.

Preston D, Mattson A, Holmbers E, Shore R, Hildreth NG and Brice JD (2002) Radiation effects on breast cancer risk: a pooled analysis. *Radiation Research* 158(2): 220–235.

Royal College of Nursing (2002) *Issues in Nursing and Health: Breast Palpation and Breast Awareness – Guidance for Practice*. London: Royal College of Nursing. Online. Available http://www.rcn.org.uk.

Sellers TA, Kushi LH, Potter JD *et al.* (1992) Effect of family history, body fat distribution and reproductive factors on the risk of post-menopausal breast cancer. *New England Journal of Medicine* 326: 1323–1329.

Slamon DJ, Clark GM, Wong SG, Lewin WJ, Ullrich A and McGuire WI (1987) Human breast cancer: correlation of relapse and survival with amplification of the Her-2 /neu oncogene. *Science* 235: 177–182.

Slamon DJ, Godolphin W, Jones LA *et al.* (1989) Studies of the HER-2/neu oncogene in human breast cancer and ovarian cancer. *Science* 244: 707–712.

Smith-Warner SA, Spiegelman D, Yaun SS *et al.* (1998) Alcohol and breast cancer in women – a pooled analysis of cohort studies. *JAMA* 279(7): 535–540.

Smith-Warner SA, Spigelman D, Yaou SS *et al.* (2001) Intake of fruit and vegetables and risk of breast cancer. *JAMA* 285(6): 769–776.

Sobin LH and Wittekind CH (2002) *TNM – classification of malignant tumours* (6th edn.). New York: John Wiley and sons.

Travis LB, Hill D, Dores GM *et al.* (2005) Cumulative absolute breast cancer risk for young women treated for Hodgkin's lymphoma. *Journal of the National Cancer Institute* 97(19): 1428–1437.

Van den Brandt PA, Spiegelman D, Yaun SS *et al.* (2000) Pooled analysis of prospective cohort studies on height, weight and breast cancer risk. *American Journal of Epidemiology* 152(6): 514–527.

Winchester DP (1985) ACP consensus statement: the relationship of fibrocystic disease to breast cancer. In: Hughes LE, Mansel RE and Webster DJT (2000) *Benign Disorders and Disease of the Breast: Concepts and Clinical Management*. London: W.B. Saunders.

Ziegler RG, Hoover RN, Nomura AM *et al.* (1996) Relative weight, weight change, height, and breast cancer risk in Asia–American women, *Journal National Cancer Institute* 88: 650–660.

2 The Histopathology of Breast Cancer

Helen E. Froyd and Victoria Harmer

INTRODUCTION

Breast cancer is a heterogeneous disease that encompasses a number of distinct biological characteristics and clinical behaviour. Breast cancer is often curable, particularly if diagnosed at an early stage. This requires early detection and a knowledge and awareness of all types of the disease, including the rarer forms of breast cancer.

TYPES OF BREAST CANCER

Breast cancer is not a single disease, but rather there are different types of breast cancers with different prognostic features (Fig. 2.1). Breast cancers arise in the terminal duct lobular unit. They are classified according to the type of tissue from which they arise and their appearance under the microscope. When making treatment decisions, the type of breast cancer may affect the choice.

In situ disease

Carcinoma cells confined within the terminal duct lobular unit and adjacent ducts, but which have not invaded the basement membrane, are known as carcinoma in situ. Two types have been identified: ductal carcinoma in situ (DCIS) and lobular carcinoma in situ (LCIS). DCIS arises from the ducts and is more common than LCIS, which arises from the lobules.

DCIS

DCIS is commonly diagnosed via the National Health Service Breast Screening Programme, as it tends to present as microcalcifications that are identifiable on mammography (20–25% of screen-detected cancers). Patients with symptomatic DCIS (3–4% of symptomatic cases) present with a breast mass, nipple discharge or Paget's disease (Page *et al.*, 2001).

DCIS is characterised by ducts and ductules expanded by large irregular cells with large irregular nuclei (Page *et al.*, 2001).

Breast Cancer Nursing Care and Management, Second Edition, Edited by Victoria Harmer
© 2011 by Blackwell Publishing Ltd.

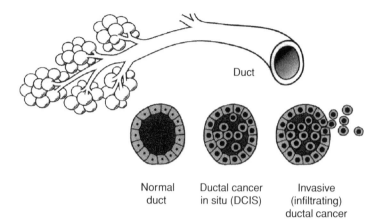

Normal   Ductal cancer   Invasive
duct   in situ (DCIS)   (infiltrating)
                                ductal cancer

Fig. 2.1   Types of breast cancer.

Several classification systems are used to describe DCIS. In the UK, the United Kingdom Coordinating Group for Breast Screening Pathology classifies DCIS according to nuclear grade into high, intermediate and low grade (NHS Breast Screening Programme, 1995).

High-grade (comedo) DCIS

High-grade (comedo) DCIS is the most common type of DCIS, accounting for 85% of all lesions. It presents as linear, branching microcalcification on the mammogram or as an ill-defined mass or Paget's disease of the nipple (Chinyama and Wells, 1998). It tends to have a high proliferation rate, HER2 gene amplification or protein over-expression, and is clinically more aggressive (Silverstein, 1999).

Low-grade (non-comedo) DCIS

Low-grade (non-comedo) DCIS is often an incidental finding when biopsying a benign lesion. It rarely presents as a palpable lesion and mammographically appears more granular (Chinyama and Wells, 1998). According to Silverstein (1999), non-comedo DCIS is less aggressive.

Intermediate-grade DCIS

Intermediate-grade DCIS is a grouping of DCIS that does not fall easily into the above two categories. Its features lie midway between the two.

Natural course of DCIS

Studies have shown that approximately 40% of DCIS cases progress into an invasive cancer over a 30-year period, with the majority of these developing within the first decade (Page *et al.*, 2001).

LCIS

LCIS is a high-risk marker of invasive cancer, but is not itself classed as a pre-malignant lesion. First described by Foote and Stewart in 1941, it is often an incidental finding as it tends to have no specific mammographic or clinical features. Seventy per cent of women with LCIS are pre-menopausal, and the condition is present in 1% of screen-detected lesions and 0.5% of symptomatic cases (Page *et al.*, 2001). LCIS tends to be multifocal and bilateral and predisposes to invasive carcinoma (Chinyama and Wells, 1998). Frykberg (1999) calculates the relative risk for developing invasive cancer to be up to 12 times that of the general population. LCIS presents as an expansion of the whole lobule by smaller regular cells with regular, round or oval nuclei.

Natural course of LCIS

There is convincing evidence demonstrating that 10–20% of patients identified with LCIS, if left untreated, develop breast cancer 15–25 years after initial diagnosis (Simpson *et al.*, 2003). Haagensen *et al.* (1978) and Andersen (1974) describe an increase of 1–2% per year after a diagnosis of LCIS, or a 30–40% increased lifetime risk.

Approximately 15–20% of women with LCIS will develop breast cancer in the ipsilateral breast; a further 10–15% will develop it in the contralateral breast.

Paget's disease of the nipple

Paget's disease of the nipple was first described as a sign of breast cancer in 1874 by Sir James Paget, who warned that cancer of the breast followed within 1–2 years after detection of these changes (Paget 1874). Paget's disease presents similarly to eczema of the nipple, is present with about 2% of all breast cancers, and is associated with a higher frequency of multicentric breast cancers (Underwood, 2004).

Diagnosis of Paget's disease

The most common features of Paget's disease are changes to the nipple, associated with a rash, eczema, scaling, bleeding, itching, or ulceration. If a patient presents with any eczematoid-type lesion of the nipple, mammography should be performed to determine whether there is a lesion that cannot be felt, and its degree of involvement with the rest of the breast. However, in many patients mammography is entirely normal. Some 40–50% of patients are diagnosed with Paget's disease without a clinical lump (Maier *et al.*, 1969; Ashikari *et al.*, 1970). The most reliable method of obtaining a diagnosis is by skin biopsy.

Treatment of Paget's disease

Historically, the standard treatment has been a mastectomy, because the goal is ensuring that surgical excision margins of the cancer are clear. However, there are increasing reports of successful use of breast-conservation techniques involving removal of the nipple and areola. Radiotherapy alone or partial central excisions of the breast and nipple have also been used (Fourque *et al.*, 1987; Bulens *et al.*, 1990; Stockdale *et al.*, 1989; Pierce *et al.*, 1997). Dixon *et al.* (2000) suggested that, in Paget's disease that presents without a lump in both males and females, wide local excision followed by radiotherapy produces good

Table 2.1   Histological types of invasive breast cancer and their relative incidence for palpable tumours.

Tumour	Percentage incidence
Infiltrating ductal	75%
Infiltrating lobular	10%
Mucinous	3%
Medullary	2–3%
Tubular	2%
Papillary	2%
Others	5%

Adapted from Underwood (2004).

results. If the nipple is removed, the breast care nurse can arrange for a prosthetic nipple to improve the cosmetic result. Possibilities for later-stage nipple reconstruction such as grafting or tattooing can be discussed.

Invasive ductal carcinoma

Invasive ductal carcinoma is the most common type of invasive breast cancer, accounting for approximately 75% of all breast cancers (Table 2.1).

Biological features

Invasive ductal carcinoma usually presents as a palpable lump or an irregular spiculated soft-tissue density on mammography. Invasive ductal carcinomas arise from the ductal epithelium and break out of the ducts into the surrounding breast tissue. There it meets with the blood and lymphatic systems, and it has the potential to invade into these vessels (vascular and lymphatic invasion) and metastasise to a secondary location (King, 1996). Invasive ductal carcinoma shows no specific features, but rather is diagnosed when the tumour does not fit into any other category, e.g. lobular or tubular. Some therefore call this tumour 'no special type' (NST).

Invasive ductal carcinomas are diagnosed as others are, using triple assessment. The tumour cells are arranged in groups, cords and gland-like structures. A well-differentiated (grade I) infiltrating ductal carcinoma will have lower numbers of mitotic figures than a poorly differentiated (grade III) tumour (Underwood, 2004).

Treatment of invasive ductal carcinoma

Surgery is the usual first treatment for invasive ductal carcinoma (see Chapter 5) although chemotherapy, radiotherapy or endocrine treatment can be delivered prior to surgery if indicated.

Invasive lobular carcinoma

Invasive lobular carcinoma is less common than invasive ductal carcinoma, accounting for approximately 10% of breast cancers in the UK. The tumour tends to infiltrate the breast stroma in single files ('Indian files') and, more often than ductal carcinoma, manifests as asymmetrical thickening or nodularity rather than a discrete lump. As a result, patients presenting with invasive lobular carcinoma symptomatically have much larger tumours when compared to patients with symptomatic ductal cancers. A characteristic feature is that these cells lack the cell adhesion molecule E-cadherin (Underwood, 2004). They are less likely to include microcalcification and thus may not be picked up on mammography.

Inflammatory carcinoma

Inflammatory carcinomas are a sub-type of ductal cancers that occur in approximately 1% of breast cancers (Harris *et al.*, 2010).

Biological features

Inflammatory breast cancer has specific clinical features. These include: skin dimpling, oedema of the skin or peau d' orange (where the skin is thick and indurated). Other characteristics include a warm, red colour of the breast, and dermal lymphatic involvement by tumour, the latter being present in at least 80% of women (Page and Anderson, 1987). These cancers are associated with a clinical picture mimicking inflammation and are most likely to be high grade (poorly differentiated cancers). They are biologically very aggressive, and therefore present frequently as locally advanced disease.

Treatment of inflammatory breast cancer

Inflammatory cancers usually involve a large area of the breast, including the skin. Breast-conservation surgery is often not appropriate where the cancer involves the skin. There is evidence that, in locally advanced disease, primary medical treatment (chemotherapy prior to surgery) is recommended to induce shrinkage of the cancer (Israel *et al.*, 1986), as inflammatory breast cancer has been shown to be associated with reduced survival rates (Buzdar *et al.*, 1982).

Following a course of chemotherapy, mastectomy with an axillary clearance is considered the safest option. Radiotherapy is normally given to reduce local recurrence rates.

Mucinous carcinoma

Mucinous carcinoma is also referred to as mucoid, gelatinous or colloid cancer, because these cancers contain abundant mucin (jelly-like material). They represent about 2–3% of invasive breast cancers and occur mainly in older women (Page and Anderson, 1987).

Biological features

Mucinous cancers arise in the ductal tissue. They comprise of small nests and cords of tumour cells, which show little pleomorphism, embedded in large amounts of mucin. Due to the absence of dense stroma, these cancers usually have a well-defined, rounded edge (Underwood, 2004). Compared with other breast cancers, pure mucinous carcinomas have a good prognosis, with survival of 70–90% at 10 years.

Medullary carcinomas

Medullary carcinomas usually occur in post-menopausal women and have a significantly better survival rate than invasive duct carcinomas.

Biological features

Medullary cancers are circumscribed and often large, and are very cellular with little stroma. The edges are often more rounded and discrete; when palpated they feel softer. They have large tracts of confluent cells with little stroma in between. Mitotic figures are many and the cells show marked nuclear pleomorphism. An infiltrate of lymphocytes surrounds the large groups of tumour cells (Underwood, 2004).

Tubular carcinomas

Tubular carcinomas represent about 2% of breast cancers but constitute a higher number of screen-detected lesions.

Biological features

Tubular carcinomas are well-differentiated, with their cells arranged as tubules. They are often small with gritty, firm and irregular outlines. The cells show little mitotic activity and lie within a dense stroma. These tumours carry better prognostic factors than invasive ductal cancers (Underwood, 2004).

Intracystic papillary carcinoma

Intracystic papillary cancers are rare tumours that occur in post-menopausal women.

Biological features

Intracystic papillary carcinoma is a distinct entity. Current controversy exists over whether this is an in-situ or invasive tumour. It should be clearly distinguished from in situ or DCIS papillary carcinoma. Intracystic papillary cancer is an invasive tumour within a thick cyst cavity. Usually these cancers are small (between 1 and 3 cm in size). Mucin secretion may or may not be seen. Pure types behave in very low-grade fashion and rarely metastasise.

Invasive papillary carcinoma

Invasive papillary carcinoma is a distinct entity that is extremely rare and carries a relatively good prognosis.

Cribriform carcinoma

Cribriform carcinoma shares some morphological features with tubular carcinoma and is also associated with a favourable prognosis.

Biological features

Cribriform carcinomas are characterised by tumour cells that invade the stroma in a cribriform or fenestrated growth pattern. There is usually a mixture of histological patterns although, to be defined as cribriform, there needs to be more than 50% of cribriform features within the tumour. Most invasive cribriform carcinomas are associated with an abundant component of cribriform carcinoma in situ (Harris *et al.*, 2010).

Phylloides tumours

Phylloides tumours are rare fibroepithelial neoplasms that range from benign to malignant in behaviour.

Biological features

Behaviour of phylloides tumours varies according to size and certain microscopic features, including cellularity, atypia, and mitoses. Although similar to fibroadenoma, they present as mixed epithelial stromal tumours which, unlike fibroadenomas, show overgrowth. There are three subtypes of phylloides: benign, borderline and frankly malignant, and they can vary in size from 2 to 10 cm but are normally over 5 cm and may grow rapidly. They mainly occur in middle-aged or elderly women, or in those who are 10–15 years older than those who develop fibroadenomas. Microscopically they are characterised by stromal components forming leaf like structures.

It is often difficult to distinguish between a fibroadenoma, a common benign breast tumour, and benign phylloides. On mammography, phylloides present as benign masses and may contain large calcifications. Cytology is usually suspicious if increased numbers of cellular stromal elements or isolated abnormal cells are present. A core biopsy may provide a definitive diagnosis, but excision biopsy is often necessary. This is one reason why most breast specialists advise excision of large 'fibroadenomata.'

Treatment of phylloides tumours

Since these lesions pose a threat of local recurrence (about 20%), it is important that there are clear surgical margins, thus a wide local excision with negative margins is the principal approach to the management of these tumours (Schnabel, 1993).

As with other stromal cancers such as sarcomas, the preferred pathway of spread is through the blood vessels to the liver or bones (Kessinger et al., 1972). These tumours rarely affect the lymphatics, which mean there is no indication for axillary node surgery.

Basal phenotype

Basal-like breast cancer refers to a subtype of breast tumours found in micro-array studies of DNA to have overlapping gene-expression patterns and to display a basal/myoepithelial gene-expression profile (Diaz et al., 2007). Basal cytokeratins are expressed in basal-like cancers, and cytokeratin 5 and 6 (Cleator et al., 2007) in the basal cells of squamous or glandular epithelium (Chu and Weiss, 2002).

Biological features

Basal-like cancers are characterised by high histological grade, high mitotoic index, area of central necrosis and lymphatic infiltrate (Bocker et al., 2002; Rakha et al., 2006). Sortie et al. (2001) reported that basal-like breast cancers were associated with poor prognosis.

Approximately 90% of basal-like breast cancers are negative for ER, PR, and HER2 or Triple Negative phenotype (Perou Sorlie Eisen et al., 2000; Nielsen et al., 2004), and have been shown to have a high rate of epithelial growth factor (EGFR); also called HER1 (Korsching et al., 2002). These tumours carry a higher rate of visceral metastases such as brain and lung rather than bone and liver (Osbourne *et al.*, 2005). They are associated with a high rate of local relapse (Rodriguez-Pinella *et al.*, 2006) and tend to occur in pre-menopausal women (Osbourne *et al.*, 2005).

They exhibit high p53 protein expression. P53 acts as a check-point in the cell cycle to trigger molecular responses to cell damage, including repair and apoptosis. These tumours are associated with *BRCA1* mutations (Foulkes *et al.*, 2004).

Treatment of basal phenotype

At present, there is no specific treatment regimen for basal-type breast cancers. One study has shown a complete response to primary paclitaxel chemotherapy, when given sequentially with cyclophosphamide, doxorubicin and fluorouracil (Rouzier *et al.*, 2005). Cleator *et al.* (2007) suggests that basal-like cancers are likely to be more chemosensitive subtypes of breast cancer.

Randomised clinical trials are underway to test the efficacy of differing combinations of chemotherapy for basal-type cancers.

Reis-Filho and Tutt (2008) suggest that basal-like cancers have been shown to express EGFR in up to 66% of cases. Clinical trials are underway to assess anti-EGFR monoclonal antibodies such as cituximab.

Apocrine carcinoma

Apocrine carcinoma is defined as a tumour of apocrine-type cells.

Biological features

The predominant architectural pattern for apocrine carcinomas is a solid growth pattern, although it can include a spectrum of patterns (Roses, 1999). Apocrine carcinoma is a rare tumour, characteristically composed of large cells with eosinophilic cytoplasm (Tsuchiya *et al.*, 1998).

Sarcoma of the breast

Sarcomas are extremely rare in the breast; the most common types are angiosarcoma and lymphangiosarcoma.

Biological features

Sarcomas of the breast arise in the stroma or connective tissue of the breast and blood vessels; they are vascular and grow quickly. They can occur 5 years post–breast radiotherapy or sporadically.

Sarcomas of the breast frequently present with a large lump that has rapidly increased in size. Mammography is usually non-specific.

Treatment of sarcoma of the breast

The surgical approach to sarcomas depends on the size of the tumour. If large, it may require mastectomy; otherwise, wide local excision is appropriate. There is some suggestion that radiotherapy may be beneficial in local control (Johnstone *et al.*, 1993). Sarcomas are usually locally aggressive and spread via the blood with a poor response to chemotherapy. Patients are usually referred from the breast team following surgery to specialist cancer units who have the expertise of managing sarcomas.

Angiosarcomas

Angiosarcomas are the commonest sarcoma cancer of the breast, most often seen following previous radiotherapy. The overall 5-year survival of only 33% is poor (Chen *et al.*, 1988).

Biological features

Angiosarcomas usually occur in patients previously treated with radiotherapy, for example for lymphoma (Zucali *et al.*, 1994).

Angiosarcomas often present as a painless lump, varying in size from 1 to 11 cm, although sometimes there is diffuse breast enlargement, without a mass, in one or both breasts. The most common sites of spread are the liver, lung, skin, and to the contralateral breast.

Lymphangiosarcoma (Stewart-Treves lesion)

Lymphangiosarcomas are associated with post-treatment lymphoedema.

Lymphangiosarcoma is a rare complication of radical mastectomy usually developing 10 years after surgery, and frequently involving only the arm. These sarcomas are very aggressive, with rapid spread producing lymphoedema in an area, followed by the disease spreading widely throughout the body. The 5-year survival rate is poor (Stewart and Treves, 1948; Martin *et al.*, 1984).

Secretory carcinoma

Secretory carcinomas are rare (less than 0.01% of all breast cancers) and were first seen in children (McDivett and Stewart, 1966) but are known in all age groups.

Biological features

Secretory carcinomas usually present as a lump measuring less than 2 cm. In children, secretory carcinoma carries an excellent prognosis, but there is limited evidence available to suggest that the outlook in adults is as favourable (Tavassoli and Norris, 1980).

Squamous cell carcinoma

Pure squamous cell carcinoma is one of the rarest tumours.

Biological features

Squamous cell carcinomas have a lack of connection with the overlying epidermis and the absence of any other coexisting breast cancer. Microscopic characteristics include stratification, intercellular bridges, keratin production and areas of acantholysis. Spindle cell metaplasia may be dominant, requiring immunohistochemical stains to determine its epithelial nature (Donegan and Spratt, 1995).

Metaplastic carcinoma

Biological features

Metaplastic carcinomas are composed of epithelial and mesenchymal cells with varying degrees of differentiation (Donegan and Spratt, 1995).

Low-grade adenosquamous carcinoma

Low-grade adenosquamous carcinoma is an unusual type of metaplastic duct carcinoma that is morphologically similar to adenosquamous carcinoma of the skin.

Biological features

Low-grade adenosquamous carcinomas are hard, yellow nodules with ill-defined boarders and have a tendency to grow between ducts and within lobules (Rosen, 2001).

UNCOMMON PRESENTATIONS OF BREAST CANCER

Breast cancer in younger women

The majority of people diagnosed with breast cancer are post-menopausal (about 80%). Pre-menopausal women who have breast cancer are usually termed 'younger women with breast cancer'.

Biological features

The literature on breast cancer in young women has largely focused on the disease being more aggressive when compared with older women, thus young age is a poor prognostic factor (Xiong *et al.*, 2001). Breast cancer found in young women is more likely to be high-grade, hormone-insensitive (ER/PR negative), have HER2/neu overexpression, and the presence of vascular invasion compared with older women (Colleoni *et al.*, 2002; Dubsky *et al.*, 2002; Kothari and Fentiman 2002). However, young age is not an independent prognostic determinant. Providing tumours are of similar grade, size and nodal status, prognosis is independent of the patient's age. The sensitivity to hormones is different in young women, since 33% of cancers in young women are oestrogen receptor–negative (ER–ve), whereas over 70% of cancers in post-menopausal women are oestrogen sensitive (ER+ve).

One of the most important features of these cancers is the increased likelihood that a genetic mutation is causing the disease (see Chapter 3). Appropriately 30% of all breast cancers in young women are caused by a genetic mutation. The option of referral to a regional cancer genetics service, which provides genetic counselling and genetic testing, should be offered. Genetic counselling should be made available for the women's siblings and female relatives who may carry increased risk or susceptibility to developing breast cancer.

Treatment of breast cancer in younger women

Chemotherapy is increasingly being considered appropriate for all women under the age of 40 years, but poses the difficult problem of infertility.

Most young women are pre-menopausal. If their cancer is oestrogen receptor–positive, there are two methods of ovarian ablation (Clive and Dixon, 2002). The permanent method involves either surgical removal with oophrectomy, or radiotherapy.

If the woman wishes to conserve her fertility, the most common method is to use a LHRH analogue (luteinising hormone-releasing hormone) such as goserelin or leuprorelin. These are injections given monthly for 2 years, either by the general practitioner, practice nurse or by a member of the hospital team.

Breast cancer associated with pregnancy

Breast cancer associated with pregnancy occurs with an incidence of 1–2% of all breast cancers (Dixon *et al.* 2006). According to Petrek *et al.* (1991), the standard definition of pregnancy-associated breast cancer (or PABC) is defined as being diagnosed with breast cancer during pregnancy or within 1 year after delivery.

Biological features

Breast cancers that present during pregnancy have a low incidence (less than 25%) of ER sensitivity.

The breast undergoes enormous changes in pregnancy, including an increase in volume, dilation of ducts, increasing hormonal levels of oestrogen, progesterone, prolactin, lobular growth and cell proliferation. Blood flow increases by up to 180% by the time the baby is at full term (Hughes *et al.*, 1989). These changes present a challenge to the clinician as the breasts are often dense, and may double in size (hypertrophy), so masking clinical features of an underlying breast cancer.

Diagnosis

Mammography is of limited value in pregnancy and does expose the foetus to some radiation.

Ultrasound is by far the safest radiological tool during pregnancy. Together with ultrasound, all palpable breast masses should be biopsied. To achieve accurate diagnosis, fine-needle aspiration cytology (FNAC) is required. FNAC is technically more difficult to perform when the breast is engorged with milk. A study by Gupta (1997) showed that FNAC in pregnancy and in lactating women could be very accurate. In one cancer centre in the USA, Keleher *et al.*, (2001) preferred the use of image-guided core biopsy

Treatment of breast cancer associated with pregnancy

The treatment sequence for each patient is individualised. It is important that treatment is not postponed because of pregnancy. The management of the breast cancer and the different treatment options follow the same principles as in a non-pregnant woman. However, the risks to the foetus and its protection are important considerations in planning treatment. Close monitoring of the foetal development by an obstetrician is important throughout the pregnancy.

Although termination of the pregnancy is not recommended, it may be considered an option under some circumstances.

Breast surgery can be performed at any time during pregnancy, with little risk to the foetus (Gianopoulos, 1995). The delivery date is usually brought forward to 30–32 weeks, and labour-induced to enable prompt commencement of treatment. Usually immediate breast reconstruction is avoided during pregnancy as subjecting a foetus to elongated anaesthetic gases is not recommended.

Breast-conservation therapy, which includes wide local excision with axillary surgery followed by a course of radiotherapy, is acceptable in a selection of patients (Kuerer *et al.*, 2002). If the diagnosis is in the third trimester, then radiotherapy can commence after delivery. Although radiotherapy in pregnancy has been reported, it is not widely accepted (Antypas *et al.*, 1998) since there is a risk of congenital abnormalities from radiation and risk of premature delivery (Willemse *et al.*, 1990). If therefore the normal radiotherapy schedule would fall within the pregnancy, then a mastectomy should be performed.At present, little is known of the effects of pregnancy on the lymphatic spread. Dixon *et al.* (2000) reported that 65% of all breast cancers in pregnancy involved axillary lymph nodes. It is likely that surgeons perform axillary clearance of the glands, since the use of sentinel node biopsy is not recommended, the main reason being that the safety of the radioactive isotope, and blue dye, in pregnancy has yet to be determined. However, pregnant women should not be excluded from clinical trials (Moirta *et al.*, 2000).

Chemotherapy is not given during the first trimester of pregnancy, to prevent damage to the development of the foetus. Chemotherapy should be avoided during three weeks before delivery to avoid myelosuppression in the baby, with the possible consequences of bone marrow depression, increased risk of infection, and death (Giacalone *et al.*, 1999).

If the cancer is large (more than 3.5 cm), the treatment considered is primary chemotherapy. Breast cancers in pregnancy are frequently oestrogen-negative, and therefore insensitive to hormonal therapy. No studies of tamoxifen in pregnant women are likely since the drug can cause vaginal bleeding, spontaneous abortions, birth defects and foetal death. Therefore hormonal therapy is never commenced until after delivery.

Breast-feeding issues

Radiotherapy to the breast can cause fibrosis of the ducts, consequently reducing the amount of milk produced. Women should be advised that future breast-feeding is rare. Although future milk production may be compromised, breast-feeding is possible on the affected side, depending on the area of breast tissue treated.

Breast cancer in men

Approximately 1% of all breast cancers occur in the male breast, equating to approximately 300 new cases diagnosed annually (Cancer Research UK, 2009) and 70 deaths in 2000 (Office of National Statistics, 2000). The average age of male breast cancer is between 60 and 70 years old – 10 years older than in women.

Biological features

The pathology is similar to that of breast cancer found in women, with infiltrating ductal carcinoma the most common type, and DCIS well described. Lobular carcinoma has not been described in men. Inflammatory carcinoma and Paget's disease have also been seen in men. Breast cancer can develop following radiotherapy for previous cancers such as lymphoma. In 75% of men, the tumour presents as a mass under the nipple. Since men have less breast tissue than women, skin infiltration is more likely (Donegan, 1991). Overall survival has been reported as similar to that of women (Borgen et al., 1992; Cutuli et al., 1995).

The causes of breast cancer in men remain largely undetermined. However, it is known that men with family history of the disease are at a higher risk that men who have no such history. Two breast cancer genes (*BRCA1* and *BRCA2*) have been mapped and maybe responsible for as much as 20% of all male breast cancers (Vetto et al., 1999) (see Chapter 3).

Treatment of breast cancer in men

Current treatments for breast cancer in men are the same as those for women with the same disease (Fenlon, 1996). The main treatment for men with breast cancer is surgery, with most commonly modified mastectomy (Borgen et al., 1992; Jaiyesimi et al., 1992; Ravandi and Hayes, 1998). In a recent study comparing breast cancer treatment between men and women, men were more likely to have a mastectomy combined with radiotherapy than women (Scott-Corner et al., 1999).

A higher percentage of male breast cancers are hormone-dependent than in women (Rosen et al., 1976), which means they are responsive to adjuvant hormonal therapy such as tamoxifen. Anelli et al. (1994) reported that the side effects of tamoxifen in 24 men with breast cancer were decreased libido, weight gain, hot flushes, mood alteration and depression.

Research on systemic therapy with chemotherapy in men with breast cancer has not been well established over the past decade and is based largely on anecdotal or retrospective reports (Bunkely et al., 2000).

CONCLUSION

Breast cancer is not only one disease, but many. To improve a patient's cancer journey, we need to improve our understanding of the histopathology of this cancer, deliver accurate and timely information, and recognise how our practice can make a difference.

REFERENCES

Andersen JA (1974) Lobular carcinoma in situ. A long-term follow-up in 52 cases. *Acta Pathologica et Microbiologica Scandinavica (A)* 82(4): 519–533.

Anelli TF, Anelli A, Tran KN, Lebwohl DE and Borgen P (1994) Tamoxifen administration is associated with a high rate of treatment-limiting symptoms in male breast cancer patients. *Cancer* 74(1): 74–77.

Antypas C, Sandilos P, Kouvaris J et al. (1998) Fetal dose evaluation during breast cancer radiotherapy. *Internal Journal Radiation Oncology Biology and Physics* 40: 995–999.

Ashikari R, Park K, Huvos AG and Urban JA (1970) Paget's disease of the breast. *Cancer* 26: 680–685.

Bocker W, Moll R, Poremba C et al. (2002) Common adult stem cells in the human breast give rise to glandular and myoepithelial cell lineages: a new cell biological concept. *Laboratory Investigation* 82: 737–746.

Borgen PI, Wong GY, Vlamis V et al. (1992) Current management of male breast cancer: a review of 104 cases. *Annals of Surgery* 215(5): 451–417.

Bulens P, Vanuytsel L, Rjinders A and van der Schueren E (1990) Breast conserving treatment of Paget's disease. *Radiotherapy Oncology* 17: 305–309.

Bunkley DT, Robinson JD, Bennett NE and Gordon S (2000) Breast cancer in men: emasculation by association? *Journal of Clinical Psychology in Medical Settings* 7(2): 91–97.

Buzdar AU, Smith TL, Powell KC, Blumenschein GR and Gehan EA (1982) Effect of timing of initiation of adjuvant chemotherapy on disease-free survival in breast cancer. *Breast Cancer Research Treatment* 2(2): 163–169.

Cancer Research UK (2009) *Statistical Information Team*. Online. Available http://info.cancerresearchuk.org/cancerstats/types/breast/incidence/#Lifetime.

Chen KT, Kirkegaard DD and Bocian JJ (1988) Angiosarcoma of the breast. *Cancer* 46: 368–371.

Chinyama CN and Wells CA (1998) Pre-malignant, borderline lesions, ductal and lobular carcinoma in situ. In: MWE Morgan, R Warren and G Querci della Rovere (eds) *Early Breast Cancer – from Screening to Multidisciplinary Management*. Amsterdam: Harwood Academic Publishers.

Chu PG and Weiss LM (2002) Keratin expression in human tissues and neoplasms. *Histopathology* 40: 403–430.

Cleator S, Heller W and Coombes RC (2007) Triple-negative breast cancer: therapeutic options. *The Lancet* 8: 235–243.

Clive S and Dixon JM (2002) The value of adjuvant treatment in young women with breast cancer. *Drugs* 62(1): 1–11.

Colleoni M, Rotmensz N, Robertson C et al. (2002) Very young women (<35 years) with operable cancer features of disease at presentation. *Annals of Oncology* 13(2): 273–279.

Cutuli B, Lacroze M, Dilhuydy JM et al. (1995) Male breast cancer: results of the treatments and prognostic factors in 397 cases. *European Journal of Cancer* 31A(12): 1960–1964.

Diaz LK, Cryns VL, Symmans F and Sneige N (2007) Triple negative breast carcinoma and the basal phenotype: from expression profiling to clinical practice. *Advances in Anatomic Pathology* 14(6): 419–430.

Dixon JM, Sainsbury JRC and Rodger A (2006) Breast cancer: treatment of elderly patients and uncommon conditions. In: JM Dixon (ed.) *ABC of Breast Diseases*, 3rd edn. London: BMJ Books, Blackwell Publishing. Ltd.

Donegan W (1991) Cancer of the breast in men. *CA-A Cancer Journal for Clinicians* 41(6) Nov/Dec: 339–354.

Donegan WL and Spratt JS (1995) *Cancer of the Breast*. Philadelphia: W.B. Saunders.

Dubsky PC, Gnant MF, Taucher S et al. (2002) Young age as an independent adverse prognostic factor in premenopausal patients with breast cancer. *Clinical Breast Cancer* 3(1): 65–72.

Fenlon D (1996) Endocrine therapies for breast cancer. In: S Denton (ed.) *Breast Care Nursing*. London: Chapman and Hall.

Foote FW and Stewart FW (1941) Lobular carcinoma in situ: a rare form of mammary cancer. *American Journal of Pathology* 17: 491–496.

Foulkes WD, Brunet JS, Stefansson IM et al. (2004) The prognostic implication of the basal-like (cyclin E high/p27 low/p53+/glomeruloid-microvascular-proliferation+) phenotype of BRCA1-related breast cancer. *Cancer Research* 64(3): 830–835.

Fourquet A, Campana F, Vielh P, Schlienger P, Jullien D and Vilcoq JR (1987) Paget's disease of the nipple without detectable breast tumor: conservative management with radiation therapy. *International Journal of Radiation Oncology Biology Physics* 13(10): 1463–1465.

Frykberg ER (1999) Lobular carcinoma in situ of the breast. *Breast Journal* 5: 296–303.

Giacalone PL, Laffargue F and Benos P (1999) Chemotherapy for breast carcinoma during pregnancy. A French national survey. *Cancer* 86: 2266–2272

Gianopoulos JG (1995) Establishing the criteria for anaesthesia and other precautions for surgery during pregnancy. *Surgical Clinics of North America* 75: 33–43.

Gupta RK (1997) The diagnostic impact of aspiration cytodiagnosis of breast masses in association with pregnancy and lactation with the emphasis on clinical decision making. *Breast* 3: 131–134.

Haagensen CD, Lane N, Lattes R and Bodian C (1978) Lobular neoplasia (so-called lobular carcinoma in situ) of the breast. *Cancer* 42 (2): 737–769.

Harris JR, Lippman ME, Morrow M and Kent Osborne C (2010) *Diseases of the Breast*, 4th edn. Philadelphia: Lippincott Williams & Wilkins.

Hughes LE, Mansel RE, Webster DJT and Gravelle IH (1989) *Benign Disorders and Diseases of the Breast*. Philadelphia: Baillere Tindall.

Israel L, Breau JL and Morore JF (1986) Two years of high dose cyclophosphamide and 5-fluorouracil followed by surgery after 3 months for acute inflammatory breast carcinomas: a phase II study of 25 cases with a median follow-up on 35 months. *Cancer* 57(1): 24–28.

Jaiyesimi IA., Buzdar AU, Sahim AA and Ross MA (1992) Carcinoma of the male breast. *Annals of Internal Medicine* 117(9): 771–777.

Johnstone PA, Pierce L, Merino MJ, Yang JC, Epstein AH and DeLaney TF (1993) Primary soft tissue sarcomas of the breast: local-regional control with post-operative radiotherapy. *International Journal of Radiation Oncology Biology Physics* 27(3): 671–675.

Keleher AJ, Theriault RL, Gwyn KM *et al.* (2001) Multidisciplinary management of breast cancer concurrent with pregnancy. *American College of Surgeons* 194(1): 54–64.

Kessinger A, Foley JF, Lemon HM and Miller DM (1972) Metastatic cystosarcoma phyllodes: A case report and review of the literature. *Journal of Surgical Oncology* 4(2): 131–147.

King RJB (1996) *Cancer Biology*. Harlow: Longman.

Korsching E, Packeisen J, Agelopoulos K *et al.* (2002) Cytogenetic alterations and cytokeratin expression patterns in breast cancer: integrating a new model of breast differentiation into cytogenetic pathways of breast cytogenesis. *Laboratory Investigation* 82(11): 1525–1525.

Kothari AS and Fentiman IS (2002) Breast cancer in young women. *International Journal of Clinical Practice* 56(3): 184–187.

Kuerer HM, Gywn T, Ames FC and Theriault RI (2002) Conservative surgery and chemotherapy during pregnancy for breast carcinoma. *Surgery* 131(1): 108–110.

Maier WP, Rosemond GP, Harasym EL, Al-Saleem TI, Tasoni EM and Schor SS (1969) Paget's disease in the female breast. *Surgery Gynecology & Obstetrics* 128: 1253–1263.

Martin MB, Kon ND and Kawamonto EH (1984) Post mastectomy angiosarcoma. *American Journal of Surgery* 10: 541–545.

McDivett RW and Stewart FW (1966) Breast carcinoma in children. *Journal of the American Medical Association* 195: 388–390.

Moirta ET, Chang J and Leong S (2000) Principles and controversies in lymphoscintigraphy with emphasis on breast cancer. *Surgical Clinics of North America* 80: 1721–1737.

NHS Breast Screening Programme (1995) *Pathology Reporting in Breast Cancer Screening: National Co-ordinating Group for Breast Screening Pathology*. Sheffield: NHSBSP Publication No 3 2nd edn.

Nielsen TO, Hsu FD, Jensen K *et al.* (2004) Imunohistochemical and clinical characterisation of the basal-like subtype of invasive breast carcinoma. *Clinical Cancer Research* 10(160): 5367–5374.

Office of National Statistics (2000) *Annual Reference Volume: Mortality Statistics, Causes* 2000 (Series DH2, no. 27).

Osbourne CR, Kannan I, Ashfaq R *et al.* (2005) Clinical and pathological characterization of basal-like breast cancer. *Breast Cancer Research Treatment* 118.

Page DL and Anderson TJ (1987) *Diagnostic Histopathology of the Breast*. London: Churchill Livingstone.

Page DL, Steel CM and Dixon JM (2001) Carcinoma in situ and patients at high risk of breast cancer. In: M Dixon (ed.) *ABC of Breast Diseases*. London: BMJ Publishing.

Paget J (1874) On the disease of the mammary areola preceding cancer of the mammary gland. *St. Bartholomew's Hospital Reports* 10 87

Perou CM, Sorlie T, Eisen MB *et al.* (2000) Molecular portraits of human breast tumours. *Nature* 406: 747–752.

Petrek JA, Dukoff R and Rogatko A (1991) Prognosis of pregnancy associated breast cancer. *Cancer* 67(4): 699–672.

Pierce L, Haffty B, Solin L *et al.* (1997) The conservative management of Paget's disease of the breast with radiotherapy. *Cancer* 80(6): 1065–1072.

Rakha EA, Putti TC, Abd El-Rehim DM *et al.* (2006) Morphological and immunophenotypic analysis of breast carcinomas with basal and myoepithelial differentiation. *Journal of Pathology* 208: 495–506.

Ravandi-Kashani F and Hayes TG (1998) Male breast cancer: a review of the literature. *European Journal of Cancer* 34(9): 1341–1347.

Reiss-Filho JS and Tutt AN (2008) Triple negative tumours: a critical review. *Histopathology* 52: 102–118.

Rodriguez-Pinella SM, Sarro D, Honrado E *et al.* (2006) Prognostic significance of basal-like phenotype and fascin expressin in node negative invasive breast carcinomas. *Clinical Cancer Research* 12(5): 1533–1539.

Rosen PP (2001) *Rosen's Breast Pathology*. Philadelphia: Lippincott Williams & Wilkins.

Rosen PP, Menendez-Botet CJ, Nisselbaum JS, Schwartz MK and Urban JA (1976) Estrogen receptor protein in lesions of the male breast: a preliminary report. *Cancer* 37(4): 1866–1868.

Roses, DF (1999) *Breast Cancer*. New York: Churchill Livingstone.

Rouzier R, Perou CM, Symmans WF *et al.* (2005) Breast cancer molecular subtypes respond differently to preoperative chemotherapy. *Clinical Cancer Research* 11: 5678–5685.

Schnabel FR (1993) Cytosarcoma phyllodes. *Surgical Oncology Clinics of North America* 2: 107–119.

Scott-Corner CEH, Jochimsen PR, Menck HR and Winchester DJ (1999) An analysis of male and female breast cancer treatment and survival among demographically identical pairs. *Surgery* 126(4): 775–781.

Silverstein MJ (1999) Ductal carcinoma in situ of the breast – can we tailor treatment to pathological findings? In: *Fentiman in Breast Cancer*. Oxford: Blackwell Science.

Simpson PT, Gale T, Fulford LG, Reis-Filho JS and Lakhani SR (2003) The diagnosis and management of pre-invasive breast disease: pathology of atypical lobular hyperplasia and lobular carcinoma *in situ*. *Breast Cancer Research* 5(5): 258–262.

Sortie T, Perou CM, Tibshirani R *et al.* (2001) Gene expression patterns of breast carcinomas distinguish tumor subclasses with clinical implications. *Proceedings National Academy of Sciences USA* 98:(19): 10869–10874.

Stewart FW and Treves N (1948) Lymphangiosarcoma in post mastectomy lymphoedema. A report of six cases in elephantiasis chirurgica. *Cancer* 1: 64–81.

Stockdale AD, Brierly JD, White WF, Folkes A and Rostom AY (1989) Radiotherapy for Paget's disease of the nipple: a conservative alternative. *The Lancet* 2:(8664): 664–666.

Tavassoli FA and Norris HJ (1980) Secretory carcinoma of the breast. *Cancer* 45: 2404–2413.

Tsuchiya A, Rokkaku Y, Nihei M, Nomizu T, and Abe R (1988) Apocrine carcinoma of the breast –a case report. *Surgery Today* 18(6): 714–717.

Underwood JCE (2004) *General and Systemic Pathology*. London: Churchill Livingstone.

Vetto J, Jun S-Y, Padduch D, Eppich H and Shih R (1999) Stages at presentation, prognostic factors and outcome of breast cancer in males. *American Journal of Surgery* 177(5): 379–383.

Willemese PHS, vd Sijde R and Sleijfer DT (1990) Combination chemotherapy and radiation for stage IV breast cancer during pregnancy. *Gynecological Oncology* 36: 281.

Xiong Q, Valero V, Kau V *et al.* (2001) Female patients with breast carcinoma age 30 years and younger have a poor prognosis. *Cancer* 92(10): 2523–2528.

Zucali R, Merson M, Placucci M, Di Palma S and Veronesi U (1994) Soft tissue sarcoma of the breast after conservative surgery and irradiation for early mammary cancer. *Radiotherapy Oncology* 30(3): 271–273.

3 Genetic Factors in Breast Cancer

Audrey Ardern-Jones

INTRODUCTION

In the UK, one in three people develop cancer in their lifetime, and there are approximately 45 500 cases of breast cancer and just over 6000 cases of ovarian cancer diagnosed per year (Cancer Research UK, 2010). The majority of cancer cases occur by chance alone. Therefore, clustering of cancer cases in a family is not uncommon. In a small proportion of cases, this may be due to the familial inheritance of a piece of genetic damage (mutation) in a gene responsible for cellular growth control or DNA repair. Cancer is always genetic at the cellular level, in that a cancer is the end result of a series of genetic changes.

INHERITED BREAST CANCER: BIOLOGICAL EXPLANATION

Mutations or changes within a gene accumulate in every somatic cell during the course of an individual's lifetime. Somatic cells are the cells in the body that are not the sex cells. Not all mutations occur in somatic cells. Mutations also occur in the ova and spermatocytes. Some of these mutations can be inherited via the germline to cause an inherited cancer predisposition.

There is a long process of cumulative genetic changes that take place in a single breast cell before it becomes malignant. The malignant cell divides many times before an outward physical change is noted as a lump in a breast.

All cells in the human body contain a chemical substance called deoxyribonucleic acid (DNA). Chromosomes are structures that contain DNA and are arranged in pairs. In the human body, there are 23 pairs, or a total of 46 chromosomes, and the sex chromosomes are the 23rd pair. Males have one X and one Y chromosome, and females have two X chromosomes. The reason why chromosomes are arranged in pairs is due to the fact that one set of the 23 chromosomes comes from the mother in the egg and the other set comes from the father in the sperm. When a sperm and an egg unite, they form a new cell with 46 chromosomes. The fertilised egg then divides, and all 46 chromosomes are copied and passed on to every cell, where DNA is arranged in sequences or units that are known as genes. Genes direct the growth, development and function of the human body; everything from the colour of our hair, to our height and to how often cells divide. Metaphorically speaking, genes are like a booklet of complex instructions. A gene is a sequence of DNA.

Breast Cancer Nursing Care and Management, Second Edition, Edited by Victoria Harmer
© 2011 by Blackwell Publishing Ltd.

As we have inherited half our chromosomes from our mother (via the egg) and half from our father (via the sperm), this means that we have two copies of every gene – one copy from each parent.

Sometimes a gene is altered (or has a mutation), so that it does not function correctly. This is not a problem if one copy of the gene works and provides the cell with the correct instruction. Some alterations in a gene do not effect change, and these are called variants of unknown significance. Currently, scientists are interested in these variants or polymorphisms and, following the initiation of the Human Genome Project, much work is being done to try and identify genes in relation to disease and treatment. This work is ongoing and promises new horizons for medicine.

Each gene has a specific function in the body. One of the main functions of the cell is to replicate itself, and therefore some genes control cell division. When mutations occur in these genes, a cell may begin to divide without control. Such a cell, once altered and therefore not functioning in a normal manner, may then change to a cancer cell. Thus all cancers are the result of gene mutations. Mutations may be caused by ageing, environmental exposure to radiation, chemicals or hormones, or to other factors such as smoking and alcohol. Over time, a number of mutations may occur in a particular cell, thus allowing the cell to divide and grow in a way that may turn into a cancer. This usually takes many years, and this therefore explains the fact that the older a person is, the higher is their risk of developing cancer. Thus the population risk that one in three people (Cancer Research UK, 2010). will develop cancer in our Western Society relates to an older population. The older we become, the greater the chance we have of developing cancer.

If an individual has inherited a copy of an altered gene (known as a mutation), then this means that every single cell in his/her body has the mutation. This mutation may or may not pass down to the offspring (Fig. 3.1). Fig. 3.1 reflects the premise that there is always a 50/50 chance of the offspring inheriting or not inheriting the faulty copy of the gene. Each circle represents a person's two copies of a gene. The copy with the mutation is darkened and has a line through it.

An individual who has inherited the gene mutation has a higher chance than a person without a mutation of developing cancer. We do not fully understand why, in some families, some people who carry mutations in a gene do not develop cancer and others do. It may well be linked with environmental issues, such as carcinogens, and with other moderator genes that the individual has that make the difference. Research is ongoing in gene carriers to try and understand these differences in families (Eeles *et al.*, 2004). Inherited gene mutations explain why, in some families, there are more cases of cancer throughout the different generations. Particularly in inherited cancer, you find bilateral disease, younger onset of cancer and the same types of cancer throughout the generations, i.e. breast.

About 5–10% of breast cancer cases are thought to be due to heritable genetic influences. This means that most breast cancers are not hereditary. However, if a woman outlines her family history, there is sometimes an explanation as to why breast cancer may have developed in her family. It is important to note that currently there is limited knowledge to explain the reasons why some families seem prone to developing breast cancer. The most likely cause relates to a combination of environmental exposures interacting with various genes that are yet to be identified. Indeed, any woman who has a first-degree relative who has developed breast cancer under the age of 50 years has an increased risk compared with other women who do not have such a relative. Very often, the increased risk is marginal, and extra screening is not recommended for these women, other than the UK National Screening Programme (www.nice.org.uk).

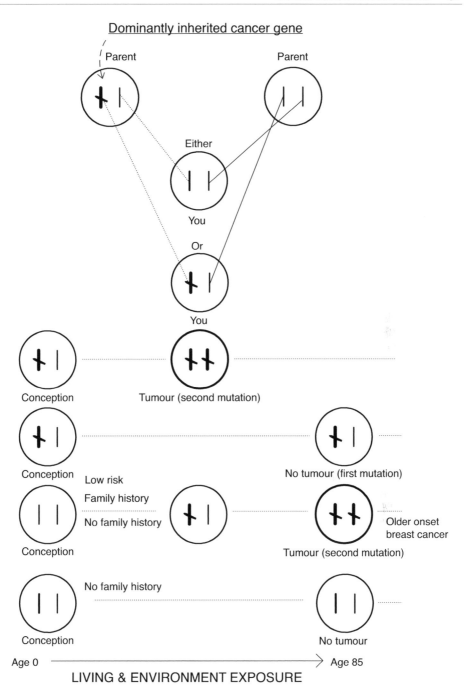

Fig. 3.1 Mode of inheritance.

FAMILY CONCERN

If a woman develops breast cancer, she may well be concerned about the risk for her daughters. Studies have shown the profound effect of the impact of a mother's breast cancer diagnosis on a daughter. These fears need to be translated into the reality of relative risk for the daughter (Wellisch *et al.*, 1996). Family contacts and dynamics are an important part of the counselling process and, sadly, many family members have experienced young-onset cancer relatives who may have died. Time needs to be taken to understand these families and to help them, as many of these families have a distorted perception of their risk (Ardern-Jones, 1997).

Many family members are under the illusion that, if they look like their relative, they will automatically develop cancer (Richards *et al.*, 1995). Genetic counselling seeks to explain simply the basics of genetic inheritance to dispel these beliefs and elucidate information about family members so that cancer cases can be independently confirmed, and cancer risk should be explained in a way that is comprehensible to everyone involved (Ardern-Jones and Mitchell, 1999).

CONFIRMING A CANCER FAMILY HISTORY

Talking about the past with a person who is bereaved of loved ones is sometimes very upsetting. It is imperative that the health professional collecting the family history is sensitive to the past experience of the client. For some families, it is hard to know what sort of illness a relative may have had. It takes a considerable amount of work to search through hospital records and collect histological evidence of different cancer illnesses. There are methods of collecting information that are not too problematic if a person is dead, and these include writing to Cancer Family Registers that exist all around the UK. However, not all registries are complete and, in some areas, were only started in the 1970s. Collecting a death certificate is possible if the family member is prepared to pay and submit accurate information on the relative that relates to their birth and death. This can be done nowadays via the website. Not all cancers are recorded, particularly if a person developed cancer many years before he/she died. If a relative is alive, it is essential to receive written consent before searching for information.

DOMINANTLY INHERITED BREAST CANCER SUSCEPTIBILITY GENES

The gene *BRCA1* (**br**east **ca**ncer 1 gene) for breast cancer is located on Chromosome 17, and was the first breast cancer–predisposition gene characterised after many years of research (Miki *et al.*, 1994). *BRCA1* mutations are linked with more than 45% of inherited breast cancers and 90% of families with broth breast and ovarian cancer. Statistical evidence shows that up to 80% of women who carry *BRCA1* mutations develop breast cancer by the age of 80 years and have an estimated 15–60% risk of ovarian cancer, the risk increasing from the early thirties for breast cancer and from the age of 40 years for ovarian cancer (Eeles *et al.*, 2004). The important information for a family is to know that this risk is carried over time. Thus, the presence of a cancer-predisposition gene increases cancer risk, but does not mean that cancer will definitely develop.

The *BRCA2* gene is located on Chromosome 13 and is another breast cancer–predisposition gene (Wooster *et al.*, 1994). This gene also confers an increased risk of breast cancer and ovarian cancer. Both genes are dominantly inherited and can be passed down through the germline, either through the mother or the father.

RISK ASSESSMENT

Risk assessment may be divided into 'absolute risk' and 'relative risk'.

Absolute risk

Absolute risk refers to the frequency with which a particular disease occurs in a particular group. For example, one in ten women will develop breast cancer if they live to 85 years of age in the UK.

Relative risk

Relative risk compares the risk of the disease among the people who have a certain risk factor with the people that do not have this risk factor. For example, a woman with a maternal history of breast cancer in several relatives is compared with a woman of the same age who has no family history of breast cancer.

The determination of what risks are meaningful, and therefore contribute towards the disease, depends on the latest research findings published in peer-review journals. The question remains as to how many factors, such as the use of the use of the oral contraceptive in high-risk breast cancer younger women, ethnicity and age of onset of menarche, alter the risk of breast cancer. True associations between risk factors and the disease being questioned are usually answered by large case-control studies analysed for statistical significance (Claus *et al.*, 1994).

The chance that breast cancer is inherited is determined by assessing the family history pattern. Both males and females can carry cancer-predisposition genes, and so multiple cases of breast and other cancers may occur either on the maternal or paternal sides of the family. Risk estimates for the presence of a cancer-predisposition gene in a family depend on the number of cases, with the ages of diagnosis of cancer and the age of the person who is seeking advice for risk. For example, if a mother or a sister develops breast cancer at the age of 35 years (only one person), there is a 30% chance that this is because of a genetic susceptibility. If both the mother and sister developed breast cancer at the age of 35 years, this then increases the chance that this was due to a gene to approximately 90%. This estimate does not identify the predisposition genes involved. The predisposition genes can be identified by factoring in the epidemiological data and conferring with the risk-assessment tool developed by Claus in 1994 (Claus *et al.*, 1994). This model does not include Ashkenazi ancestry or the risk of ovarian cancer. Many other newer models are now involved in assessing risk.

The breast cancer risk for a female in a high-risk family starts at the age of 30 and steadily rises until they reach 75 years of age. In rare families, this may start at an earlier age if there are younger cases. The older that a family member is without developing cancer, the less likely it is that she has inherited the cancer-predisposition gene. In other words, the person 'lives through their risk period' and does not develop breast cancer.

The other model used to measure breast cancer risk is the Gail model (Costantino *et al.*, 1999). This model evaluates a woman for risk factors that include: current age, age at first live birth, number of primary relatives with breast cancer, number of breast biopsies, biopsy with hyperplasia and age at first menstruation. It does not take into account other cancers. Interestingly, Amir *et al.* (2003) debated the different models of risk assessment and concluded that the Tyrer–Cuzick model, which looks at breast cancer risk and includes Jewish ancestry and ovarian cancer, is the most consistently accurate model for prediction of breast cancer.

At this point in time, there are computer programs being developed for use in GP surgeries and general clinics to estimate breast cancer risk for an individual with regard to their family history.

Both the *BRCA1* and *BRCA2* genes are associated with an increased risk for individuals who are carriers of germline mutations. This estimate varies according to ethnic group and age of the individual. However, there is a significant risk of developing breast and or ovarian cancer, and family members need to be counselled accordingly

IN SUMMARY

Definitions of hereditary, familial and sporadic breast cancers

Hereditary breast cancer

With hereditary breast cancer, there is evidence of high-incidence breast cancer in the first- and or second-degree relatives in several generations. Typically, early age at onset (under 45 years) bilateral disease is associated with cancer of the ovary and may sometimes be associated with other tumours. More recently, there is evidence to suggest that women who develop breast cancer under the age of 35 years and who have triple-negative tumours (TNT = tumour negative for oestrogen receptor [ER], progesterone receptor [PR] and HER2 expression) are more susceptible to being a *BRCA* carrier (Lakani *et al.*, 2002). In some centres, women are offered genetic testing if it may alter their management, the reason being that, if a woman who is a *BRCA* carrier has a significant risk of a contralateral tumour (up to 65%), she may wish to consider bilateral preventative breast surgery if appropriate. This option of offering genetic testing at diagnosis is controversial. A small qualitative research project discussed this option, which involved both medical professionals and *BRCA* patients under the age of 40 years (Ardern-Jones *et al.*, 2005). Interestingly, most of the women in this small study felt that the prospect of having the genetic diagnosis at the same time as the breast cancer diagnosis would be too much to cope with. The professionals had mixed views about these developments.

Familial breast cancer

With familial breast cancer, there is evidence of breast cancer involving one or more first- or second-degree relatives but which does not fit the definition of hereditary breast cancer.

Sporadic breast cancer

Sporadic breast cancer shows limited family history of breast cancer through two generations, including both sets of grandparents, parents, aunts and uncles and siblings and offspring. Sporadic breast cancer is breast cancer that develops by chance and is not associated with a genetic predisposition. This accounts for most breast cancers.

Classifications of hereditary breast cancers

Classifications of hereditary breast cancers all involve pre-menopausal onset of the disease and increased risk of bilateral disease.

1   Site-specific hereditary breast cancer: Predominantly breast involvement. No other tumours present.
2   Breast/ovarian syndrome: Association of breast and ovarian cancer and *BRCA* genes.
3   Li-Fraumeni syndrome: Association of breast cancer with sarcoma, brain tumour, leukaemia and adrenocortical cancers. Li-Fraumeni syndrome may be associated with a mutation in the *TP53* gene. It is very important to refer any young woman with this sort of family history to a Genetics Specialist Unit for clinical advice.
4   Cowden's syndrome: Association of breast cancer with mouth and skin lesions and thyroid tumours. Cowden's syndrome is associated with a mutation in the *PTEN* gene. If a patient with a family history of thyroid and or endometrial tumours is seen, she should be referred to Clinical Genetics for advice.
5   Breast/gastrointestinal syndrome: Association with cancers of the stomach, colon and pancreas. Breast/gastrointestinal syndrome could be associated with a mutation in the hereditary non polyposis gene. The chance of breast cancer being linked with breast/gastrointestinal syndrome is much rarer, but if a patient with the above-stated family history is seen, then she should be referred to Clinical Genetics for advice.
6   Some people question as to whether or not in situ cancer, such as DCIS and LCIS should be included and managed in the same way as invasive breast cancer in assessment of mammographic follow-up and genetic testing. Currently, they are included, but possibly this may change in the future.

Screening and prevention options for at-risk women

There is uncertainty regarding the efficacy of screening women with a family history of breast cancer. These women may understandably have increased anxiety levels, and false-positive screens may increase their fears. Reasonable screening for women in high-risk hereditary families includes the following:

Breast self-examination

The evidence that breast self-examination (BSE) is an effective screening technique is weak in the general population. Several studies have failed to demonstrate that it impacts on mortality, stage or tumour size (Thomas *et al.*, 1997; Semiglazov *et al.*, 1996). There is limited evidence to suggest that that it is an effective option in high-risk women (Gui *et al.*, 2001) Women should be educated about BSE and choose whether they practise it. If done, it should be performed monthly, preferably 5–10 days after a period has finished. A trained breast care nurse should teach the procedure.

Clinical breast examination

There is debatable evidence that clinical breast examination is effective. However, it is generally considered a key component of screening, and young women at risk should have this available from a trained health professional in a screening centre if they are at high risk. Indeed Gui *et al.* (2001) reports, in his study on younger women, the effectiveness of both clinical breast examination and mammography screening.

Mammography screening

Data regarding the efficacy of mammography screening come from a series of randomised trials that were conducted in the general population. It is known that, in women over the age of 50 years, regular mammography screening reduces breast cancer by about one third. Mammography as a screening tool under the age of 50 years has a lower overall accuracy. The subject of screening and its value is controversial, but Fieg (1996) suggests that the benefit of mammography screening far outweighs any recorded risk of radiation-induced cancer. Furthermore, there have been recent papers that suggest that screening younger women (40–50 years) has been found to be beneficial for those with a family history (Kollias *et al.*, 1998; Lallo *et al.*, 1998). In the UK, mammography screening in high-risk women does not usually start until a woman reaches the age of 40 years. However, in rare cases where there are very young–onset cases, screening may occur at an earlier age. It is recommended that mammography screening should begin no earlier than the age of 30 years. More recently, National Institute for Health and Clinical Excellence (NICE) guidelines have stratified those who should have mammography screening. NICE has divided the guidelines into women who are low-, moderate- and high-risk screening (NICE, 2006). Digital mammographic screening is considered further in the Chapter 4. More recently, units have used a combination of two mathematical models – Manchester scoring (Antoniou *et al.* 2007) and BOADICEA (Antoniou 2006) to define protocols for management and decisions regarding breast screening and *BRCA* genetic testing.

Ultrasound and MRI

Ultrasound and MRI are currently used for investigations of symptoms. Ultrasound plays a role when an abnormality is detected, in order to differentiate cystic from solid. Not enough evidence exists to support the use of these tools as effective screening options, however. Following recent published research (Warner, 2009), MRI screening has been recommended for carriers of both *BRCA1* and *BRCA2* genes, and for *TP53* gene carriers and for those who are at 50% risk of inheriting one of these genes. These carriers are recommended MRI breast screening on annual basis from the age of 30 years, along with mammography screening until the age of 50 years and thereafter annual mammography screening until the age of 70 years.

Ovarian screening

Ovarian screening and its efficacy and who is eligible for screening is currently being evaluated in a National UK Study for efficacy in high-risk women. This study is called UKFOCSS and is supported by Cancer Research UK. Current practice is for women to have a one-off ovarian screen.

Prophylactic surgery

The role of prophylactic surgery in high-risk breast cancer gene carriers is unproven. However, a recent study reported that prophylactic bilateral total mastectomy reduces the incidence of breast cancer at 3 years follow-up (Meijers-Heijboer *et al.*, 2001). The Hartman *et al.* (1999) study suggested a risk reduction of breast cancer of at least 90% after prophylactic mastectomy. More recent studies have supported this level of risk reduction (Narod, 2006). Although there are no long-term studies looking at survival, the psychological impact of surgery is profound, and it is highly recommended that sufficient time is given to discussion of psychological issues related to body image. These sessions should be shared with a partner at an appointment with a clinical psychologist. The breast nurse plays a pivotal role with these patients, and very often it is therapeutic to meet others who have undergone the procedure.

Prophylactic oophorectomy

Prophylactic oophorectomy in high-risk women is thought to reduce the risk of ovarian cancer considerably from a range of 16–60% to approximately 2–3%. The risks are not reduced to exactly those of the general population because of the 2–3% risk of peritoneal adenocarcinomatosis. The impact of this surgical procedure on reduction of breast cancer risk, as well as of ovarian cancer risk, has been highlighted by Rebbeck *et al.* (2002) in a study of women with *BRCA1* and *BRCA2* mutations. This risk reduction persisted beyond 10 years of follow-up and is encouraging. As this surgical procedure can be keyhole, many women at high risk are opting for this procedure, as a preventative option, after full counselling. Many women have hormone therapy following this intervention as they have menopausal symptoms following surgery. Psycho-social research on high-risk women who have had prophylactic surgery highlights the depths of emotional feelings that are present in some women following this option for reduction of cancer risk (Hallowell *et al.*, 2004).

Preventive measures rely on screening procedures to reduce death from breast cancer by picking up a tumour at its early stage of development and treating it accordingly. Familial breast cancer is usually associated with breast cancer occurring at a young age. Guidelines about cancer risk and pedigree drawing may be accessed via http://www.geneticseducation.nhs.uk. (See also Standardization Task Force, 1995.)

Guidelines about who should have screening are on the NICE website and, as protocols change, it is important that nurses are informed of up to date recommendations. These recommendations are the results of research findings in high-risk women, and are another good source for up-to-date recommendations on screening and genetic testing.

GENETIC TESTING AND COUNSELLING

The most likely individuals to be carrying a breast cancer–predisposition gene are those with a dramatic family history of breast and ovarian cancer. Those at highest risk are women with a family history of young-onset breast cancers in a family as well as multiple cases under the age of 60 years and women with a family history of breast and ovarian cancers (Eeles *et al.*, 2004). Others who are at high risk and may wish to be tested are families with two cases of breast cancer and one case of ovarian cancer; families with male and female breast cancers or Ashkenazi Jewish women with breast cancer in a single family member (at 40 years of age), with or without a family history. Normal *BRCA1* and *BRCA2* genes control cell growth. Mutations in these genes, which are more common among Ashkenazi Jewish women (Jewish women of Eastern European descent) than in the general population, increase the risk of breast and ovarian cancers. This makes genetic testing for unaffected persons possible in this population as the search is for the three founder mutations in *BRCA1* and *BRCA2*. It is still better to test an affected member of a family first, and then unaffected people coming forward for testing can have a clear-cut result if a mutation is identified.

For high-risk women, several options are open to them. They may wish to consider genetic counselling and to discuss, in a private and confidential setting, the pros and cons of genetic testing. If they choose the genetic-testing option, an affected person with cancer in the family must be tested first, to search for the mutation that is specific to that particular family.

Testing the cancer patient

In order to start the process of genetic testing, it is the current practice to look for the alteration in the gene in the affected person. The reason for this is that only by looking in the DNA make-up of an individual who has already developed cancer is it possible to interpret the results of the genetic test for the whole family.

If an alteration in the gene is found in the affected member, unaffected family members may then be tested. The process of genetic counselling for the affected individual is essential to give the cancer patient the chance to consider all the implications of the test. It is sometimes thought that a patient who has already developed cancer may not need time to discuss all the issues. However, this is not the case, and it is essential that the individual seeking counselling fully understand the risks. These risks include the development of other cancers, in particular ovarian cancer. Furthermore, there is the knowledge that, if he/she is a gene carrier, there is 50/50 chance that each of their offspring may carry the same alteration. The test for the cancer patient may take anything up to 3 months to screen the gene in a National Health Service (NHS) laboratory, and screens the whole coding area of the *BRCA1* and *BRCA2* genes. The Department of Health's initiative to promote efficiency in genetic testing (2003) has improved the process, and laboratories only test families where there is a probability of at least 20% of finding a pathogenic mutation in a gene (http://www.icr.ac.uk/fbcprotocols). Test results can sometimes be 'uninformative', and this can be falsely reassuring for some women. This then means that other members in their families cannot have testing, and managing these women so as to make best use of further prevention options can be confusing for the professionals looking after them (Ardern-Jones *et al.*, 2008, 2010).

If a mutation is not picked up in the genetic test, several reasons may be to blame:

- The wrong gene is being tested.
- The test may have missed the mutation, as it is present in a region of the gene as yet not coded for, i.e. the regulatory part of the gene.
- The person undergoing the genetic test developed cancer by chance alone and was unlucky, rather than having an inherited a gene fault despite a strong family history. This may happen in high-risk families but of course is very rare.

The individual with cancer is given his/her genetic test result and, if no mutations were identified in the test, they are informed that the test is negative, and the family must continue with the guidelines for appropriate screening as advised at the time of counselling. More recently, women who test negative for *BRCA* mutations and were having ovarian screening are reassured that the risk for ovarian cancer is very low. They do not need ovarian screening. Some women find the information that no mutation has been found confusing (Hallowell *et al.*, 2002) and need further time to reflect on the limits of the test with a health professional. If a mutation is identified, the individual returns to meet with the counsellor and is informed. The counsellor always follows up this session. Individuals vary as to how they handle the information and to whom in the family they divulge it. This may be problematic in some families. Confidentiality is paramount within the genetic-counselling programme, and a professional is unable to inform the family other than through the index case. This may present problems for some families where communication has broken down.

OPTIONS AVAILABLE FOR CANCER PATIENTS WITH A MUTATION

Prophylactic surgery for risk reduction is a possibility, as well as further screening if needed. The prophylactic surgery option needs to be carefully considered with the specialists caring for the patient, taking into consideration the status of the cancer patient and balancing the patient's needs with regard to any further surgery.

It is essential that all carriers of genetic mutations should be followed up annually for the rest of their lives (Ardern-Jones and Eeles, 2002).

Predictive genetic testing

Predictive genetic testing is usually arranged for someone in the family who wishes to know their genetic status and has not developed cancer. In this case, the affected person has been tested and a mutation has been identified. The test usually takes 4 weeks before results are given in the NHS Clinical Testing Programme. The individual has a session which includes outlining all the possible risks, and taking time to consider all the implications of undergoing such a test, including mention of insurance issues. Fear of discrimination may exist for people who are known to be high risk. The Association of British Insurers (ABI) has agreed with the Government, through the Code of Practice on Genetic Testing and the Concordat and Moratorium, that no predictive genetic test results for breast cancer risk be requested by ABI insurance companies. The Moratorium has been extended to 2014 (http://www.abi.org.uk).

Time is taken to discuss the emotional implications of undergoing such a test and to check whom the individual will have to share their concerns with and how they will cope following their results. Follow-up support is always offered. Communication may well be a problem for some families, as family members do not always feel comfortable informing other relatives about their gene test result (Foster *et al.*, 2002).

The number of sessions that are arranged for a person considering predictive genetic testing vary. For some people where testing has taken place in other family members, they may know about many of the risk estimates as well as the impact of a positive result. Each case is considered in the multidisciplinary meeting and, for some people, it is practical and helpful to have the test on the first visit. However, in many other cases, the first session informs the individual about all the risk estimates associated with the mutation in the family gene, and discusses the options that are available to that individual should they find out that they are a carrier of the gene. Currently, the lifetime risk of developing breast cancer for those who carry either the *BRCA1* or *BRCA2* genes ranges from 50% to 85% (Breast Cancer Linkage Consortium, 1999). The risk starts at the age of 30 years and is very low. The risk for ovarian cancers varies between 15% and 60% (Breast Cancer Linkage Consortium, 1999) depending on the gene, ethnic group and previous medical history, i.e. oral contraceptives taken for more than 3 years may reduce the risk of developing ovarian cancer. These risks are altered for Ashkenazi Jewish women.

It is important for the individual to be aware of potential problems such as depression and anxiety, which may occur following disclosure of the genetic status. It may be that a further session is arranged before a blood sample is taken. The final session is when the results are given, and this will depend upon the turnaround time for mutation analysis after the blood was taken. It is recommended that another person should attend the clinic with the patient to provide support. In rare cases, this test may need to be accelerated, as the results may alter clinical management (Mitchell *et al.*, 2001).

If a predictive test is negative, the person undergoing the test is then informed that their risk for cancer is that of the general population. It is not necessary for a woman who does not carry the family gene alteration to continue with early screening unless there is a history on the other side of the family. All women should practise breast awareness and arrange to take part in the National Screening Programme for those over the age of 50 years. If a woman or man does not carry the gene, it means that they cannot pass it on to their children. In particular, some of the gene-negative persons undergoing testing express disbelief or an emotion called 'survivor guilt'. These emotions need time to heal and should be followed up by the nurse (Ardern-Jones *et al.*, 2010).

Men do seek predictive testing as they have the same chance of inheriting the gene as women in the same family. It has been reported that their uptake is lower: they are sometimes keen to have the test and then consider the issues, and this can be problematic for their families (Hallowell *et al.*, 2004) This may be due to many factors, including the fact that men do not attend health appointments so readily as women. If a person tests positive, they may become depressed and anxious.

ETHICAL ISSUES

Ethical issues can be considered in three different categories:

1   Individual rights;
2   Obligations of health professionals;
3   Likely conflicts between the rights of the individual and the rights of others.

Individual rights

It is straightforward that an individual seeking genetic testing should have the nature of the tests and the implications of the results explained to them before they give consent. The individual should be prepared well for the results, and for the impact that the results may have on his or her psychological wellbeing. Furthermore, the discussion of confidentiality and the consequences associated with the result should be made clear before testing (Hallowell, 2003).

Rights of other individuals

Should a woman or man be obligated to inform her family about her genetic status? Should she or he inform her/his partner and medical doctor about the test? There are major consequences to the family in terms of emotional burden and the implications of the risk for all first-degree relatives. The individual's right to the confidentiality of test results may conflict with the interests of employers and insurance companies. For these reasons, some people refuse the test. Currently, legislation to protect gene carriers from possible discrimination does not exist in the UK. A great deal has been debated in the literature about the problems of family communication (Forest *et al.*, 2003) and the difficulties in informing others.

The obligation of health care professionals

There are important ethical obligations for health care providers and policymakers with regard to the criteria for testing. These ethical obligations include identifying those who test positive and providing systems, personnel and training.

One of the principles of an appropriate screening test is that an effective preventative strategy is available for those testing positive for the condition. It could be argued that it is unethical to test unless one can do something about it. Currently, there are no proven preventative measures, other than the use of screening modalities as already described. Furthermore, it is welcoming news that prophylactic surgery has benefits, although little is known about the long-term effects.

When should genetic testing be undertaken? The age of adult consent in the UK is 18 years, so this could be an appropriate time if a young person is interested in this option. However, there are no screening programmes available for young persons of this age. It would ethically be essential for the young persons to be counselled that they are not eligible for screening at this age, and to take time to remind them of the normal levels of risk and the appropriate ages of screening.

Psychological assessment of the individual choosing testing is essential. The counsellor caring for high-risk women must be aware that mood disorders, anxiety and depression are common and severe in women at risk of breast cancer. Referral to a clinical psychologist or psychiatrist is essential if someone has a history of current psychiatric problems.

Thus, if genetic testing is chosen, then genetic counselling must be provided. This is a multidisciplinary practice where the individual may be seen by a Nurse Specialist or Genetic Counsellor and, in some cases, may meet the Medical Consultant and have access to psychological care if needed. It is essential that health professionals consider the ethical issues of consent and disclosure to help support their families (Duggan *et al.*, 2003)

VIGNETTES: BREAST CANCER GENETIC COUNSELLING

All the family trees for the purpose of this chapter are fictional (see Fig. 3.2).

Family 1

The family tree comprises of a woman aged 41 years who has developed unilateral breast cancer, as has her sister who developed breast cancer aged 35 years. Her father is well and healthy at the age of 70. However, it transpires that his sister developed bilateral breast cancer aged 44 and 51, respectively. Another aunt developed breast cancer aged 56 years. The paternal grandmother developed ovarian cancer at 49 years of age and is now dead.

Question:

Does the family history represent any known syndrome?

Answer:

Family 1 represents a family with a high chance of a *BRCA* mutation.

Question:

Are there any significant issues?

Answer:

If this family has a significant risk of both breast and ovarian cancer, have all the histologies been checked? For example, if the ovarian cancer was uterine cancer and if the breast cancers in one of the younger cases were not cancers but benign disease, this would then lower the risk of there being a gene mutation present in the family.

Question:

If the cancers in the family are confirmed by histology, what are the options?

Answer:

All the females in the family should have both breast and ovarian screening on an annual basis. Mammography screening starts at 40 years for high-risk families such as these; however, if a gene is identified in the family, it is recommended at 30 years along with MRI screening. Genetic testing may be arranged after full counselling on a person who has developed cancer. The person most likely to carry the mutation is the youngest person in the family. However, this depends on the person wishing to know their status. The person with cancer having the test must appreciate that, if she is a mutation carrier, she has a significant risk of another cancer developing in the other breast. If she is a *BRCA* carrier, she has a significant risk of ovarian cancer. Ovarian screening starts at the age of 35 years. If, after testing, a mutation is identified, then unaffected members of the family may come forward for genetic testing, and there is a 50/50 chance that they may or may not have inherited the gene mutation that exists in the family.

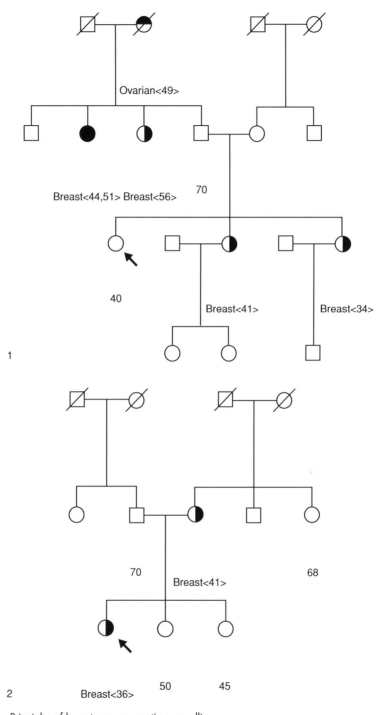

Fig. 3.2   Principles of breast cancer genetic counselling.

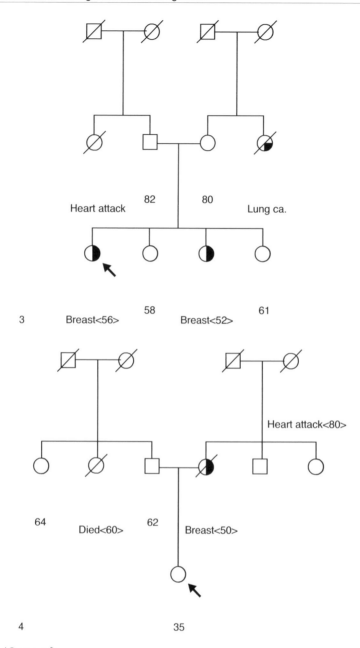

Fig. 3.3 (Continued).

Question:

What are the ethical and social implications associated with this family?

Answer part 1:

It may well be that the person seeking advice with regard to genetic testing does not fully appreciate that other family members may need to be informed regarding the advice for screening. In some families where communication is problematic, revealing information can become difficult and unexpected. The genetic nurse may have difficulty in obtaining accurate information from live affected members of the family, as written consent may not be forthcoming due to barriers in the family communication system.

Answer part 2:

If one person has developed breast cancer and is very ill, then the partner of that particular person may be very reluctant to involve the family member in genetic testing. It may then become a sensitive and very traumatic time for other members in the family, who may be feeling desperate to find out more information.

Answer part 3:

Men may not realise that their offspring are at risk of developing both breast and ovarian cancer.

Answer part 4:

There may be concerns about future effects on insurance despite the current ABI moratorium.

Answer part 5:

The father of the daughter seeking counselling may not realise that he is a potential carrier of a gene mutation, and may then become devastated if he finds that he is the carrier in the family that has put his daughters at high risk of developing cancer. This may be problematic in a relationship. He would have a risk of breast and prostate cancer if *BRCA2*-positive and would need to be informed. Research is currently taking place in many centres, looking at the risk of prostate cancer and involving men in PSA screening. Called IMPACT, this study is supported by Cancer Research UK.

 If the father is tested and does not carry the gene then none of his offspring are at risk and do not need screening or testing.

Answer part 6:

There may be issues surrounding further surgery for the person who is only 41 years old; i.e. if she is a gene carrier, should she then have prophylactic surgery on the other breast with possible reconstruction, and perhaps her ovaries removed? All these are very serious issues, and the consideration of surgery in the light of current health status, i.e. lymph node status and the possibility of recurrence and of course the individual choice of the patient and quality of life, is a complex and difficult decision for someone in this situation.

Answer part 7:

The worry that relates to the children and their risk is always stressful for the person who has developed cancer, which is exacerbated if an experience with another family member has been traumatic and frightening. Despite being assured that young children are not at risk, these family members find it hard sometimes to appreciate this knowledge in a factual light.

Family 2 – Ethical and social issues

In Family 2, the person seeking advice developed breast cancer at the age of 36 years and her mother developed breast cancer at 41. There are no other recorded cancers in this family, and several other women in the family have not developed cancer. This family has a high risk of there being a genetic factor that is causative towards the development of breast cancer.

However, although there is a high genetic risk, the pattern of the cancers may not reflect a *BRCA1* or *BRCA2* gene mutation. It is highly likely that there is another gene(s) not currently identified to explain the development of these two cancers. However, if the family have a Jewish background, there is significant risk of there being a *BRCA* mutation Struewing *et al.*, 1997).

Question:

Would you test this family for *BRCA*?

Answer:

Yes, according to current guidelines we would test this family for *BRCA*. This is classed as a high-risk family. It is unclear as to whether or not we would find a mutation. We would be more likely to find a positive result if the person tested was of Ashkenazi Jewish descent. Again, it the person had a family history of bilateral disease or ovarian cancer then this would increase the chances of identifying a mutation. We normally test the youngest person in the family and, if the person was triple-negative tumour (oestrogen receptor–negative, progesterone receptor–negative and HER-2–negative) again, this person would be more likely to be a *BRCA1* carrier.

Question:

How do the unaffected women in this family ask their relatives to do the test?

Answer:

Many people want straight answers and, if a mutation were to be identified, then this is easy. In a family where there is no diagnosis of ovarian cancer, then the news that there is a significant increased risk of developing ovarian cancer may be overwhelming for a breast cancer patient. If the test shows nothing, it is called an 'uninformative or negative genetic test. result can be confusing both for professionals and patients (Ardern-Jones *et al.*, 2008, 2010) and their families. The problem is if the family misinterpret the information if the test is 'uninformative' and think that their risk is lowered because there is no identified mutation.

Question:

What would you recommend if the person available for testing (i.e. the young-onset cancer patient) does not want to be involved in testing?

Answer:

It would be possible to store a sample from an affected person as, in the future, this may become informative for the family if further genes are identified. This option very often satisfies both the family and the person not wanting the test. Sometimes, at a later stage, the person changes their mind.

Question:

What issues would be concerning for the unaffected members in the family?

Answer:

The main issues are related to the appropriateness of preventative surgery and screening. As there is a 90% chance of there being a gene in the family, other family members would be informed that there is a high risk of developing the disease. Some relatives may wish to choose the option of preventative surgery without knowing whether they harbour the high-risk gene. This is a very difficult time for individuals, who need psychological support and information. High-risk breast screening starts at 30 years for other females in this family who test positive for the *BRCA* gene or are at 50% risk of inheriting the gene as recommended by the NICE guidelines (2006). Earlier screening can be arranged in some families after discussion. If no mutation is identified, the high-risk breast screening starts at 40 years of age unless there is a specific reason to start earlier.

Family 3

In Family 3, two sisters have developed unilateral breast cancer at the age of 56 and 52 years, respectively. Two other sisters have not developed breast cancer, and neither has the mother. This family represents a moderate-risk family. There is a low chance that the two women in this family developed breast cancer due to an inherited genetic predisposition, and this predisposition may be polygenic. Thus there may well be several genes involved in the chance that there is an inherited predisposition. Therefore, there is a 50% chance that both these women developed cancer by chance alone, and are not linked with an inherited genetic predisposition.

One would not arrange genetic testing for unaffected members in the family as there is a low likelihood of there being a *BRCA1* or *BRCA2* mutation in the family. There may well be worried people in this family who need explanation, but early breast screening of unaffected family members would not be appropriate. This would be reconsidered for Jewish families who do have the option of genetic testing due to their increased susceptibility to having a *BRCA* mutation.

Question:

The daughter of one of the women in the above case who has breast cancer is convinced that she will develop breast cancer and she wishes to have her breasts removed as a prevention option. What advice would be given to the daughter?

Answer:

With the lower level of level of risk for this daughter for the development of breast cancer, this would need very careful discussion with the breast surgeon and consultant geneticist.

She would not be eligible for early mammographic screening, despite having two first-degree relatives with breast cancer (http:/www.icr.ac.uk/fbcprotocols). Evidence of the cancer diagnosis would need to be proved in the family and time given to explain the genetic risk and the possibility of the chance occurrence of cancer in the family. The long-term effects of surgery are unknown, and the psychological factors underlying the fear of developing breast cancer need to be addressed. Appropriate psychological counselling may be needed to help the worried person cope with her cancer fear. Some centres may consider testing a relative in the research setting despite the low level of risk that it is a *BRCA* family, if someone was seriously considering preventative surgery.

Question:

Are there any other reasons why my mother and her sister both developed cancer at the age of around 50 years?

Answer:

If both these women were exposed to high levels of radiation for reasons of treatment, this may increase the chances that environmental reasons contributed to the development of breast cancer (Shore *et al.*, 1986).

If there are other familial influences, i.e. obesity, high-fat diet and early menarche, there may be an increased risk.

If they had their children late and did not breast feed and took oral contraceptives for many years, there may be a small increased risk.

There are many reasons that may not relate to a high-risk gene, but which may cause two members in one family to develop breast cancer. Other genes may be responsible, and recent research by Easton *et al.* (2007) has identified several lower-penetrance genes that confer a lower increased risk to an individual. So, theoretically, it is possible that someone may have several copies of these genes, which increases their risk. More information will be forthcoming in the future when chip technology becomes more available.

Family 4

In Family 4, only one relative – the young woman's mother – developed breast cancer (unilateral breast cancer) at the age of 50 years and sadly died 2 years later. The young woman has two sisters who are well, and no other members of the family have developed cancer except an uncle, who was a smoker and developed lung cancer at the age of 63.

Aged 35 years, the young woman underwent a very traumatic experience looking after her mother for many years and is very worried about her risk of developing breast cancer. As the only girl in the family, she feels very vulnerable. In this case, early-onset breast screening would not be recommended for a very worried person – only the three-yearly National Screening Programme for women over the age of 50 years. Careful explanation with regard to risk and psychological support is needed to help a woman in this situation. The nurse would need to take time to understand and help this person through a very difficult time.

CONCLUSION

Risk interpretation may well be subjective, and the nurse caring for a worried family relative may need to spend time with the person, exploring the many contextual reasons as to why the individual is very worried about his/her risk. It is essential not to focus on statistics, but to consider the social and cultural implications to help women make decisions. In today's climate of rapidly developing new technology, families with high genetic risk should have the opportunity to receive in-depth genetic counselling from experts. Thus referrals should be made to the local genetics service. Furthermore, gene carriers should be followed up annually for the provision of support and advice in a suitable clinic, with both oncological and genetic expertise (Ardern-Jones and Eeles, 2002).

Risk management and advice for screening is a changing area of knowledge, and nurses should be able to confidently reassure some women regarding their risk and refer others onto either screening services or to the local Regional Genetics Service for advice. More nurses need to be educated to a level that will enable them to support genetic testing at the time of a breast cancer diagnosis. The reason for this relates to the ever-increasing developments that are being made in the molecular biology of tumours. It may well be evident at the time of diagnosis that the individual being diagnosed is highly likely to be a *BRCA* carrier due to the tumour diagnosis. Treatment for gene carriers may be different to that of sporadic cases, and nurses are very often the most trusted and sensitive people to manage and help these women and their families. An excellent website regarding breast cancer and genetic testing and questions often asked is here http:/www.icr.ac.uk/fbcprotocols).

The Genetics Education Centre in Birmingham is involved in the education of nurses and, in the very near future, is launching Knowledge Skills and Framework competencies appropriate to this work. The Genetics Education Centre can be accessed on http://www.geneticseducation.nhs.uk/about_us/events.asp.

REFERENCES

Amir E, Evans D, Shenton A, Lalloo F, Moran A *et al.* (2003) Evaluation of breast cancer risk assessment packages in the family history evaluation and screening programme. *Journal of Medical Genetics* 40: 807–814.

Antoniou A, Hardy R, Walker L, Evans DG, Shenton A *et al.* (2007) Predicting the likelihood of carrying a *BRCA1* or *BRCA2* mutation: validation of BOADICEA, BRCAPRO, IBIS, Myriad and the Manchester scoring system using data from UK genetics clinics. *Journal of Medical Genetics* Advance online publication 15 April 2008 (doi:10.1136/jmg.2007.056556).

Antoniou AC, Durocher F, Smith P, Simard J, INHERIT *BRCA*s program members and Easton D (2006). *BRCA1* and *BRCA2* mutation predictions using the BOADICEA and BRCAPRO models and penetrance estimation in high-risk French-Canadian families. *Breast Cancer Research* 8(R3): doi:10.1186/bcr1365.

Ardern-Jones A (1997) *The Experience of Hereditary Cancer in the Family*. MSc thesis, London University.

Ardern-Jones A and Eeles R (2002) Cancer genes – management of carriers of breast cancer genes who have already developed cancer: the Carrier Clinic Model *European Journal of Cancer Care* 11(1): 63–68.

Ardern-Jones A and Mitchell G (1999) Family inheritance. *Journal of Women's Health* 7–9.

Ardern-Jones AT, Kenen R and Eeles R (2005) Too much too soon? Patients and health professional's views concerning the impact of genetic testing at the time of breast cancer diagnosis in women under the age of 40 *European Journal of Cancer Care (England)* 14: 272–281.

Ardern-Jones AT, Kenen R, Lynch E, Doherty R and Eeles R (2010) Inconclusive genetic test results in *BRCA2* and *BRCA2* from patients and professionals' perspectives. *Hereditary Cancer Clinical Practice* 8(1): 1.

Ardern-Jones A, Thomas S, Doherty R and Eeles R (2008) Hereditary cancer. In: J Corner and C Baily (eds) *Cancer Nursing.* Oxford: Blackwell Publishing Ltd.

Breast Cancer Linkage Consortium (1999) Cancer risks in *BRCA2* mutation carriers. *Journal of the National Cancer Institute* 91(15): 1310–1316.

Cancer Research UK (2010) Cancer Incidence – UK Statistics. http://www.stats.team@cancer.org.uk.

Claus EB, Risch N and Thompson WD (1994) Autosomal dominant inheritance of early onset breast cancer. Implications for risk prediction. *Cancer* 73: 643–651.

Costantino JP, Gail MH, Pee D, Anderson S, Redmond CK *et al.* (1999) Validation studies for models projecting the risk of invasive and total breast cancer incidence. *Journal of the National Cancer Institute* 91(18): 1541–1548.

Department of Health (2003) *Our Inheritance, Our Future.* London: HMSO.

Dugan RB, Wiesner GL, Juengst ET, O'Riordan M, Matthews AL and Robin NH (2003) Duty to warn at-risk relatives for genetic disease: genetic counselors' clinical experience. *American Journal of Medical Genetics. Part C, Seminars in Medical Genetic* 119(1): 27–34.

Easton DF, Pooley KA, Dunning AM, Pharoah PD, Thompson D *et al.* (2007) Genome-wide association study identifies novel breast cancer susceptibility loci. *Nature* 447(7148): 1087–1093.

Eeles RA, Ponder BAJ, Easton DF and Eng C (2004) *Genetic Predisposition to Cancer,* 2nd edn. London: Arnold.

Fieg SA (1996) Assessment of radiation risk from screening mammography *Cancer* 77(5): 818–822.

Forest K, Simpson SA, Wilson BJ, van Teijlingen ER, McKee L *et al.* (2003) To tell or not to tell: barriers and facilitators in family communication about genetic risk. *Clinical Genetics* 64(4): 317–326.

Foster C, Watson M, Moynihan C, Ardern-Jones A and Eeles R (2002) Genetic testing for breast and ovarian cancer predisposition: cancer burden and responsibility *Journal of Health Psychology* 7(4): 469–484.

Gui G, Hogben R, Walsh G, A'Hern R and Eeles R (2001) The incidence of breast cancer from screening women according to predicted family history risk: does annual clinical examination add to mammography? *European Journal of Cancer* 37: 1668–1673.

Hallowell N, Foster C and Ardern-Jones A (2002) Genetic testing for women previously diagnosed with breast/ovarian cancer: examining the impact of *BRCA1* and *BRCA2* mutation searching. *Genetic Testing* 2(6): 79–87.

Hallowell N, Foster C, Eeles R, Ardern-Jones A, Murday V and Watson M (2003). Balancing autonomy and responsibility: the ethics of generating and disclosing genetic information. *Journal of Medical Ethics* 29: 74–79; discussion 80–83.

Hallowell N, Mackay J, Richards M, Gore M and Jacobs I (2004) High-risk premenopausal women's experiences of undergoing prophylactic oophorectomy: a descriptive study. *Genetic Testing* 8(2): 148–156.

Hartmann LC, Schaid DJ, Woods JE, Crotty TP, Mpyers JL *et al.* (1999) Efficacy of bilateral prophylactic mastectomy in women with a family history of breast cancer. *New England Journal of Medicine* 340(2): 77–84.

Kollias J, Sibbering D, Blamey RW, Holland PA, Obuszko Z *et al.* (1998) Screening women aged less than 50 years with a family history of breast cancer. *European Journal of Cancer* 34(6): 937–940.

Lakhani SR, van de Vijver M, Jacquemier J, Anderson TJ, Osin PP *et al.* for the Breast Cancer Linkage Consortium (2002) The Pathology of familial breast cancer: predictive value of immunohistochemical markers estrogen receptor, progesterone receptor, HER-2, and p53 in patients with mutations in *BRCA1* and *BRCA2. Journal of Clinical Oncology* 20: 3752–3753.

Lalloo F, Boggis CRM, Evans DG Shenton A, Threlfall AG and Howell A (1998) Screening by mammography: women with a family history of breast cancer. *European Journal of Cancer* 34: 937–940.

Meijers-Heijboer H, van Geel B, van Putten WL, Henzen-Logmans SC, Seynaeve C *et al.* (2001) Breast cancer after prophylactic bilateral mastectomy in women with a *BRCA 1* or *BRCA 2* mutation *New England Journal of Medicine* 345(3): 159.

Miki Y, Senesen J, Shattuck-Eidens D, Futreal PA, Harshman K *et al.* (1994) A strong candidate for the breast and ovarian cancer susceptibility gene, *BRCA1. Science* 226: 66–71.

Mitchell G, Kissen M, Ardern-Jones A, Tayor R and Eeles RA (2001) Urgent genetic testing – a paradox. *Familial Cancer* 1: 25–29.

Narod, SA (2006) Re Overview: modifiers of risk of hereditary breast cancer. *Oncogene* 25: 5832–5836.

National Institute for Health and Clinical Excellence, NICE (2006) *Clinical Guidance: Familial Breast Cancer: The Classification and Care of Women at Risk of Familial Breast Cancer in Primary, Secondary and Tertiary Care* (partial update of CG14).

Rebbeck T, Lynch H, Neuhausen S, Narod S, van't Veer L *et al.* (2002) Prophylactic oophorectomy in carriers of *BRCA1* or *BRCA2* mutations *New England Journal of Medicine* 346(21): 1616–1622.

Richards MPM, Hallowell N, Green JM, Murton F and Statham H (1995) Counselling families with hereditary breast and ovarian cancer: a psychosocial perspective *Journal of Genetic Counseling* 4(3): 219–233.

Semiglazov VF, Sagaidak VN, Moiseenko VM and Protsenko SA (1996): Preliminary results of the Russia (St Petersberg)/WHO program for the evaluation of the effectiveness of breast self-examination. *Voprosy Onkologii* 42: 49–55.

Shore RE, Hildreth N, Woodard E, Dvoretsky P, Hempelmann L and Pasternack B (1986) Breast cancer among women given X-ray therapy for acute postpartum mastitis. *Journal of the National Cancer Institute* 77(3): 689–696.

Struewing JP, Hartge P, Wacholder S, Baker SM, Berlin M *et al.* (1997) The risk of cancer associated with specific mutations of *BRCA1* and *BRCA2* among Ashkenazi Jews. *New England Journal of Medicine* 336: 1401–1408.

Standardization Task Force (1995) *American Journal of Human Genetics* 56: 745–752.

Thomas DB, Gao DL, Self DG, Allison CJ, Tayuo Y *et al.* (1997) Randomized trial of breast self-examination. Cancer in Shanghai: methodology and preliminary results. *Journal of the National Cancer Institute* 89: 355–365.

Warner E (2009) A prospective study of breast cancer incidence and stage distribution in women with a *BRCA1* or *BRCA2* mutation under surveillance with and without magnetic resonance imaging. Proceedings of the 32nd CTRC-AACR San Antonio Breast Cancer Symposium. San Antonio, Texas. Abstract 26.

Wellisch DK, Schain W, Gritz ER and Wang H-J (1996) Psychological functioning of daughters of breast cancer patients. Part 111: Experiences and perceptions of daughters related to mother's breast cancer. *Psycho-Oncology* 5: 271–281.

Wooster R, Neuhausen S, Mangion J, Quirk Y, Ford D *et al.* (1994) Localisation of breast cancer suscepti-bility gene to *BRCA2* to Chromosome 13Q 12–13 *Science* 265: 2088–2090.

4   Breast Screening

Ann-Marie Fretwell (previous contribution by Linda Lee)

INTRODUCTION

Wilson and Junger (1968) first devised the principles of screening for the World Health Organization. Any proposed national screening programme should be considered against these criteria before it is implemented. In order to consider the role of a breast-screening programme for England, Scotland, Wales and Northern Ireland, a report was commissioned by the Health Ministers of the time, which was chaired by Sir Patrick Forrest. Two previous studies were particularly to influence the out come of the enquiry (Tabar *et al.*, 1985; Shapiro *et al.*, 1982). At the time of the Forrest enquiry, the evidence, which supported the implementation of the programme against the criteria, was as detailed below (Forrest, 1986)

THE EVIDENCE

The condition being screened for should pose an important health problem

At the time of the Forrest enquiry, 24 000 new cases of breast cancer were diagnosed every year. Annually, there were 15 000 deaths from breast cancer.

The natural history of the disease should be well understood

Breast cancer was known to be a progressive disease, with early cancer development confined to the ductal system. This was followed by an early invasive stage, when the cancer cells break through the basement membrane of the ducts, with the potential to spread to other parts of the body and to produce metastases.

Breast Cancer Nursing Care and Management, Second Edition, Edited by Victoria Harmer
© 2011 by Blackwell Publishing Ltd.

There should be a recognisable early stage

At the time of the Forrest report, it was well established that 20% of cancers were too small to be identified by clinical examination, either by the woman or by a clinician, but these cancers were evident on mammography.

Treatment of the disease at an early stage should be of more benefit than treatment started at a later stage

Previous studies had indicated that there was a reduction in mortality when comparing women who had attended a screening programme compared to those who had not been invited.

A suitable screening test should exist

The aim of a screening test is to identify those who are normal and those who may have mammographic signs of possible breast cancer. The test should be able to maximise the number of true positives (high sensitivity) and to minimise the number of false positives (high specificity). Evidence indicated a range of 80–90% sensitivity and 95% specificity for mammography.

The test should be acceptable to the population

A test is deemed acceptable if attendance is high, particularly on repeat visits. Attendance of 60% had been achieved in previous studies, but these had covered a greater age range than that intended for the UK programme. It was in women over 65 years of age that attendance had been limited.

There should be adequate facilities for the diagnosis and treatment of abnormalities detected

Staff and facilities to provide a screening and assessment service varied across the UK. It was noted that these would need to be developed to address the needs of the programme on a national basis.

For diseases of insidious onset, screening should be repeated at intervals determined by the natural history of the disease

Evidence at the time of the Forrest enquiry varied, and previous screening studies and trials had different intervals, ranging from 12 to 33 months.

The chance of physical or psychological harm should be less than the chance of benefit

Although the test involved ionising radiation, the dose delivered for mammography was felt to be small enough not to pose any significant threat to the women. Concern was also expressed that women who did not have breast cancer might require an excision biopsy to establish their normality. Women might also receive treatment for a cancer that would not become invasive and would therefore not be life-threatening in their lifetime. Finally, there was a risk of psychiatric morbidity. There was little evidence to suggest that women who were returned to normal screening suffered any long-term psychological sequelae.

The cost of the screening programme should be balanced against the benefits it provides

Many factors were considered by the Forrest enquiry. Financial cost was considered in terms of the cost of life years gained and the Quality Adjusted Life Year (QALY) gained. Compared to other costs within the National Health Service (NHS), breast cancer screening equated to the QALY of kidney transplantation, whilst being more costly than hip replacement and less costly than heart transplantations. Other factors considered were the psychological costs to the women invited and the cost of time and travel.

RECOMMENDATIONS

As a result of their deliberations, the Forrest committee, in their report of 1986, recommended the following proposal for a national programme:

- Women should be invited for screening once every 3 years.
- Women attending should have one view taken of each breast.
- The age range of the women invited should be from 50 to 64 years of age.

The Forrest report recognised that further work needed to be undertaken to develop and refine the national programme. They therefore recommended continued research into five specific areas:

- Number of views;
- Screening age group;
- Screening frequency;
- Natural history and treatment;
- Risk factors.

UK wide, the number of women expected to be invited within the 3-year programme was 4857 000. The recommendations of the report were accepted and, in 1988, the National Health Service Breast Screening Programme (NHSBSP) was implemented. Similar programmes were agreed and implemented in both Wales and Scotland. Throughout the history of the national breast-screening programme, Wales and Scotland have acted independently of the NHS, but in the main they mirror the service in the NHS.

   The aim of the programme was to reduce morality from breast cancer in the screening age group. In 1992, the Department of Health made this target more specific by stating that the programme should reduce mortality by 25% by 2000 (Department of Health, 1992). It was against this background that later discussions about the success or otherwise of the programme would occur. It has been estimated since that 119 000 cancers have been detected in women since the introduction of the service and that 1400 lives per year have been saved in England alone (Madan and Rawdin, 2008) (Fig. 4.1).

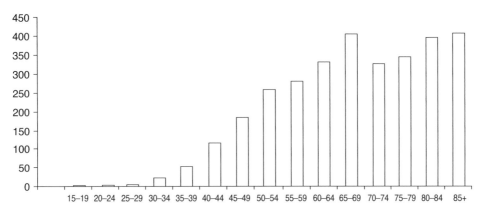

Fig. 4.1   Illustration of breast cancer incidence according to age.

INTRODUCING THE NHS BREAST SCREENING PROGRAMME

The first screening mammogram was performed in England towards the end of 1988. The first centres to take part were those that had already been offering a mammography service for women with breast symptoms and had both equipment and skilled personnel in place. As was noted in the Forrest report (1986), the implications for training and educating the workforce were considerable, and the supply of good quality equipment would take some time to be put in place. Many programmes were therefore unable to commence until staff had been trained and equipment put in place. It was not until 1993 that every programme had commenced screening, and it was not until 1995 that every woman in the programme had received an invitation. This was later to have an impact on how the effectiveness of screening would be demonstrated in breast cancer mortality data.

SCREENING IN ACTION

Identifying eligible women

Screening procedures differ from the normal route to investigation when a patient reports a symptom to the GP. With the breast-screening process, women who perceive themselves as being well are invited. Lists of women eligible within the relevant age group are obtained by the screening service. The list is then sent to the general practices so that they can identify those who have undergone a bilateral mastectomy, those who may have recently died or those who are wheelchair users and may require any additional time. This is sometimes seen as arduous, but it is nevertheless an important task. The introduction of information technology for patient records at the surgery has meant that, in recent years, the lists provided are more easily kept up to date and accurate.

It is important to note that women can only be removed from the lists temporarily. Women who are unable to attend at the time of invitation due to ill health can request an appointment for breast screening as soon as they are well enough to attend. They also should automatically receive an invitation at the next round of screening in 3 years. In some cases, women who are on follow-up for breast cancer are removed from the screening list, but this is due to the fact that they are on routine follow-up with the surgical/oncological team.

Invitations and written information

All women receive a letter of invitation for screening. Women are invited for an appointed time, usually approximately 3 weeks ahead. They are able to request a change of time and date, and occasionally may request an alternative site as they may work near one unit but live near another. The design of the letter will vary to some degree between units, but each should contain essential, and clearly presented, information about the invitation (Austoker and Ong, 1994). Additional information about the screening process is provided by the inclusion of a leaflet, *Breast Screening, the Facts 2010*. The current format of this nationally agreed leaflet is based on research into several factors affecting women's anxiety associated with an invitation to be screened, as well as the issue of informed consent (Austoker, 1999). After their examination, women are given a leaflet detailing how and when they will receive their results.

Results

Quality Assurance Guidelines for Breast Cancer Screening (NHSBSP, 2005) set a minimum standard that 90% women attending for a mammogram must receive their results within 2 weeks and that invitations to an assessment clinic must be within 3 weeks from the initial examination. The results letter will either state that the mammogram was normal and that no further action is required or that the woman is requested to return to an assessment clinic on a specified date for further imaging. A *Being Breast Aware* leaflet will also accompany any normal-result letter.

Liaison with general practitioners

Throughout the screening process, general practices are kept informed of the key information. Whenever women are recalled for further tests, the practice is informed and advised of the likelihood of malignancy. The practice is then able to respond if women enquire about the reasons for recall. The practice is also informed when a woman is being referred for treatment. Usually the woman is referred to the local specialist breast surgical team but, if it is felt – by either the women or the GP – that another referral pathway is more appropriate, they have the right to seek a change of referral. Since the development of highly specialised breast care teams within the locality, changes of referral pattern are now rare. At the end of a screening round, practices are advised of those women who have not responded to their invitation, and a note is attached to the practice notes. This alerts health professionals within the practice team, and the issue can be raised when the woman next attends the surgery.

Non-attenders

In order for any screening programme to remain viable, a high acceptability is necessary. NHSBSP guidelines set a minimum attendance standard of 70% of all women invited to attend, with a target of 80% (NHSBSP, 2005). The 2007 NHSBSP Annual Review stated that 84% of all women invited in 2005/2006 attended (NHSBSP, 2007). London was the only region where the average first attendance was 55%, followed by 75% for subsequent visits. This could be explained partly by the diverse and transient population.

There are many reasons why women choose not to attend for breast screening. Fear of the procedure and the results appear to be the most common explanation. Many of the non-attendees appear to possess flawed knowledge about breast cancer, treatment and the screening process. A large majority of the studies carried out reported that an incorrect address was the main reason for non-attendance, and this highlights the importance of keeping up-to-date patient records. The Exeter software system allows direct access by the screening office to a GP surgery's address database, and this then should reduce the potential for posting invitations to the wrong address. To date, this software is only in use in the East Midlands. An increased understanding of the screening process could be achieved through the use of letters/poster campaigns and direct intervention. A study by Hoare *et al.* (1992) looking at reasons for non-attendance for breast screening by Asian women found that there was a 70% increase in uptake after direct personal intervention. Leaflets are now available in a variety of languages and dialects. Other successful methods have included placing a 'flag' in the patient's notes, enabling the matter to be discussed when the patient attends for other appointments, or sending a letter directly from the GP surgery. Direct intervention can be a costly but effective method.

It is important, however, to remember that mammography is a procedure that requires informed consent, and the woman has the right to choose without pressure or judgement.

The screening unit

Each breast-screening unit delivers the mammography service in different ways according to the geographical area and population density. To achieve the target attendance of 80%, the service needs to be easily accessed by the women invited. Most centres now combine a static unit based within a local Acute Trust, with a mobile service that can be taken to rural or socially deprived areas. Mobile units are only used for the basic screening mammogram. Women with potential abnormalities will all need to attend the static screening unit for assessment (Fig. 4.2).

The basic screening method – mammography

Mammography is the name given to X-ray imaging of the breast. At the present time, mammography is based on the use of X-ray film and cassettes (film container). The cassette contains a fluorescent screen which, when hit by X-rays, converts this into light. X-ray film is very similar to photo film and, although it does respond to X-rays to produce a latent image, the film responds more effectively to light. The use of an intensifying screen can reduce the dose received by patients considerably. The use of cassettes, and screens in combination with film, is standard practice for all basic radiographic imaging.

The use of digital imaging is becoming widespread in radiology departments and mammography is no different. The majority of Breast Units use digital equipment for X-ray–guided biopsies and, where possible, assessment clinics. There is an enthusiastic move towards digital imaging within the NHSBSP given the advantages of image manipulation, storage (no hard copies) and fewer technical recalls. Although research suggests that image quality for the screening population is no different on analogue or digital, the main benefits

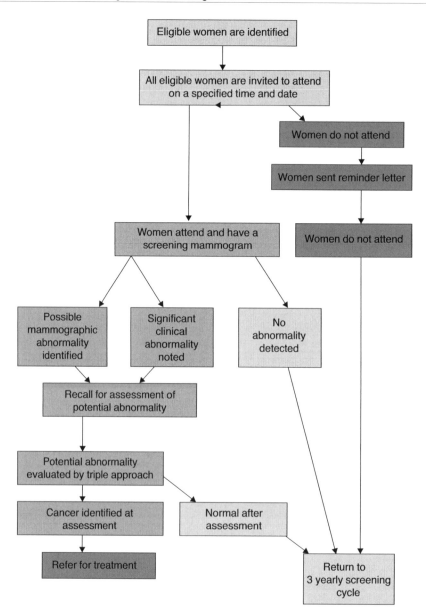

Fig. 4.2 Screening process.

are for the younger symptomatic/family history patients. These patients generally have much denser breasts for which film-screen mammography is less sensitive. More on this subject will be referred to later in this chapter.

In mammography, X-ray equipment is used to produce the image, whether analogue or digital, and is highly specialised. In mammography, the system needs to enhance areas of minimal contrast, i.e. the difference between fat and the breast parenchyma. The inherent contrast differences between these areas are minimal when compared to differentiating between bone and soft tissue as in the majority of plain film imaging.

The mammography equipment is designed for ease of use, both for the women attending and the radiographer. The machine is designed to rotate through 360 degrees and is able to be raised and lowered by counterbalanced and electronic drives in order to adjust the height of the machine to suit the stature of the individual woman being screened.

Screening mammography clinics are very labour-intensive. The norm is for approximately 70 appointment slots to be made available each day. One woman is invited every 5–6 minutes. These screening sessions take place on one machine, with two radiographers performing the examination in turn. In a static unit, the radiographer who is not performing the examination will put the films through the film processor and check the resultant images for quality and accurate patient-identification marking. Whilst on a mobile screening service, the non-examining radiographer will perform reception duties, and the films will be processed at the end of the day back at the base unit. Where more than one machine and sufficient radiography staff are available, additional screening sessions can scheduled each day.

The radiographer needs to produce a high-quality examination and must also ensure the woman feels welcome, unembarrassed and able to make an informed choice about proceeding with the examination (Lee *et al.*, 1995). The radiographer must also make sure that the compression to the breast is sufficient to produce a good examination on which a diagnosis can accurately be made, but also that the compression is not painful for the woman. If women experience extreme discomfort or pain, they are less likely to return for the subsequent examination.

Compression

All mammographic examinations of the breast require that the breast be compressed during the procedure. The benefits of compression cannot be underestimated (Lee *et al.*, 1995). Application of compression to the breast:

- Reduces movement and therefore the risk of motion blur;
- Brings the breast tissue nearer to the film, which increases the detail of breast tissue demonstrated;
- Reduces the radiation dose required;
- Ensures even X-ray penetration of the breast by equalising the depth of the majority of tissue;
- Spreads and separates the tissue to improve visualisation of potential abnormities.

Positioning

As a general rule, women are positioned in the erect position, which helps with patient mobility and speed of examination (which is of significance in an NHS-funded programme of this type). This does not preclude, however, the possibility of imaging women who are seated. Mammography positioning requires that the whole body of the woman is placed in the appropriate position to facilitate the accurate positioning of the breast on the machine. With patients who are seated, this flexibility of position can occasionally be compromised, with the result that films may not be of optimal quality.

The two views used for the NHS Breast Screening Programme, and for any attendance at a symptomatic service, are the cranio-caudal projection and the medio-lateral oblique projection. The cranio-caudal projection means that the X-ray beam is sent from the superior

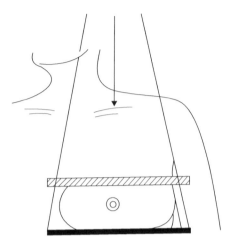

Fig. 4.3   Positioning for the cranio-caudal projection. Reprinted from *Fundamentals of Mammography*, 2nd edn. Lee, Stickland, Evans and Wilson (2003) by permission. Copyright 2003 Elsevier.

surface of the breast though to the inferior surface of the breast on to the film below. This position can demonstrate the majority of the breast tissue, but with a very small amount excluded form both the lateral and medial borders (Fig. 4.3 and Fig. 4.4).

The medio-lateral oblique projection has the X-ray beam coming from an angle of 45 degrees from the medial side (upper-inner quadrant of the breast) through to the lateral

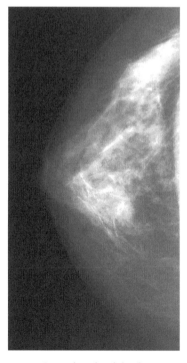

Fig. 4.4   Cranio-caudal mammogram. Reproduced with kind permission of Nottingham University Hospital NHS Trust.

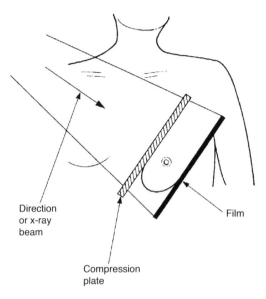

Direction
or x-ray
beam

Film

Compression
plate

Fig. 4.5 Positioning for the 45-degree medio-lateral oblique projection. Reprinted from *Fundamentals of Mammography*, 2nd edn. Lee, Stickland, Evans and Wilson (2003) by permission. Copyright 2003 Elsevier.

(lower-outer quadrant). This view is the one most likely to demonstrate the whole breast tissue and, in particular, the upper-outer quadrant of the breast. (The upper-outer quadrant of the breast is excluded form the cranio-caudal projection, and it is also the most common site for cancers to be found (Fig. 4.5 and Fig. 4.6).

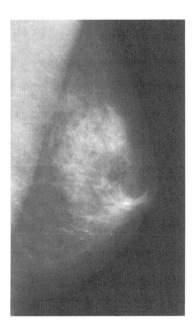

Fig. 4.6 Oblique mammogram. Reproduced with kind permission of Nottingham University Hospital NHS Trust.

Film reading

When the mammograms have been completed and checked for diagnostic quality, they will all need to be examined for potential abnormalities. The mammography films are loaded on to a multi-viewer, which has the capacity to hold between 70 and 150 mammographic examinations, depending on the manufacturer. Two film readers review all the screening mammograms, with any discordant cases given a third reading, in a procedure known as double reading with arbitration, which was introduced in the NHSBSP in 2002, following comprehensive research published on the accuracy of single and double reading. A film reader can either be a radiologist or a non-medically trained member of staff who has undertaken post-graduate advanced practice. The film-reading process is designed to identify the women who are normal and those who have a possible abnormality. This is not a definitive report but will enable women to be:

- Returned to routine screening invitation;
- Recalled for further assessment.

Each examination is identified as being within the one of five categories:

1 Benign;
2 Probably benign;
3 Indeterminate;
4 Probably malignant;
5 Malignant.

Women in category 1 will not require recall. More than 90% of women attending for screening should be in this category. Women who are in categories 2 to 5 will be recalled for screening assessment. The categorisation will also help in identifying the pathway of care on reaching the screening-assessment clinic.

Computer-aided detection

For those units with digital equipment, images are reported from sophisticated computer workstations rather than hard-copy film. Computer-aided detection (CAD) uses computer software to place prompts on areas of concern on a mammogram to draw the reader's attention to possible abnormalities. CAD systems are very effective in correctly marking cancers on a mammogram, and can identify around 98% of cancers manifesting as micro-calcifications and 87% of mass lesions. The problems with CAD tend to be associated with specificity, with CAD marking many areas on a mammogram which ultimately prove to be normal. It is estimated that the film reader will have to ignore in the region of 2000 of these false prompts for every correctly placed mark (Fenton et al., 2007).

The use of CAD in the interpretation of screening mammograms remains controversial (Fenton et al., 2007). In the USA, where single reading rather than double reading is the norm, around 25–30% of mammograms are now read with the aid of CAD (Lindfors, 2006). Some studies have shown an improvement in cancer detection rates, whereas others have shown little benefit. Any improvement in cancer detection can be associated with increases in recall rates.

It is well established that double reading of mammograms improves cancer detection by between 4 and 14% over that which is achievable with single reading (Astley and Gilbert, 2004). Double reading is always going to be more expensive and can be difficult to achieve due to manpower issues. The question that needs answering before CAD is adopted into UK practice is whether CAD can achieve the same cancer detection rates as double reading and whether it is cost effective compared to other strategies that have been successfully adopted by the NHS Breast Screening Programme, such as the training of non-medically qualified staff to read mammograms.

To try and address some of these issues, the Computer-Aided Detection Evaluation Trial II (CADET II) was set up (Gilbert *et al.*, 2008). This large prospective randomised trial recruited over 30 000 women in the UK. The study found that a single reader using CAD performed as well as double reading, with equal numbers of cancers being detected by both reading regimens. Although cancer detection rates were equivalent, the use of CAD did lead to a 15% relative increase in recall rates. Consequently, a single reader using CAD is an alternative to double reading, but double reading remains the best method of film reading to achieve high cancer detection and to maintain low recall rates. Further work is ongoing to look at the cost effectiveness of the different reading methods. In countries where single reading is the norm, the CADET II study provides good evidence for the use of CAD to improve performance up to levels achieved with double reading.

Screening assessment

There should be only two outcomes from screening assessment:

- Return to routine screening invitation;
- Refer for treatment.

In the early days of the screening programme, the use of early recall (between 6 and 12 months) was comparatively common. Research indicated that the psychiatric morbidity associated with early recall was detrimental to the well being of women attending, and all screening units are encouraged to eliminate this as an outcome (Ong and Austoker, 1997; Ong *et al.*, 1997a; Ong *et al.*, 1997b). There will inevitably be one or two cases where this will occur, but these should be less than 1% of women screened.

When the Forrest (1986) and Pritchard (1989) reports were published, the role of the multidisciplinary team and the use of the triple approach was recommended. The triple approach refers to the use of the three modalities employed to accurately differentiate between benign and malignant – imaging (mammography and ultrasound), clinical examination and cyto-histopathology.

When a woman is recalled for screening assessment, the imaging characteristics of the abnormality will define which investigative techniques will be employed to determine the nature of the abnormality. Various procedures can be performed, and these are outlined below.

Additional mammography

Within the assessment clinic, one of the options available for patient work-up is additional mammography, which can comprise additional views, paddle views and magnification views. A paddle or localisation view will require the replacement of the normal full-field compression plate with one of approximately 3 inches in diameter. The potential abnormality is measured from the film, and compression is applied to the appropriate area

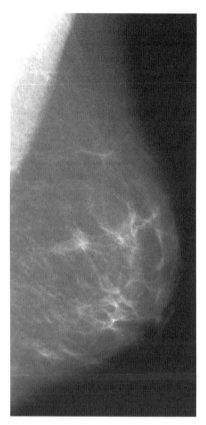

Fig. 4.7   Potential solid mass. Reproduced with kind permission of Nottingham University Hospital NHS Trust.

of the breast. If an abnormality is real, it should be demonstrated on the resultant film. If it appeared coincidentally, it should disappear on compression (Fig. 4.7 and Fig. 4.8). It is now common practice to use ultrasound on all areas that require paddle views, whether the result is positive or not. If the resulting ultrasound is also negative, the woman can be confidently discharged; otherwise a biopsy can be performed.

Magnification views are mainly used to examine areas or specks of microcalcification more closely, as these can signify early malignant disease or ductal carcinoma in situ (DCIS), or can be produced by normal breast processes. The differentiation between these two is obviously critical. Magnification can also be combined with the use of the 3-inch compression device, which will clarify the situation where there is a potential parenchymal deformity with associated microcalcification. The numbers of magnification views carried out are being reduced as more units use digital systems. A lateral view is usually requested instead at assessment, thereby allowing image manipulation such as digital zoom/contrast enhancement/polarity reversal to magnify any calcifications of concern. Only definite benign 'tea-cup' calcifications will be discharged; any discordance will be sampled. It is hoped that the number of recalls for benign calcification will reduce in the future, as the breast-screening service becomes fully digital, allowing the film reader to manipulate the initial image.

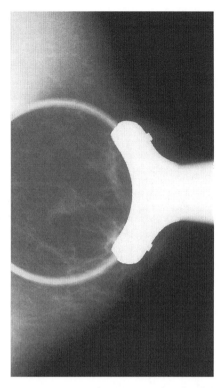

Fig. 4.8 Mass spread by compression – normal tissue. Reproduced with kind permission of Nottingham University Hospital NHS Trust.

Ultrasound

Ultrasound is a non-invasive procedure that is painless and that does not utilise ionising radiation. It is an invaluable tool for work-up of a potential abnormality in breast screening and in the symptomatic service. A mass can be examined to determine whether it is solid, fluid filled or mixed. Appearances on ultrasound are not definitive, and any mass confirmed as solid will require cytology or histopathology. Ultrasound is particularly useful for estimating the size of a lesion as accurate measurements can be taken.

As the quality and sensitivity of ultrasound equipment has improved, it has become very useful in identifying invasive disease including both masses and parenchymal deformities. High-frequency ultrasound can also demonstrate calcification, but this is a coincidental finding, and ultrasound has not yet been demonstrated to be sufficiently sensitive to be able to detect DCIS. Ultrasound cannot be used as a screening tool, as examining both breasts thoroughly is time consuming and lacks specificity.

Clinical examination

Not all women attending the assessment clinic receive a full clinical examination. Women who have a potential abnormality on mammography, which proves to have been superimposition shadowing on paddle compression and ultrasound, will be discharged after imaging. The role of clinical examination in the screening situation is two-fold.

1   To examine all women who are about to undergo needle biopsy. Examination of women post–needle biopsy is compromised by haematoma.
2   To examine women who have reported a significant clinical sign to the radiographer or when the radiographer has noticed a significant clinical sign whilst performing the original screening mammogram.

Approximately 5% of cancers are occult and are not demonstrated on a mammogram. The noting of symptoms is therefore a small, but significant, factor within the programme.

Image-guided biopsy methods

Two techniques are regularly used in screening assessment to establish the nature of a confirmed abnormity. Initially, fine-needle aspiration cytology was widely used in the first years of the programme, but this has gradually been usurped by automated core and vacuum-assisted mammotomy biopsy devices. Core-biopsy devices have now become the primary choice for ultrasound-guided biopsies. Fine-needle aspiration is still used on occasion in difficult situations, e.g. where the lesion is close to the nipple or a patient has implants.

Methods of biopsy under X-ray guidance have also changed with the development of vacuum-assisted biopsy systems. Vacuum-assisted biopsy systems use an 11–8-gauge needle to obtain a larger sample and require only a single insertion into the breast, giving a more accurate pre-operative diagnosis of DCIS and invasion. A multicentre study of 2874 patients showed that twice as many patients had their initial atypical ductal hyperplasia (ADH) diagnosis upgraded to DCIS/invasion at surgery if a core biopsy, compared with a vacuum-assisted biopsy, had been taken (Kettritz *et al.*, 2004). An accurate X-ray–guided 14-gauge core-biopsy needle can require 5–10 insertions. Although the calcification retrieval rate is much the same whether a core or vacuum-assisted biopsy is used, the re-biopsy rate when vacuum-assisted biopsy is used can be half that of the core biopsy (Liberman, 2000). The degree of use of these tests will vary according to local practice. The main benefits of using either core or vacuum-assisted biopsy are that they can indicate invasive disease, and their use helps in deciding on the treatment required and, in cases of microcalcification, will demonstrate inclusion of the calcification, thereby confirming the accuracy of the test.

Methods of core-biopsy and vacuum-assisted mammotomy

Even in the case of women who have been recalled for a reported clinical abnormality, the lesion will be sampled by imaging whenever possible, to ensure accuracy as the site of the needle can be identified. Ultrasound is the more desirable technique, as women are supine throughout the procedure, thereby reducing the risk of syncope. The abnormality and the needle can be seen in real time, providing greater accuracy of sampling. Ultrasound is therefore used for palpable abnormalities, parenchymal deformities and masses detected in mammography.

In the case of microcalcification, stereotactic (X-ray–guided) localisation will be used and requires a special add-on attachment to be placed on the mammography machine. This attachment enables images to be taken whilst the woman is seated at the machine, and the images can be checked whilst the sampling is taking place. In the past, this equipment was film-based, requiring additional time whilst images were processed. Digital imaging systems have been developed for this procedure, reducing the time during which women are seated at the machine. The images are produced on a monitor within the mammography room almost instantaneously, allowing adjustment of the needle position and increased accuracy of sampling. The samples taken from the breast are also imaged to ensure that calcification has been included in the specimen.

A few units within the UK have a prone-table biopsy system, which is beneficial for the patient as, if she is prone throughout, she cannot see the procedure as it is being performed and is therefore less likely to suffer from syncope. However, these units are extremely expensive and they also take up a large amount of space with a machine that cannot be used for anything except invasive procedures. The upright add-on system more commonly used means that the equipment can be used both for screening and assessment. Bearing these factors in mind, it is unlikely that prone tables will be adopted throughout the service. A compromise has been to use a couch, where the women can lie on her side and can be positioned against the X-ray machine. It is for use with lateral or vertical add-on biopsy systems and provides easier access to lesions close to the pectoral muscle.

Diagnostic excision biopsy

The screening process can proceed up to the point of diagnosis; this means that if a pre-operative diagnosis is not achievable by needle-biopsy technique, it will be necessary for women to undergo a diagnostic excision biopsy. Due to the recent aggressive sampling of identified lesions with core-biopsy techniques, the potential to accurately identify a malignant lesion is greatly improved, and the need to resort to operative procedures is reduced. The target for benign biopsy is less than four per 1000 women screened. In the NHS Breast Screening Programme Annual Review (NHSBSP, 2009) for the years 2007/2008, the achieved benign biopsy rate was 0.1%.

Therapeutic excision

The larger sampling size from vacuum-assisted mammotomy allows for the therapeutic excision of benign lesions such as fibroadenomas, radial scars and papillomas (except those with atypia). This can be done as an outpatient procedure, requiring only 10–15 ml of local anaesthetic and usually taking an hour. A pressure dressing is applied afterwards, with minimal scarring as a result. This is a much less invasive option, the alternative being an open surgical procedure.

Quality assurance

Subsequent to the Forrest report (1986), another document was produced called the Pritchard report (1989). The Pritchard report outlined the need for extensive training and education for the radiographers and radiologists and that the programme should be based on several quality assurance (QA) principles. The QA mechanism is one of the great strengths of the programme and, in the Calman Hine report (Department of Health, 1995), QA in the NHSBSP was raised as being an indicator of good practice, which should be applied in a wider health service arena. There are now numerous NHSBSP publications to underpin the quality of the service, and these relate to the technical aspects of the programme, the call and recall system, guidance for quality-assurance visits and guidance for each professional group involved in the programme. All these publications should be available within each breast-screening unit, at the local Quality Assurance Reference Centre and from the National Coordinating Office in Sheffield (http://www.cancerscreening.nhs.uk).

The programme is subject to rigorous and regular monitoring of a variety of factors. The full details of the standards and targets for the programme are available in the majority of NHSBSP publications (e.g. *Clinical Guidelines for Breast Cancer Screening Assessment*, 2001). Each standard relates to one of the domains defined in *The New NHS Modern and Dependable* (Department of Health, 1988)

- Fair access;
- Effective delivery of appropriate health care;
- Efficiency;
- Patient/user experience;
- Health outcomes of NHS care.

UPDATING THE BREAST-SCREENING PROGRAMME

Screening age group

Currently, all women between the age of 50 and 70 years are eligible for breast screening. Initially, the age group selected by the 1986 Forrest Report (after due consideration of the evidence) was 50–64 years. In the previous studies, women aged 65 years and over had not attended when invited for breast screening. In the NHSBSP, women over 65 years of age were not excluded from breast screening, but were not sent a specific invitation to be screened. Women over 65 years of age were able to refer themselves to the screening unit for an appointment via their GP.

Following a study published in 2001 (Moss *et al.*, 2001), establishing that attendance for women in the age group 65–70 years was 71%, the *NHS Cancer Plan* stated the intention to extend invitations for routine screening to women up to 70 years of age (Department of Health, 2000). Women over the age of 70 years are now encouraged to self-refer once they have been discharged from the screening programme. Somewhat controversial extensions to the age range will be discussed later in this chapter, under 'Contentious issues'.

Number of views

The Forrest Report (1986) suggested a one-view screening technique, based on the results of the previous studies. The NHS Breast Screening Programme was therefore funded on this basis. Some centres, however, adopted two views at the first visit, the prevalent screen, and whilst others opted to perform two views at both prevalent and incident screens. The units who took this path had to identify the additional funding locally.

In 1995, research (Wald *et al.*, 1995) indicated that the number of cancers detected at the prevalent round was increased in units that used two views at each visit. As a result of this research the NHSBSP was adjusted so that all women had two views at the prevalent screen. Further research ensued (Blanks *et al.*, 1997; Blanks *et al.*, 1998) and in the *NHS*

Cancer Plan a two-view policy was announced for all women at all visits. This change has been implemented across the country (Department of Health, 2000).

Contentious issues

Over the years, several aspects of the breast-screening programme have been subject to adverse comment.

It has been suggested (Baum *et al.*, 1995; Baum, 1996) that the cost of the programme far outweighs any benefits and that the money would be better spent on improving treatment. The process of detection would then rely solely on reported symptoms via the GP. Treatment has improved considerably and is improving life expectancy for women, but the paper by Blanks (2000) clearly demonstrates that screening is beginning to have a direct impact on mortality rates. As some programmes did not complete their first screening round until 1995, the full benefit of breast screening on mortality did not become apparent until 2005.

Over-treatment

Within the screening programme, a large number of cases of DCIS are detected. The detection of DCIS in the screening programme can lead to a mastectomy in patients where those who are demonstrated to have small invasive tumours may have a wide local excision. DCIS may, or may not, ultimately lead to invasive disease depending on its grade, and the sojourn time. Women who are treated with a mastectomy for low-grade DCIS may never develop invasive disease, but will live with the knowledge that they have cancer for their lifetime. The nature and progression of DCIS into invasive disease is not clear and continues to be the subject of considerable research.

Interval cancers

Interval cancers are detected between the three-yearly screening invitations. There are three main categories of interval cancers:

- The true interval which, despite a review of previous mammography examinations, shows no evidence at the previous visit.
- The false negatives which, on review of the previous examinations, showed some evidence of a malignant process, which was not detected at the previous visits.
- The occult cancer, which is detected after referral from the GP, and confirmed on clinical examination alone, and which is not evident on the current or previous mammographic examinations.

The majority of interval cancers occur in the third year after screening. A research study, referred to as the Frequency Trial (Breast Screening Frequency Trial Group, 2002) examined the issue of the screening interval. The conclusions of this trial were that the NHSBSP has the correct interval between screening and invitations. Many of the amendments to the programme implemented in recent years should have an impact on the number of interval cancers. Research continues into the false-negative mammogram, which will inform clinical practice (McCann *et al.*, 2001).

Age extension

At 40–49 years

The incidence of breast cancer within this age group is lower than that of women of 50 years and above (see Fig 4.1). The breast is more likely to be dense mammographically, and identifying a small cancer would more difficult. Several studies have been reviewed and further studies have been undertaken, regarding a screening programme in this age group. Initial data from the Age Trial, published in 2005 (Moss *et al.* 2005), suggest that a reduction in breast cancer mortality is likely to be observed in women invited for annual mammography between the ages of 40 and 49 years. However, the numbers are uncertain, with no definite results apparent until the 10-year follow-up. Broadly to date, there is insufficient evidence to suggest that a national programme would bring similar benefits to those offered by the current programme for women aged between 50 and 70 years. Research continues in this area.

At 47–49 and 71–73 years

In 2007, the NHS Cancer Reform Strategy (Department of Health, 2007) announced a proposed extension to the NHS Breast Screening Programme to include those women aged 47–49 and 71–73 years, to be implemented by 2012. There are significant differences at either end of this extension in terms of incidence, compliance, treatment options and relapse rates. The ScHARR Initial Assessment Report (Madan and Rawdin, 2008) is assessing the merits of screening the 47–50 years and 70–73 years cohorts. There is controversy over the proposed extension, as there is some doubt as to its effectiveness in terms of breast cancer mortality. Traditionally, the attendance is poorer in the 70–73 years age group and, although the incidence may be higher, the grade/risk is likely to be lower. In the younger (47–50 years) cohort, the incidence is likely to be lower, but is likely to be of a higher grade/risk. Initial analysis from the ScHARR report suggests that it is more likely to be cost effective in the older cohort due to a higher incidence of breast cancer in this age group. At present, women are encouraged to self-refer at their final screening appointment, and some centres are investigating increasing the number of self-referrals through individual interviews/leaflets. Although the current age range is 50–70 years, in reality many women are not invited until they are 53 years and have their last screen at 68 years old. Targeting this shortfall first might be an appropriate use of resources.

ANXIETY ASSOCIATED WITH THE SCREENING PROCESS

A large number of papers have examined the issue of anxiety caused by the invitation to screening attendance (Ellman *et al.*, 1989; Fallowfield *et al.*, 1990; Sutton *et al.*, 1995; Steggles *et al.*, 1998; Aro *et al.*, 1999), and anxiety relating to recall for assessment (Sutton *et al.*, 1995; Scaf-Klomp *et al.*, 1997; Rimer and Bluman, 1997; Steggles *et al.*, 1998; Brett *et al.*, 1998; Pisano *et al.*, 1998; Ong and Austoker, 1997; Aro *et al.*, 2000). It is clear that anxiety does exist. and it is the responsibility of every member of staff within the service and those within general practice to try to alleviate some of the symptoms of anxiety. All staff within a breast-screening unit should have excellent communication skills, in particulate those of effective listening and empathy. Each member of the clinical team needs to have an awareness of the potential impact of the screening and assessment process on the women attending.

NURSE'S ROLE

Breast care nurses

Since the commencement of the programme, the need for good quality psychological support has been recognised. In the early days of the programme, specialist breast care nurses were not available for the majority of services. In recent years, it has become essential practice to provide good emotional support for women attending for screening assessment (Ong and Austoker, 1997). The role of the breast care nurse has developed over this time, and all units have the benefit of a breast care nurse to a greater or lesser degree.

In the assessment clinics, breast care nurses are those who have been trained to have a greater understanding of the psychological impact of recall and, in particular, are well versed in the impact of a malignant diagnosis and options available to women in terms of treatment and psychological support. In many assessment clinics, nurses come into contact with the woman attending at the commencement of the clinic. They are therefore a familiar face when women receive the final results of their diagnosis, and can not only provide emotional support and guidance at that time, but continue to be available for women on an ongoing basis throughout their treatment. Many women are affected by the diagnosis of cancer some time after initial treatment, as well as at the point of diagnosis. Continuity of patient care is invaluable, and role of the breast care nurse will continue to influence that care for the women who attend the programme.

Ward nurses

Nurses on a general ward may be asked about the programme, or women in the ward for other clinical problems may be unable to attend their screening appointment. The ward nurse can provide information on how to rearrange this appointment after the current episode of care is complete.

Nurses in general practice

Nurses in all areas of practice can be a source of valuable information on the NHSBSP. The practice nurse needs to be well informed so that she can discuss the programme with women who attend nurse-led clinics. The practice nurse can provide these women with information on whom the programme is for and for whom it is not, can explain why the NHSBSP is aimed at this group and not others, and can encourage those who have not attended an invitation to reconsider their decision.

When women are recalled for assessment, the nurse may be approached for information on why this is the case. The nurse can explain that being recalled may not signify the presence of malignant disease, but may simply be because the situation is unclear.

CONCLUSION

In national terms, the NHS Breast Screening Programme can be considered successful in achieving its aim of reducing mortality in those women invited for screening. However, locally, in deprived and multi-ethnic communities, uptake is noticeably poorer. Expertise in language skills, and cultural knowledge on the part of practice teams, are useful forces for change, but they require resources (Atri *et al.*, 1997). Health care professionals need to act as an effective resource for people, championing the idea of a healthy lifestyle, which can hopefully only increase the public's personal responsibility of their own health, resulting in them attending screening and being more open to adopting better lifestyle choices. Breast screening is of imperative importance (Harmer, 2009).

REFERENCES

Aro AR, de Koning HJ, Absetz P and Schreck M (1999) Psychological predictors of first attendance for organised mammography screening. *Journal of Medical Screening* 6(2): 82–88.

Aro HR, Polvikki Absetz S, van Elderen TM *et al.* (2000) False positive findings in mammography screening induces short-term distress – breast cancer specific concern prevails longer. *European Journal of Cancer* 36(9): 1089–1097.

Astley S and Gilbert F (2004) Computer aided detection in mammography. *Clinical Radiology* 59(5): 390–399.

Atri J, Falshaw M, Gregg R, Robson J, Omar RZ and Dixon S (1997) Improving uptake of breast screening in multiethnic populations: a randomised controlled trial using practice reception staff to contact non-attenders. *British Medical Journal* 315: 1356–1359.

Austoker J (1999) Gaining informed consent for screening is difficult – but many misconceptions need to be undone. *British Medical Journal* 319(7212): 722–723.

Austoker J and Ong G (1994) Written information needs of women who are recalled for further investigation of breast screening: results of a multi-centre study. *Journal of Medical Screening* 1(4): 238–244.

Baum M (1996) The breast screening controversy. *European Journal of Cancer* 32A(1): 9–11.

Baum M, Querci della Rovere G *et al.* (1995) Screening for breast cancer, time to think-and stop? *The Lancet North American Edition* 346(8972): 436–439.

Blanks RG (2000) Effect of the NHS breast screening programme on mortality from breast cancer in England and Wales, 1990–8: comparison of observed with predicted mortality. *British Medical Journal* 321: 665–669.

Blanks RG, Given-Wilson RM and Moss SM (1998) Efficiency of cancer detection during routine repeat (incident) screening: two view versus one view mammography. *Journal of Medical Screening* 5(3): 141–145.

Blanks RG, Moss SM and Wallis MG (1997) Use of two view mammography compared with one view in the detection of small invasive cancers: further results from the National Health Service Breast Screening Programme *Journal of Medical Screening* 4(2): 98–101.

Breast Screening Frequency Trial Group (2002) The frequency of breast cancer screening: results from the UKCCCR Randomised Trial. *European Journal of Cancer* 38: 1458–1464.

Brett J, Austoker J and Ong G (1998) Do women who undergo further investigation for breast screening suffer adverse psychological consequences? A multicentre follow-up study comparing breast screening result groups five months after their last screening appointment. *Journal of Public Health Medicine* 20(4): 396–403.

Department of Health (1992) *The Health of the Nation: a Strategy for Health in England.* London: HMSO.

Department of Health (1995) *The Calman Hine Report. A Policy Framework for Commissioning Cancer Services. A report by the Expert Advisory Group on Cancer to the Chief Medical Officer of England and Wales.* London: HMSO.

Department of Health (1998) *The New NHS Modern and Dependable: A National Framework for Assessing Performance.* London: HMSO.

Department of Health (2000) *The NHS Cancer Plan: A Plan for investment. A Plan for Reform.* London: HMSO.

Department of Health (2001) *Clinical Guidelines for Breast Cancer Screening Assessment* London: HMSO

Department of Health (2007) *Cancer Reform Strategy*. London: HMSO. Available: http://www.dh.gov.uk.

'Ellman R, Angeli N, Christians A, Moss S, Chamberlain J and Maguire PP (1989) Psychiatric morbidity associated with screening for breast cancer. *British Journal of Cancer* 60: 781–784.

Fallowfield LJ, Rodway A and Baum M (1990) What are the psychological factors influencing attendance: non attendance and attendance at a breast screening center. *Journal of the Royal Society of Medicine* 83(9): 547–551.

Fenton JJ, Taplin SH and Carney PA (2007) Influence of computer-aided detection on the performance of screening mammography. *New England Journal of Medicine* 356: 1399–1409.

Forrest APM (1986) *Breast Cancer Screening: Report to the Health Ministers of England, Wales, Scotland and Northern Ireland.* London: HMSO.

Gilbret FJ, Astley SM, Gillan MGC *et al.* (2008) Single reading with computer-aided detection for screening mammography. *New England Journal of Medicine* 359: 1675–1684.

Harmer V (2009) Breast care – awareness and screening. *Practice Nurse* 38(5): 12–14.

Hoare T, Johnson C, Gorton R and Alberg C (1992) Reasons for non-attendance for breast screening by Asian women. *Health Education Journal* 51(4): 157–161.

Kettritz U, Rotter K, Schreer L *et al.* (2004) Stereotactic vacuum assisted breast biopsy in 2874 patients. A multi-center study. *Cancer* 100: 245–251.

Lee L, Stickland V, Roebuck EJ and Wilson ARM (1995) *Fundamentals of Mammography* London: W.B. Saunders.

Liberman L (2000) Percutaeneous Image guided core breast biopsy. *American Journal of Roentgenology* 174: 1191–1199.

Lindfors KK, McGahan MC, Rosenquist CJ and Hurlock GS (2006) Computer aided detection of breast cancer: a cost effectiveness study. *Radiology* 239: 710–717.

Madan J and Rawdin A (2008) *ScHARR Initial Assessment Report.* Available: http://www.cancerscreening. nhs.uk/breastscreen/nhsbsp-appraisal-47-49.pdf.

McCann J, Britton PD and Warren RML (2001) Radiology peer review of interval cancers in East Anglian breast screening programme: what are we missing? *Journal of Medical Screening.* 8(2): 77–85

Moss S, Waller M, Anderson TJ and Cuckle H (2005) (The Age Trial) Randomised controlled trial of mammographic screening in women from age 40: predicted mortality based on surrogate outcomes. *British Journal of Cancer* 92: 955–960.

Moss SM, Brown J, Garvican L *et al.* (2001) Routine breast screening for women aged 65–69: results from evaluation of the demonstration sites. *Journal of Cancer* 85(9): 1289–1294.

National Health Service Breast Screening Programme (2005) *Quality Assurance Guidelines for Breast Cancer Screening*. NHSBSP Publication No 59. Sheffield: NHS Cancer Screening Programmes.

National Health Service Breast Screening Programme (2005) *Consolidated Guidance on Standards for the NHS Breast Screening Programme*. NHSBSP Publication No 60. Sheffield: NHS Cancer Screening Programmes.

National Health Service Breast Screening Programme (2009) *NHSBSP Annual Review.* Sheffield: NHS Cancer Screening Programmes.

Ong G and Austoker J (1997) Recalling women for further investigation of breast screening: women's expediencies at the clinic and afterwards. *Journal of Public Health Medicine* 19(1): 29–36.

Ong GJ, Austoker J and Brett J (1997a) Breast screening: adverse psychological consequences one month after placing women on early recall because of a diagnostic uncertainty. A multicentre study. *Journal of Medical Screening* 4(3): 158–168.

Ong GJ, Austoker J and Michell M (1997b) Early rescreen/recall in the UK National Health Service breast screening programme: epidemiological data. *Journal of Medical Screening* 4(3): 146–155.

Pisano ED, Earp J, Schell M, Vakaty K and Denham A (1998) Screening behaviour of women after a false positive mammogram. *Radiology* 208: 245–249.

Pritchard (1989) *Quality Assurance Guidelines for Mammography.* NHSBSP Publication No 1. Sheffield: NHS Cancer Screening Programmes.

Rimer BK and Bluman LG (1997) The psychological consequences of mammography. *Journal of the National Cancer Institute* Monographs No22.

Scaf-Klomp W, Sanderman R, van de Wiel HBM, Otter R and van den Heuval WJA (1997) Distressed or re-lived? Psychological side effects of breast cancer screening in the Netherlands. *Journal of Epidemiology and Community Health* 51(6): 7705–7710.

Shapiro S, Venet W, Strax P and Venet L (1982) Ten- to fourteen- year effect of breast screening on mortality. *Journal of the American Cancer Institute* 69: 349–355.

Steggles S, Lightfoot N and Sellick SM (1998) Psychological distress associated with organised breast cancer screening. *Cancer Prevention and Control* 2(5): 213–220.

Sutton S, Saidi G, Bickler G and Hunter J (1995) Does routine screening for breast cancer raise anxiety? Results from a three wave prospective study in England. *Journal of Epidemiology and Community Health* 49: 413–418.

Tabar L, Fagerburg CJ, Gad A *et al.* (1985) Reduction in mortality form breast cancer after mass screening with mammography. Randomised trial from the breast cancer screening working group of the Swedish National Board for Health. *The Lancet* i: 829–832.

Wald N, Murphy P, Major P, Parkes C, Townsend J and Frost C (1995) UKCCCR multicentre randomised controlled trial of one and two view mammography in breast cancer screening. *British Medical Journal* 311: 1189–1193.

Wilson JMG and Junger G (1968) *Principles and Practice of Screening for Disease.* World Health Organization Public Health Paper 34.

5 Surgery for Breast Cancer

Victoria Harmer

INTRODUCTION

The treatment of breast cancer often involves lengthy and complex procedures that require a high level of holistic nursing care. During cancer treatment, patients face a number of challenges, both physically and emotionally, some of which can be ameliorated through the use of appropriate techniques (Harmer, 2000a).

All patients should be discussed at a multidisciplinary (MDT) meeting to ensure the treatment plan suggested is the result of an informed consensus.

Most management plans for breast cancer will involve some form of surgery for local control of the disease (Harmer, 2008a). Surgery is usually the first treatment modality used, although it can follow systemic treatments – chemotherapy or hormone therapy. Surgery can be prophylactic, diagnostic, definitive (curative), reconstructive, palliative or supportive (e.g. cannula/Hickman line) (Harmer, 2008b). Surgery can also be performed after radiotherapy has been given, although this may result in slower post-operative healing.

There are clinical and pathological features of breast cancer that influence the type of surgery used. These features include the position and size of the cancer, the size of the host breast, the completeness of any initial excision, the histological grade, a young age of patient (less than 35 year sold), the presence of extensive in situ component, and lymphovascular invasion (Sainsbury *et al.*, 2006).

NEOADJUVANT CHEMOTHERAPY

Chemotherapy may be offered as the first treatment modality if the primary breast tumour is thought to be large (more than 3 cm), fixed to the skin or chest wall, or an inflammatory breast cancer (Lewis, 2005).

Following chemotherapy, there may be a sufficient reduction in the size of the breast cancer to then offer breast-conserving surgery and radiotherapy rather than mastectomy. Chemotherapy may also be recommended if the breast cancer appears inoperable at presentation, with a hope to shrink and downstage it to a size where a mastectomy is possible.

Trials have shown that neoadjuvant chemotherapy does not improve survival compared with patients who receive chemotherapy post-operatively. However, neoadjuvant chemotherapy can downstage the tumour, allowing more patients to have breast-conserving surgery, which appears to be safe and effective and increases a person's quality of life (Stebbing and Gaya, 2001).

Surgery in the axilla has often divided opinion among clinicians. With neoadjuvant chemotherapy being used more regularly and readily, the staging of the axilla again becomes a talking point. This will be discussed later in this chapter under the heading 'The axilla'.

NEOADJUVANT ENDOCRINE TREATMENT

Endocrine treatment may be offered as a treatment prior to surgery for much the same reasons that chemotherapy is offered, i.e. to downstage the disease. Endocrine treatment may also be given if a patient needs more time to adjust psychologically to the idea of an operation, or if they need a 'work up' to ensure fitness for an anaesthetic.

BREAST-CONSERVING SURGERY

With the increased understanding that people with breast cancer die not from uncontrolled local disease but from blood-borne metastases, the surgery of choice is usually breast conservation (Harmer, 2006).

Breast-conserving surgery is considered to be a more complex treatment than a mastectomy for breast cancer. This is because a separate incision is required for axillary lymph node dissection, and post-operative radiotherapy is always recommended (Butler Nattinger *et al.*, 2000).

Even if a cancer is suitable for breast-conserving surgery, a patient should be given a choice of operation. Survival rates are equal if a patient has a mastectomy, or if they have breast-conserving surgery followed by a course of radiotherapy, (providing certain pathological criteria are met). Women treated for breast cancer by breast-conserving surgery, who do not have radiotherapy, have local recurrence rates of 35% after 5 years (Fisher *et al.*, 1995; Early Breast Cancer Trialists' Collaborative Group, 1995).

Some people prefer to have the whole breast removed, and therefore do not require daily radiotherapy, lasting 3–4 weeks. For others, the thought of losing their breast when it is not necessary would seem totally alien.

Excision biopsy

If a patient has a suspicious, but non-conclusive triple-assessment examination (clinical examination, imaging and cytology) of a breast lump, an excision biopsy may be required (see Fig. 5.1a). Excision biopsy involves removing the lump under general anaesthetic.

The specimen can then be sent to the histology department and analysed. If the lump is confirmed as breast cancer, a second operation is usually necessary so that good margins can be taken from around the lump, and some form of axillary lymph node surgery may be recommended.

Needle-wire localisation for impalpable breast lumps

Some cancers are detected through screening investigations. The percentage of these screen-detected non-palpable breast cancers has risen from 5% in the early 1980s to 30% at the

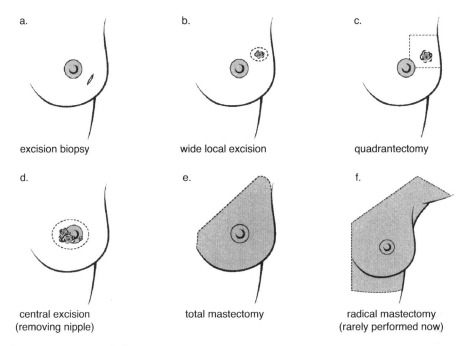

Fig. 5.1 Operations for breast cancer.

present day. This is due to the National Health Service (NHS) Breast Screening Programme, which followed the Forrest Report (1986), and also to diagnostic methods becoming more refined (Costa and Zurrida, 1998). Mammography is becoming more sophisticated with the birth of digital mammography, which results in smaller lesions being identified.

To assist in the surgical removal of these lesions (usually the first modality of treatment for screen-detected breast cancers), needle wires need to be placed to identify the location of these impalpable breast cancers. Thus the wire can guide the surgeon to the area to be removed.

Pre-operatively, a radiologist will identify the location of the breast cancer using either ultrasound waves or X-rays. The radiologist will inject local anaesthetic into the skin of the breast, so the procedure is minimally painful. The imaging locates the lesion, and the tip of the needle wire will then be inserted into the centre of the breast cancer. Accurate placement of the wire is crucial. The radiologist will have been guided by microcalcification seen on the mammogram or a suspicious shadow on ultrasound. After the wire has been securely taped, the patient can return to the ward or admission zone until the operation takes place.

The needle wire guides the surgeon and enables the correct piece of breast tissue to be removed. A specimen X-ray is often taken post-operatively of the piece of breast tissue removed, to show the tip of the wire and as proof that the cancer has been removed. Many screening units require a copy of this X-ray for their files. Some breast units localise impalpable cancer by injecting a radioactive isotope.

Importance of clear margins in breast cancer surgery

In order for breast-conserving treatment to be successful, a margin of about 1 cm of normal breast tissue around the cancer must be excised. If there is in situ or invasive disease at the margin of the specimen removed from the breast, the local recurrence rate is increased. The completeness of excision is the most important factor influencing local recurrence after breast-conservation surgery (Sainsbury *et al.*, 2006).

In some cases, a patient may require a second operation once the histopathologist has examined the specimen if the margins of normal tissue are deemed to be compromising local recurrence rates. This usually involves the surgeon opening the original excision wound, and excising a slither of breast tissue from the margin as required.

In a minority of cases, the specialist team may realise that much more breast tissue needs to be removed in order to completely excise the cancer with good margins. A mastectomy may be recommended to the patient. This mostly occurs with lobular carcinoma (see Chapter 2).

Studies that discuss the value of magnetic resonance imaging (MRI) in determining clear margins for breast cancers are currently underway. Some hospitals, within trial conditions, perform an MRI scan after the wide local excision, while the patient is still anaesthetised. By doing this, it is hoped that if there is cancer or in situ disease persisting in the breast at the margin of the excision, this will show up during the scan, thus the surgeon can remove a slither more from that margin. It is hoped that this would prevent the need for a second operation. Many hospitals recommend a pre-operative MRI scan if lobular carcinoma is diagnosed. This assists in determining the actual size of the cancer, as often the edges of lobular cancer are ill-defined. After reviewing the MRI scan, an appropriate operation can be recommended to the patient.

Wide local excision

Wide local excision involves the removal of the cancer with its surrounding tissue (see Fig. 5.1 and Fig. 5.2). Although there is no size limit for breast-conserving surgery, breast units tend not to offer this surgery to women with cancers larger than 3–4 cm due to poor cosmetic outcomes. In addition, randomised trials comparing breast-conserving surgery with mastectomy as treatments for breast cancer have never included breast cancers larger

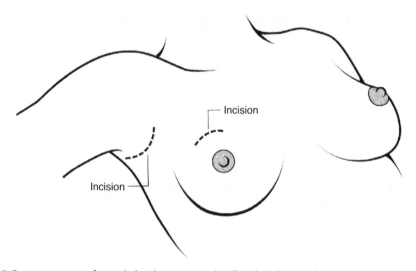

Fig. 5.2 Appearance after wide local excision and axillary lymph node dissection.

than 4 cm, and some surgeons therefore suggest that breast-conserving surgery has not been adequately tested in those larger tumours.

There is no age limit for breast-conserving surgery, and research shows that breast-conserving surgery followed by radiotherapy produces similar survival rates when compared to a mastectomy alone (Veronesi *et al.*, 2002). A possible exception for giving radiotherapy includes small low-grade node-negative cancers that have been excised with good margins, or tumours in older women (>55 years) who have undergone quadrantectomy rather than wide local excision. Radiotherapy will not be administered if a low-grade ductal carcinoma in situ has been removed (Lewis, 2005).

If the cancer is found directly behind the nipple, this operation is referred to as a central excision, which often includes removal of the nipple, thus giving a poorer cosmetic result but one that the patient may still prefer to mastectomy (see Fig. 5.1d).

Volume-displacement technique – oncoplastic breast-conservation reconstruction

Oncoplastic breast-conservation reconstruction is a reasonably recent technique and is effectively an adaptation of conventional breast-conserving surgery as it involves a simultaneous breast reduction.

In essence, oncoplastic breast-conservation reconstruction involves rearranging the remaining breast tissue once the cancer has been removed. The volume loss is absorbed over a wider area, with reshaping of the breast taking place. This reduces the size of the breast and lifts the position of the nipple, and therefore a symmetrisation procedure on the contralateral side is often requested by the patient. Oncoplastic breast-conservation reconstruction is appropriate if the patient has an inferior pole cancer (in the 3 to 9 o'clock position of the breast), or if the tumour is immediately above the nipple (Benson and Absar, 2008). The nipple can therefore be lifted and the remainder of the breast remodelled. Scars will run around the nipple and downwards into the fold under the breast (Rainsbury, 2008) (see Fig. 5.3).

Volume-replacement technique – quadrantectomy and mini-flap reconstruction

A quadrantectomy is where a quadrant of breast tissue is removed (Fig. 5.1c). At this first operation, sentinel lymph node biopsy may be performed if appropriate. Cosmetic results are usually poor, as the resulting deficit is larger than that following wide local

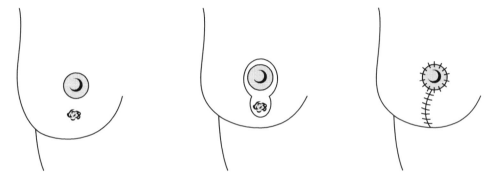

Fig. 5.3 Volume displacement technique.

excision, thus a patient may be offered a volume-replacement procedure in the form of a mini-flap reconstruction. This reconstructive operation usually takes place a few days to 1 week after the quadrantectomy, to ensure that surgical margins have been checked and are cancer-free.

During this second reconstructive operation, part of the latissimus dorsi muscle is harvested and turned with its blood supply to the front to fill breast volume, i.e. tissue is taken from a nearby site to assist in reconstructing the breast.

An axillary lymph node clearance should accompany a quadrantectomy, and this may take place at the time of the mini-flap operation as this is thought to be technically easier.

Careful selection of patients for each operation is crucial. More volume-replacement techniques will be discussed in Chapter 7, which is dedicated to breast reconstruction.

CONTRAINDICATIONS TO BREAST-CONSERVING SURGERY

Breast-conserving surgery may not be recommended by the medical team owing to a number of factors:

- If there is a large breast cancer volume–to–breast volume ratio, which would result in a poor cosmetic result and noticeable breast asymmetry;
- If radiotherapy has been given to that breast previously;
- If there are diffuse, suspicious microcalcifications over a large area of the breast;
- If the disease is multi-focal (i.e. more than one breast cancer in the same breast);
- If the breast cancer is located centrally to the breast, as the cosmetic result of breast-conserving treatment would be poor;
- If the patient with breast cancer was in the first half of pregnancy, as radiotherapy cannot be given as adjuvant treatment to the pregnant woman.

Treatment plans should always be discussed in partnership with the patient and family as requested so that an agreed trajectory can be established. Table 5.1 details the characteristics

Table 5.1 Characteristics of breast cancers that indicate an increased risk of local recurrence post–breast-conservation surgery.

Feature	Description
Extensive component in situ (ECIS)	In situ component forming >25% of main tumour mass
Involved excision margins	Histological evidence that the surgeon has cut through the cancer when excising the lump
Presence of vascular and/or lymphatic invasion	Histological evidence of cancer within the blood vessels or lymphatic system
Young age	Being diagnosed with breast cancer under the age of 40 years increases the chance of local recurrence
Positive lymph nodes	Histological evidence of cancer within the lymph nodes
High tumour grade	Histological diagnosis of a grade 3 breast cancer

Adapted from Leinster *et al.* (2000).

of breast cancers that are associated with an increased risk of local recurrence post–breast-conservation surgery.

MASTECTOMY

Approximately 30% of all breast cancers are unsuitable for breast-conserving surgery and require a mastectomy (Fig. 5.1e,f, Fig. 5.4 and Plate 3) (Sainsbury *et al.*, 2006). Some women opt for a mastectomy rather than for the 'package' of breast-conserving surgery and radiotherapy, as they feel that daily hospital treatments interfere too much with the activities of daily living.

Radiotherapy is, however, sometimes required post-mastectomy. Criteria for post-mastectomy radiotherapy vary between different centres, but generally include high-grade, large cancers with vascular involvement, and/or positive lymph nodes, (particularly a high number of positive lymph nodes).

A mastectomy is usually the recommended surgical option for men diagnosed with breast cancer since the breast is small and clearance more difficult.

The most common mastectomy is the total mastectomy.

In a modified radical mastectomy, the pectoralis minor muscle is removed or divided to enable the surgeon to clear the axillary lymph nodes fully (see Fig 5.4 for anatomy and physiology breast revision diagram).

A subcutaneous mastectomy that leaves the nipple intact may be performed, especially as part of a reconstructive operation. If this is the case, there can be no guarantee that all of the breast tissue has been removed as some can remain behind the nipple. The procedure is therefore not commonly recommended for most breast cancer patients (Leinster *et al.*, 2000).

Mastectomy should always be combined with some axillary lymph node surgery.

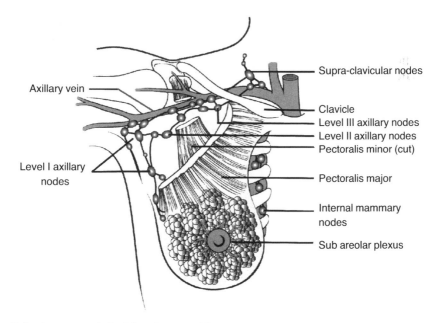

Fig. 5.4 Anatomy and physiology breast revision.

Breast cancer recurrence

If a patient presents with a recurrence, staging tests such as X-ray, bone and CT scan are usually carried out to distinguish if the breast cancer has metastasised and treatment can be titrated accordingly.

If a patient has previously had breast-conserving surgery and develops a local recurrence, a mastectomy would be the usual treatment. The breast cancer would have shown itself to be aggressive and resistant to treatment and should be dealt with accordingly. Wound healing may take longer if radiotherapy has previously been given, so sutures should remain in longer.

If the patient has previously had a mastectomy and develops a local recurrence, radiotherapy can be given to the skin flaps in addition to further surgical resection. However, radiotherapy can only be used radically once, so if it has been used previously, a re-excision of the skin flaps and systemic treatment may be offered. If the breast cancer has recurred extensively within the skin flaps, a skin graft may be required to enable closure of the wound when re-excision takes place.

Extensive recurrence within the skin flaps is a potentially serious situation and may herald systemic disease.

THE AXILLA

The method by which the axilla is treated has remained controversial for the past 50 years, and treatment has varied from hospital to hospital, with lymph nodes being sampled, cleared or irradiated.

It is probable that all surgery for breast cancer will include surgery to the axillary lymph nodes. There are about 20–30 axillary lymph nodes in each armpit, which form part of the lymphatic system draining fluid and infection from the breast. The lymph nodes do not serve as an adequate anatomical barrier to the spread of cancer and are often the first place where breast cancer metastasises (Harmer, 2000b). However treated, the cancer status of the lymph node remains the single most important and powerful prognostic factor, and one on which to base treatment decisions (Bundred *et al.*, 2000; Reintgen *et al.*, 2000; Whitworth *et al.*, 2000) as it shows the potential of the cancer to metastasise.

Sentinel lymph node sampling

Sampling four or five lymph nodes from the lower axilla was first tested in randomised controlled trials in Edinburgh in 1985. This sampling method had 100% sensitivity in their initial series of 65 patients when identifying those with a positive axilla (i.e. breast cancer that has spread through the lymphatic system to the axillary lymph nodes) (Steele *et al.*, 1985). The breast unit in Edinburgh then conducted two subsequent randomised controlled trials comparing axillary lymph node clearance with that of a four-node sampling procedure in combination with mastectomy (Forrest *et al.*, 1995) or breast-conserving surgery (Chetty *et al.*, 2000). Patients who were randomised to have four-node sampling and were lymph node–positive received radiotherapy to the axilla. Results illustrate no difference in survival or axillary recurrence.

Ahlgren *et al.* (2002) reported a similar prospective series on 552 patients in 2002. In this study, up to five lymph nodes were sampled, with axillary clearance being performed as a back-up to assess sensitivity of one-, two, three-, four- or five-node sampling. A sensitivity of 96% was reported for four-node sampling and 97.3% for five-node sampling.

Sentinel lymph node biopsy when using neoadjuvant chemotherapy

Several studies have investigated the use of sentinel lymph node biopsy, both pre- and post–neoadjuvant chemotherapy. Sentinel lymph node biopsy can take place in a day-surgery unit prior to the first cycle of chemotherapy being administered.

Although Breslin *et al.* (2000), Xing *et al.* (2006) and Manounas *et al.* (2005) suggest that post-chemotherapy sentinel lymph node biopsy is reliable in identifying the sentinel lymph node, some authors believe that the sentinel lymph node could have been rendered clear (negative) by chemotherapy, and thus the patient will be understaged. The most modern treatment has surgeons performing sentinel lymph node biopsy pre-administration of neoadjuvant chemotherapy. This is deemed more accurate as the status of the lymph nodes, i.e. whether they contain metastatic cancer, can be reliably discovered prior to any treatment. Indeed Sabel *et al.* (2003) explored the use of sentinel lymph node biopsy prior to administering neoadjuvant chemotherapy and concluded that, if this procedure is performed, it can avoid the morbidity of an axillary lymph node clearance without compromising the accuracy of axillary staging. Sentinel lymph node biopsy pre–neoadjuvant chemotherapy allows identification of node-positive patients subsequently rendered disease-free in the regional nodes, which can assist in planning additional chemotherapy or radiation.

Linking together these studies into the use of sentinel lymph node biopsy, Stearns *et al.* (2002) concluded that sentinel lymph node biopsy after chemotherapy may reliably predict axillary staging except in those patients with inflammatory breast cancer.

In conclusion, it is important to recommend individual treatment to the patient, based on the evidence provided.

Lymphatic mapping and sentinel lymph node biopsy in breast cancer

Lymphatic mapping and sentinel lymph node biopsy was first reported in breast cancer by Krag *et al.* (1993) using a radioactive isotope. Giuliano *et al.* (1994) used a blue dye to map this process and, with its development, the success at finding the sentinel lymph node has reached well over 95%.

The sentinel lymph node is identified as the lymph node that drains and receives fluid first from the area of the breast that has the tumour. It is the most likely lymph node to contain metastatic cancer. (Fig. 5.5 shows sentinel lymph node spread.)

A sentinel lymph node biopsy is minimally invasive, and its examination by frozen section is thought to be an accurate and reliable predictor in determining axillary lymph node cancer status at the time of operating (Jansen *et al.*, 1998; Rodier *et al.*, 2000; Badwe and Mittra, 2001; Veronesi *et al.*, 2001). By using this technique, it is thought that many women with primary breast cancer could avoid being overtreated by an axillary lymph node clearance, with the morbidity this carries with it (Beechey-Newman, 2002).

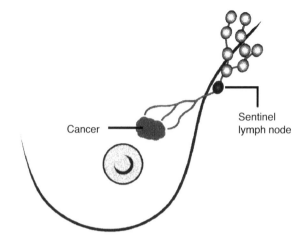

Fig. 5.5 Sentinel node spread.

An hour prior to surgery, or thereabouts, a radioactive isotope is injected around the breast cancer by the surgeon. A blue dye is also injected 5–10 minutes prior to axillary exploration. The optimal technique is the use of this combination (McIntosh and Purushotham, 1998). The theory is that, once injected, the dye and radioactive material will be drawn through the breast to the lymph nodes downstream. Thus, when the surgeon opens the axilla during the operation, a blue lymph node will be visible, which also concentrates the radioactive particles by phagocytosis (see Plates 1 and 2). This node is the sentinel lymph node; the first lymph node to receive fluid from that area of the breast where the breast cancer is. This sentinel lymph node can then be removed and sent to the histopathology laboratory for analysis as a frozen section. The surgical team, in the meantime, can be operating on the breast until they are given the pathology findings on whether cancer was found in the node. Many surgeons choose to examine the sentinel lymph node by paraffin section only.

If cancer is found in the sentinel lymph node, the surgeon may choose to perform an axillary lymph node clearance or give radiotherapy to the axilla.

Post-operatively, some care should be taken with the arm that has had the nodes sampled, to avoid trauma and prevent infection, although this need not be as militant as if the patient had all the lymph nodes removed.

If cancer is not found in the sentinel lymph node, the surgeon may remove a further three lymph nodes from around that area.

Pre-operatively, the patient must give their consent for both procedures.

Nurses should be mindful if a patient has returned from a sentinel lymph node frozen section and has required an axillary lymph node clearance. Once patients realise their cancer has spread to the lymph nodes, depression and distress may well set in as, if lymph nodes contain cancer, chemotherapy is often offered as a treatment modality.

The downside to the sentinel lymph node biopsy technique is that it demands a close working relationship between the clinical physics department, the surgical team and the histopathologist. In some hospitals, this may not be a realistic situation. The probe used to detect radioactivity is expensive, and requires use from a skilled operator, who regularly performs the technique to ensure confidence and competence.

The sentinel lymph node biopsy remains a relatively new technique, and one that is ultimately successful in identifying the 'first station' lymph node in 98.4% of patients and has a false-negative rate of 4.4%, when metastastic lymph nodes will remain untreated in the axilla (Krag *et al.*, 2001). It must also be noted that there is a variation in the institutional and individual surgeon's ability to define and identify sentinel lymph nodes. A learning curve can be illustrated.

Breast cancers that present in the inner quadrant of the breast may drain and therefore metastasise firstly to the internal mammary nodes. If this is the case, excising the axillary lymph nodes may not result in complete staging.

Although thought to be state-of-the-art at the moment, it is expected that the sentinel lymph node biopsy will take its place as standard treatment in future years (Whitworth *et al.*, 2000). It offers a major advance in treating the node-negative population, who can therefore escape needless axillary surgery (Reintgen *et al.*, 2000). However, many controversial issues need be resolved prior to this happening.

In the era of non-palpable screen-detected breast cancers, this technique allows treatment and assessment of the axilla, while sparing the potential problems associated with an axillary clearance, as most women with screen-detected breast cancers do not harbour metastasis in the downstream lymph nodes (Badwe and Mittra, 2001).

A careful selection process should be employed for patients undergoing sentinel lymph node frozen sections. People with larger-sized or multi-focal breast cancers may not be appropriate for this technique. Treatment must be individualised.

Axillary lymph node clearance

Axillary lymph node clearances are usually indicated if a patient has a large or multi-focal breast cancer, or if cytology from the lymph node has proved malignancy to be present.

Axillary clearances may be to any of the three levels of lymph nodes (see Chapter 1 and Fig. 5.4). A clearance should strip the fascia from the walls of the axilla below the axillary vein, while preserving the long thoracic nerve and thoracodorsal bundle. With a level-three clearance, the chance of significant lymphoedema is 10% (Leinster *et al.*, 2000).

If an axillary lymph node clearance has been performed, the patient should be informed that care should be taken against infection and trauma of that arm for the rest of their lives, in order to reduce the chance of lymphoedema.

It is emerging that lymphoedema is a lifelong risk for patients having undergone axillary surgery with or without radiotherapy, rather than sequelae of treatment, and this lifelong risk develops soon after initial surgery or radiotherapy (MacLaren and Harmer, 2002.

Nurses can assist greatly with a patient's compliance with 'arm care' by reminding the patient and also following recommendations. For instance, after a clearance, a patient should not have blood pressure taken on that affected arm. The patient should not have blood taken, venflons inserted or injections into that arm. Nurses can assist patients by disseminating the knowledge of what to do and what not to do. Patient education is the cornerstone of care, and it is through explanations of treatment methods that responsibility of the condition should be 'given' back to the patient (Harmer, 2009). Some hospitals give patients who have had this surgery 'credit cards', which state why invasive procedures cannot be carried out on affected arms. This is a helpful reminder and a useful piece of teaching apparatus for health-care professionals. Park *et al.* (2008) found a significantly decreased risk of lymphoedema in women who exercised regularly, received pre-treatment education of lymphoedema and who had performed preventative self-care activities.

For many patients who experience the development of lymphoedema, it heralds a lifetime of ongoing management and attention to a medical condition that can be disruptive to daily activities (MacLaren and Harmer, 2002). It is therefore vital to try to prevent it.

More information on lymphoedema and maintenance of the arm post–axillary lymph node clearance is available in Chapter 11.

Axillary recurrence

If cancer recurs in the axilla, repeat surgical axillary intervention is usually recommended. Adjuvant systemic treatment can also be appropriate, and the patient is usually re-staged for disseminated disease. Radiotherapy can also be given, although the addition of radiation to axillary surgery increases the risk of subsequent lymphoedema.

COMPLICATIONS OF BREAST SURGERY

Seroma formation

It is normal for haemo-serous fluid to collect post-operatively at the site of excision. Fluid collects, where there is a space following tissue removal, and it will continue to do so until the underlying tissues cause a vacuum and adhere. This is why post-operative closed-suction drainage is used. These drains are inserted if a patient has had an axillary clearance, a wide local excision or a mastectomy. The drains are removed at various post-operative intervals according to hospital policy, the surgeon's preference and the volume they have drained over a 24-hour period. It is quite usual, however, for serous fluid to collect post-removal of the drain. Depending on the amount that has collected, a surgeon or specialist nurse may aspirate this fluid on a regular basis, before the body then reabsorbs it. Undrained seromas could become infected and are uncomfortable. The nurse should explain that these seromas are common and, apart from the inconvenience of drainage, are not important.

Infection

As with all surgery, there is the possibility of infection after breast surgery, although infection is rare. Infection should be treated according to hospital policy and antibiotics prescribed. Care should be taken if this occurs, as patients may experience psychological problems, in addition to pain and fever, reacting to how their body image is affected by such a personal part of their body becoming infected.

Flap necrosis

Flap necrosis occurs when the skin flaps post-mastectomy become necrotic. It is rare and more often occurs in heavy smokers or older patients. Necrosis due to impaired blood supply may resolve with regular dressings; however occasionally the necrotic skin may need to be excised with the possibility of skin grafts.

Cording

Cording may occur post–lymph node surgery due to fibrosis or thickened lymph or blood vessels. Cording causes pain and a decrease in arm mobility. It is through exercise that cording can be treated (see Chapter 6).

TIMING OF SURGICAL TREATMENT FOR PRIMARY BREAST CANCER IN RELATION TO THE MENSTRUAL CYCLE

Many retrospective studies have been undertaken over the past 13 years to assess whether there is any relationship between the menstrual phase and the timing of the surgical intervention for primary breast cancer on disease-free and overall survival rates.

Much of the literature is contradictory, and there are shortcomings in the data. Therefore, there is still no real evidence to lead us to time breast surgery according to the phase of the menstrual cycle (Hortobagyi, 2002).

Some evidence suggests that survival is improved if surgery is performed during the luteal phase of the cycle (Veronesi *et al.*, 1994).

NURSING CARE

Pre-operatively

Ward nurses play a vital role in the patient's surgical experience. Ward nurses must assess the health needs of the individual and form a foundation for all decision-making and problem-solving activities concerned with care.

Nurses must continually assess how the patient's state of health may be influencing their level of dependence, giving the ability to pitch nurse intervention at the correct level.

The nurse's main aim pre-operatively must be to ensure a safe environment for the patient. This means identifying any allergies and administrating regularly required medication according to the prescription chart. The nurse must also ensure that baseline observations (temperature, blood pressure, pulse, respiration and oxygen saturation) are recorded, detecting any abnormalities which may delay the operation.

Hospitals may have a pre-operative integrated-care pathway that should be followed and filled out. This will ensure, among other things, that the patient is correctly dressed for the operation; that nail varnish, jewellery and prostheses are removed, and that the correct size of anti-thromboic stockings are worn. These stockings decrease the chance of a deep-vein thrombosis, which is a potential problem for patients undergoing surgery. Anti-thromboic stockings give legs graded compression to encourage the complete emptying of vein segments, thereby decreasing pooling of venous stasis.

Nurses must also ensure a patient undergoes a period of starvation and fluid deprivation, a medical and legal requirement prior to an anaesthetic, except in cases of emergency.

Boore (1978) demonstrated that the provision of information before surgery lowers anxiety levels, reduces stress, decreases pain and promotes a better and quicker recovery. Nurses must appreciate this and should assist patients to the best of their ability.

Post-operatively

The post-operative period presents many potential problems. The most important task is to check that the patient's airway is clear and that oxygen is given if prescribed. Mouthcare is extremely important for patient safety and comfort. Blood is often present after an endotracheal intubation. If the patient is unable to drink water, the nurse should use mouthwash and foamsticks to sweep the mouth, gums and teeth to remove any blood or debris. Petroleum jelly should be applied to dry, rough or chapped lips.

Observations (temperature, pulse, blood pressure, respiration, and oxygen saturation) should be performed regularly and according to hospital policy. Any abnormalities should naturally be reported.

Pain should be assessed regularly and analgesia administered swiftly.

Dressings should be checked regularly for post-operative bleeding and any blood on the dressing marked and monitored. Vacuum-suction drains should be labelled and regularly checked. These drainage bottles will be removed in time, according to the amount drained, the surgeon's preference, and hospital policy.

Nurses should ensure that patients are safe, clean and comfortable while they are dependent. As a patient becomes less dependent, a nurse should be guided by them as to what care is required.

It must be remembered that the nurse does not only care for the patient, although this must be the focus. Post-operatively it is vital the nurse informs the patients chosen family and friends of patient progress.

When a patient comes to a post-operative outpatient's clinic, a nurse should be sensitive, as they may not have looked at their breast post-surgery. The nurse must also be aware the patient may be receiving pathology results and awaiting discussions regarding the next step in their treatment trajectory.

AMBULATORY BREAST CANCER SURGERY

With recent increasing attention to rising health-care costs, both public and private sectors are demanding more value from the services and products they purchase (Shalowitz, 2010). With the difficult financial situation facing the NHS, and the need to save about £15–20 billion by the end of 2013/14 (NHS Institute for Innovation and Improvement, 2010), departments are changing the way they work and hospital stays are becoming shorter. Breast cancer is a common disease, affecting one million women annually worldwide; thus any strategy that can be put in place to reduce costs is attractive, with the proviso that patient safety is not compromised (Ranieri *et al.*, 2004). Most management plans for breast cancer will involve some form of surgery for local control of the disease (Harmer, 2000b). Surgery may be the first treatment modality used, or it can follow systemic treatments – chemotherapy or hormone therapy.

Ambulatory surgery (day-case setting with discharge within 23 hours post-surgery) for breast cancer is becoming more common place, resulting in a mean bed-day saving per patient of 4.7 days (Chadha *et al.*, 2004). Patients may be discharged with or without suction drains in situ. Although breast surgery, including mastectomy is increasingly being performed in this outpatient setting, there are concerns regarding whether patients receive adequate post-mastectomy care (Bian *et al.*, 2008), and whether this type of surgery is associated with a lower rate of immediate breast reconstruction (Bian *et al.*, 2008).

Investigations into this arena were carried out by a number of studies, a selection of which will be discussed.

Margolese and Lasry (2000) compared inpatient to same-day discharge surgery for breast cancer on selected patients. They report similar levels of pain, fear, anxiety, health assessment and quality of life for the two groups of patients, with the ambulatory patients manifesting a significantly better emotional adjustment and fewer psychological distress symptoms. The inpatient group returned to usual activities and felt that they had recovered from their operation about 10 days later than those patients in the ambulatory group (Margolese and Lasry, 2000).

Marchal *et al.* (2005) focused on post-operative care and patient satisfaction after ambulatory surgery for breast cancer. Here, none of the 236 patients were re-admitted during the first week, but post-operative pain presented a problem for those who had axillary dissection in addition to the surgery on the breast. Both groups scored the post-operative information given by the nurse higher when compared to the information given by the surgeon (Marchal *et al.*, 2005).

Rovera *et al.* (2008) selected patients for ambulatory surgery according to specific social, environmental, physical and oncological criteria. They discovered no intra-operative complications and, despite some post-operative complications (e.g. wound infections), they concluded that this surgery is feasible, effective, safe, cost-effective and highly appreciated by women. Tan and Guenther (1997) found neither post-operative complications nor re-admissions problematic in their study.

To drain or not to drain?

It is normal for haemo-serous fluid to collect post-operatively at the site of excision. Fluid collects, where there is a space following tissue removal, and it will continue to do so until the underlying tissues adhere. Thus post-operative closed-suction drains are traditionally used for breast surgery (Harmer, 2003). Drains are removed at various post-operative intervals. It is quite usual, however, for serous fluid to collect post-removal of the drain. Depending on the amount of fluid that has collected, a surgeon or specialist nurse may aspirate this fluid before the body then reabsorbs it (Harmer, 2003). Most outpatient breast surgery units do not use drains, although Ranieri *et al.* (2004) discharged the patient with drains in situ and found no apparent problems. Chadha *et al.* (2004) undertook a retrospective study of discharging patients with drains and found that only 6% of patients felt confident going home early from hospital, two-thirds of patients admitted feeling anxious on their first day at home, and the lack of confidence over emptying drains was worse in older patients.

A word of caution

Driving the service into the community in this way may burden district or practice nurses. There may even be a place for the breast care nurse to straddle both hospital and community settings and to make post-operative visits to the patient's home. Where this is geographically difficult, telephone calls may suffice until the patient is seen in the outpatients clinic.

Despite many potential benefits of this surgical strategy, some may instinctively feel that the patient has less psychological input from their breast nurse specialist. The breast nurse would normally visit the inpatient recovering from breast surgery daily, with an agenda to cover. Issues pertaining to body image, sexuality and a need for increased input from professionals may be missed, unless expert communication skills are present. Some may feel that the patient discharged home the same day as their operation may feel they need to 'recover' more quickly and show the family that they are able to carry on as usual. If they were inpatients, they may have protected times to enable them to psychologically adjust to having had an operation for breast cancer.

The clear financial benefit of ambulatory surgery (Simpson *et al.*, 2007), along side the freeing up of acute surgical beds, may seem advantageous for the health service, but this needs to be evaluated carefully if this service is to be offered. The time taken by the breast care nurse to visit post-operative patients on the ward needs to be evaluated in conjunction with time taken during telephone calls to these patients if they are discharged home, and any implications to the nurse's job plan should be addressed.

If ambulatory breast surgery, namely outpatient mastectomy, becomes more common-place, this may have a knock-on effect on the number of immediate breast reconstructions performed. The reconstruction is a more complex operation and, although some suggest this can be a safe and effective procedure for carefully selected patients in this ambulatory setting (Simpson *et al.*, 2007), I would suggest this is an extreme and uncommon view. Future research could investigate whether the push to perform these outpatient mastectomies denies women their immediate breast reconstructions.

BREAST PROSTHESIS

Many years ago, breast prostheses were bags filled with either bird seed or water. Thankfully, times have changed, and the range available at present is extensive. It is important for every woman who has had a mastectomy to be fitted with a breast prosthesis prior to her discharge home, so that dignity and confidentiality are upheld.

Temporary prosthesis

The first prosthesis that a woman will be fitted with is a soft, foam breast form. This temporary prosthesis will be gentle next to the skin while healing takes place. These prostheses either sit inside the empty cup of a bra or, due to their cloth cover, are pinned at the appropriate level to the inside of a vest or shirt.

The temporary breast prosthesis is often called a comfy or softy. It is obviously lighter than the natural breast, so symmetry is often a problem, and bra straps may need to be adjusted to compensate this. The bra strap on the side of the bra with the natural breast should be tightened, so that the natural breast is lifted and aligned with the lighter side with the prosthesis.

Permanent silicone breast prosthesis

Six to eight weeks post-mastectomy, an appointment is usually made to enable a more natural-looking prosthesis to be fitted. The permanent silicone prosthesis is heavier than the temporary one, so looks more natural in the bra.

A patient should bring a correctly fitting cotton bra, preferably a sport bra, and a plain-coloured, tight-fitting T-shirt, so that their profile can be seen, and a good match to the natural breast found. (Bras and swimwear will be discussed later in this chapter).

Thankfully, there are many manufacturers of breast prostheses, so the range is wide. Different companies produce different-shaped prostheses, some more ptotic, some with extra silicone at the sides to fill any deficit of tissue, and some that adhere to the chest wall.

Adhesive prostheses can be used 6 months post-mastectomy, or 6 months post-radiotherapy to the chest wall. Although they are recommended for use with a bra, some smaller-breasted women feel able to use them without a bra. The chest wall first needs to be prepared by using a toning liquid that removes dead skin cells, and provides a good surface for the prosthesis to stick. When the prosthesis loses its adhesion (some say up to 3 days later) it is removed and cleaned with a special cleanser and brush. Some companies have developed a system of stickers to adhere the prosthesis to the chest wall. Once the adhesion has gone, the sticker needs be removed, and another sticker replaced. These adhesive prostheses are especially useful for women who enjoy healthy physical lifestyles.

Breast prostheses are available in different colours, and this subject must be approached with care. Some women are most offended when faced with a darker shade of breast form, and others are upset if faced with a prosthesis for a Caucasian-coloured skin. It is a sensitive subject and one that can be most surprising.

The prosthesis appointment is an ideal opportunity to assess the patient's body image, coping mechanisms and her support network. Each time a woman has a breast prosthesis appointment, it is a perfect time to reassess her psychologically and socially.

Permanent breast prostheses should last for at least 1 year; however, if a woman's weight fluctuates, she will need to be refitted.

Made-to-measure silicone prosthesis

If a woman's chest wall is notably uneven, possibly as a result of a previous infection, a made-to-measure prosthesis may be required. An appointment will be made with a specialist from the company, when a 'normal' prosthesis will be fitted and measurements and notes of areas where extra silicone is needed will be made. This can be effective be done by 'filling in' or 'building up' parts of the chest wall. The end result is a prosthesis which has added-on parts that should fit the wearer comfortably and safely. These prostheses are more expensive than others and take about 3 months to be made.

PROSTHETIC NIPPLES

Although all breast prostheses have a nipple built into them, some women prefer to wear an additional prosthetic one. Prosthetic nipples can be bought from specialist companies or sex shops or can be made in some hospital surgical appliance departments. Those from the specialist companies tend to look generic, and are stuck onto the breast form using special adhesive. The nipples that are made in hospital departments look much more realistic, although the process of making them can sometimes be regarded as distressing. Firstly, a plaster cast of the natural nipple is taken, and silicone is used to make the shape of the nipple. The nipple will then be painted to match the natural side. These are also stuck on using adhesive.

Nipples can also be tattooed, or reconstructed (Chapter 7).

CHOOSING A BRA AFTER BREAST SURGERY

The breast care nurse should give bra advice to women who have had breast surgery. Some patients feel that they could not bear to wear a bra immediately after breast surgery, while others feel that a bra would be supportive. There are no rules for this, and each woman should do what is comfortable.

It is advisable for women to be measured correctly and to be fitted by a trained bra fitter. This would ideally take place pre-operatively although, if time does not allow for this, some department stores have fitters trained to measure women for bras post–breast surgery and some have a selection of pocketed bras. An easy solution is to advise the purchase of a bra one size larger around the middle. This will compensate for any swelling that may occur, and ensures that the bra is not too tight, where it may be painful.

Under-wired bras are really not advised, as the wire may dig into skin around the operation site which may be numb. Under-wired bras are also not advised if radiotherapy is to be given, as a reaction may be caused if the wire irritates fragile skin.

The best choice of bra is a soft cotton sports bra. The bra should ideally have wide, padded, adjustable shoulder straps, a high neckline, a wide rib-band underneath the cups, at least two hook fastenings and good separation between the cups. This not only gives support to women who have had parts of their breast removed, but can also contain a breast prosthesis safely.

A long-line bra or corselette is suitable after breast surgery.

Pocketed bras and swimwear

The majority of women post-mastectomy find they are able to wear an ordinary well-fitting bra. Some prefer the security of a pocketed bra, especially if they have a very active lifestyle.

Swimwear is slightly different. If a woman uses a breast prosthesis for swimming, she needs pocketed swimwear. As there is enough competition among manufacturers, the swimwear is elegant and fashionable. Some high street stores are also introducing a range of pocketed swimwear. Although the front of the costume/bikini needs to be firm and supportive, the backs can be stylish and flattering.

Breast prostheses used for swimming are usually of the lighter variety, so that the weight of the water behind the prosthesis does not pull the costume.

Adapting bras

Women who prefer the security of a pocketed bra can adapt their own current bras. They can buy and sew in soft cotton pockets bought from department stores or specialist companies. Bias binding or ribbon can adapt a bra, with strips sewn from top to bottom of the cup and the prosthesis sitting behind.

It is important for nurses to discuss this information with patients. The patient must feel empowered and confident in the way that they dress, as well as feeling secure and comfortable.

PALLIATIVE SURGERY

If a patient has a systemically advanced or locally advanced breast cancer, surgery may still be required. Palliative surgery is mainly the case for patients with fungating lesions. Fungating lesions are breast cancers that have grown extensively, ulcerating the breast with usually little systemic spread. Mastectomy is the operation of choice, although skin-flap coverage is often an issue, as much of the skin of the breast will need to be removed. Clearance of the cancer by mastectomy for a fungating lesion is usually short-lived, as recurrence may quickly occur on the chest wall. Radiotherapy may be an option at this point. The relief from debulking a fungating lesion is intense, preventing bleeding and smelling, and removing the necessity for dressings. (More information on fungating wounds can be found in Chapter 12).

PSYCHOLOGICAL ISSUES AND BREAST CANCER SURGERY

There are many potential psychological issues that someone with a breast cancer diagnosis could experience at any time during their cancer journey. Care and support should be given to enable patients to cope with this huge potentially life-threatening diagnosis, as well as with the treatment modalities and their side-effects.

Much literature exists that is confusing and contradictory regarding the psychological issues of surgery for breast cancer. Women may feel disfigured after surgery, or may feel euphoric that treatment has begun, seeing life in a different way after 'a brush with death'. Pre-operative preparation of the patient is paramount, and the shape and size of the scar, body-image issues and the side effects of surgery (e.g. arm movement) should be discussed (Harmer 2008b)

Information has demonstrated that, in some cases, women who have breast-conserving surgery may be less affected psychologically and may be quicker to resume sexual relationships than those who have had a breast removed. Other research shows no difference in psychological issues in women who have had breast-conserving surgery to those post-mastectomy, underlining the fact that survival from cancer is the major concern.

Women can be extremely worried about the response of their partner to their surgery. Partners are also anxious about how they will respond. On the one hand, a partner may want to initiate sex, and this may be considered insensitive, whereas, if a partner does not initiate sex then the person with breast cancer may feel unattractive and undesirable (Love, 2000).

In spite of the varied responses, nurses can help people psychologically post-surgery for breast cancer. There is no way of telling when people with breast cancer will choose to voice their deepest concerns, although this is strangely sometimes to the most junior nurses who lack experience. The nurse must know her limitations and be aware that expert help is available.

Hopefully this chapter, along with Chapter 15, will give information to nurses about this treatment modality and its possible psychological effects.

CONCLUSION

Breast cancer treatment is multi-modal and is often given over a number of years (Harmer, 2008c). Surgery has proved a crucial role in the treatment of breast cancer. All practitioners should be continually striving to achieve the highest possible standard in the delivery of care. It is with the involvement of the multidisciplinary team that the individual treatment trajectory is planed and executed in partnership with the patient and carers.

Nurses must be vigilant and should ensure that they offer appropriate support throughout this treatment, as the effects of support can have a tremendous personal impact on patients.

Over the past decade, more superior treatments alongside the NHS Breast Screening Programme, and better awareness of cancer, have started to contribute to a reduction in the death toll from this disease.

The excellent treatments that we have to treat breast cancer are only a starting block. As health-care professionals, we must ensure excellent communication with patients undergoing these treatments. It is with excellent communication skills, paired with relevant up-dated medical knowledge regarding policies and procedures, that we must direct our services. The focus must be the patient, and we must strive to give quality care in partnership with the patient, dovetailing care with their chosen support structures.

REFERENCES

Ahlgren J (2002) Five node biopsy of the axilla: an alternative to axillary dissection of levels I-II in operable breast cancer. *European Journal of Surgical Oncology* 28(2): 97–102.

Badwe RA and Mittra I (2001) Sentinel node biopsy in breast cancer. The Lancet *357 (June 23)*: 2054

Beechey-Newman N (2002) Sentinel node biopsy in primary breast cancer. *International Journal of Clinical Practice* 56(2): 111–115.

Benson JR and Absar MS (2008) Volume replacement and displacement techniques in oncoplastic surgery. *Advances in Breast Cancer* 5(1): 3–9.

Bian J, Krontiras H and Allison J (2008) Outpatient mastectomy and breast reconstructive surgery. Annals of Surgical Oncology 15(4): 1032–1039.

Boore J (1978) *Prescription for Recovery*. London: RCN.

Breslin TM, Cohen L, Sahin A *et al.* (2000) Sentinel lymph node biopsy is accurate after neoadjuvant chemotherapy for breast cancer. *Journal of Clinical Oncology* 18(20): 3480–3486.

Bundred NJ, Morgan DAL and Dixon, JM (2000) Management of regional nodes in breast cancer. In: Dixon JM (ed) *ABC of Breast Cancer*, 2nd edn. London: BMJ Publishing Group.

Butler Nattinger A, Hoffmann RG, Kneusel RT and Schapira MM (2000) Relation between appropriateness of primary therapy for early-stage breast carcinoma and increased use of breast-conserving surgery. *The Lancet* 356(30): 1148–1153.

Chadha NK, Cumming S, O'Connor R and Burke M (2004) Is discharge home with drains after breast surgery producing satisfactory outcomes? *Annals of the Royal College of Surgeons of England* 86(5): 353–357.

Chetty U, Jack W, Prescott RJ *et al.* (2000) Management of the axilla in operable breast cancer treated by breast conservation. *British Journal of Surgery* 87: 163–169.

Costa A and Zurrida S (1998) The future of breast cancer surgery. *Oncology in Practice* 3: 8–10.

Early Breast Cancer Trialists' Collaborative Group (1995) Effects of radiotherapy and surgery in early breast cancer: an overview of the randomised trials. *New England Journal of Medicine* 333: 1444–1455.

Fisher B, Anderson S, Redmond C, Wolmark N, Wickerham DL and Cronin WM (1995) Re-analysis and results after 12 years of follow-up in a randomised clinical trial comparing total mastectomy with lumpectomy with or without irradiation in the treatment of breast cancer. *New England Journal of Medicine* 333: 1546–1561.

Forrest APM (1986) *Breast Cancer Screening: Report to the Health Ministers of England, Wales, Scotland and Northern Ireland*. London: HMSO.

Forrest APM, Everington D, McDonald CC *et al.* (1995) The Edinburgh randomized trial of axillary sampling or axillary clearance after mastectomy. *British Journal of Surgery* 82: 1504–1508.

Giuliano AE, Kirgan DM, Guenther JM and Morton DL (1994) Lymphatic mapping and sentinel lymphadenectomy for breast cancer. *Annals of Surgery* 220(3): 391–398.

Harmer V (2000a) Symptom control for breast cancer. *Nursing Times* 96(50): 38–39.

Harmer V (2000b) The surgical management of breast cancer. *Nursing Times* 96(48): 34–35.

Harmer V (2003) Surgery as a treatment for breast cancer. In: Harmer V *Breast Cancer Nursing Care and Management*. London: Whurr Publishers.

Harmer V (2006) Breast cancer treatments – a synopsis. *Practice Nurse* 31(8): 33–38.

Harmer V (2008a) Breast Cancer. Part 2: present and future treatment modalities. *British Journal of Nursing* 17(16): 1028–1035.

Harmer V (2008b) Breast cancer. Part 3: advanced cancer and psychological implications. *British Journal of Nursing* 17(17): 1088–1098.

Harmer V (2008c) Supporting patients during breast cancer care. *Practice Nurse* 35(12): 21–26.

Harmer V (2009) Breast cancer related lymphoedema: implications for primary care. *British Journal of Community Nursing* 14(10): S15–S19.

Hortobagyi G (2002) The Influence of menstrual cycle phase on surgical treatment of primary breast cancer: have we made any progress over the past 13 years? *Journal of the National Cancer Institute* 94(9): 641–643.

Jansen L, Nieweg OE, Valdes Olmos RA *et al.* (1998) Improved staging of breast cancer through lymphatic mapping and sentinel node biopsy. *European Journal of Surgical Oncology* 24(5): 445–446.

Krag DN, Harlow S, Weaver D and Ashikaga T (2001) Radiolabelled sentinel node biopsy: collaborative trial with the National Cancer Institute. *World Journal of Surgery* 25(6): 823–828.

Krag DN, Weaver DC, Alex JC and Fairbank JT (1993) Surgical resection and radiolocalization of the sentinel lymph node in breast cancer using a gamma probe. *Surgical Oncology* 2(6): 335–339.

Leinster SJ, Gibbs TJ and Downey H (2000) *Shared Care for Breast Disease*. Oxford: Isis Medical Media Ltd.

Lewis J (2005) *Your Guide to Breast Cancer*. Hodder: London.

Love SM (2000) *Dr Susan Love's Breast Book*, 3rd edn. USA: Perseus.

MacLaren J and Harmer V (2002) Breast cancer related lymphoedema: a review of evidence based management. *CME Cancer Medicine* 1(2): 56–60.

McIntosh SA and Purushotham AD (1998) Lymphatic mapping and sentinel node biopsy in breast cancer. *British Journal of Surgery* 85(10): 1347–1356

Mamounas EP, Brown A, Anderson S *et al.* (2005) Sentinel node biopsy after neoadjuvant chemotherapy in breast cancer: results from National Surgical Adjuvant Breast and Bowel Project Protocol B-27. *Journal of Clinical Oncology* 23(12): 2694–2702.

Marchal F, Dravet F, Classe JM *et al.* (2005) Post-operative care and patient satisfaction after ambulatory surgery for breast cancer patients. *European Journal of Surgical Oncology* 31(5): 495–499.

Margolese RG and Lasry JC (2000) Ambulatory surgery for breast cancer patients. *Annals of Surgical Oncology* 7(3): 181–187.

NHS Institute for Innovation and Improvement (2010) The Leadership Qualities Framework. Available: http://www.nhsleadershipqualities.nhs.uk.

Park JH, Lee WH and Chung HS (2008) Incidence and risk factors of breast cancer lymphoedema. Journal of Clinical Nursing 17(): 1450–1459.

Ranieri E, Caprio G, Fobert MT *et al.* (2004) One-day surgery in a series of 150 breast cancer patients: efficacy and cost-benefit analysis. *Chirurgia Italiana* 56(3): 415–418.

Rainsbury D (2008) Reconstruction after partial mastectomy. In: Rainsbury D and Straker V *Breast Reconstruction. Your Choice*. London: Class Publishing pp. 102–114).

Reintgen D, Giuliano R and Cox CE (2000) Sentinel node biopsy in breast cancer: an overview. *Breast Journal* 6(5): 299–305.

Rodier JF, Routiot T, Mignotte H *et al.* (2000) Lymphatic mapping and sentinel node biopsy of operable breast cancer. *World Journal of Surgery* 24(10): 1220–1225.

Roses DF (1999) Breast Cancer. Philadelphia: Churchill Livingstone.

Rovera F, Ferrari A, Marelli M *et al.* (2008) Breast cancer surgery in an ambulatory setting. *International Journal of Surgery* 6(1): S116–118.

Sabel MS, Schott AF, Kleer CG *et al.* (2003). Sentinel node biopsy prior to neoadjuvant chemotherapy. *The American Journal of Surgery* 186(2): 102–105.

Sainsbury JRC, Ross GM and Thomas J (2006) Breast cancer. In Dixon JM (ed) *ABC of Breast Diseases*, 3rd edn. Blackwell Publishing: London, 36–41.

Shalowitz J I (2010) Implementing successful quality outcome programs in ambulatory care: key questions and recommendations. *Journal of Ambulatory Care Management* 33(2): 117–123.

Simpson SA, Ying BL, Ross LA *et al.* (2007) Incidence of complications in outpatient mastectomy with immediate reconstruction. *Journal of the American College of Surgeons* 205(): 463–467.

Stearns V, Ewing A, Slack R, Penannen MF, Hayes DF and Tsangaris TN (2002) Sentinel lymphadenectomy after neoadjuvant chemotherapy for breast cancer may reliably represent the axilla except for inflammatory breast cancer. *Annals of Surgical Oncology* 9: 235–242.

Stebbing JJ and Gaya A (2001) The evidence-based use of induction chemotherapy in breast cancer. *Breast Cancer* 8(1): 23–37.

Steele RJ, Forrest AP, Gibson T *et al.* (1985) The efficacy of lower axillary sampling in obtaining lymph node status in breast cancer: a controlled randomized trial. *British Journal of Surgery* 72(5): 368–369.

Tan LR and Guenther JM (1997) Outpatient definitive breast cancer surgery. *The American Surgeon* 63(10): 865–867.

Veronesi U, Cascinelli N, Mariani L *et al.* (2002) Twenty-year follow-up of a randomized study comparing breast-conserving surgery with radical mastectomy for early breast cancer. *New England Journal of Medicine* 347(16): 1227–1232.

Veronesi U, Galimberti V, Zurrida S *et al.* (2001) Sentinel lymph node biopsy as an indicator for axillary dissection in early breast cancer. *European Journal of Cancer* 37(4) 454–458.

Veronesi U, Luini A, Mariani L *et al.* (1994) Effect of menstrual phase on surgical treatment of breast cancer. *The Lancet* 343(8912): 1545–1547.

Whitworth P, Mc Masters KM, Tafra L and Edwards MJ (2000) State-of-the-art lymph node staging for breast cancer in the year 2000. *American Journal of Surgery* 180(4): 262–267.

Xing Y, Foy M, Cox DD, Kuerer HM, Hunt KK and Cormier JN (2006) Meta-analysis of sentinel node biopsy after pre-operative chemotherapy in patients with breast cancer. *British Journal of Surgery* 93: 539–546.

6 Physiotherapy for Patients with Breast Cancer

Helen Macleod and Pauline Koelling

INTRODUCTION

Chapter 6 will examine the role of the physiotherapist in the management and treatment of the patient with breast cancer. Particular attention will be paid to the input that the physiotherapist has in the acute phase following certain types of breast surgery. Increases in survivorship mean that more patients are living with the impact of their disease and its treatments, and there may be an increased role for the physiotherapist with these patients. The latter part of this chapter will focus on physiotherapy for patients with metastatic breast disease.

Physiotherapists may be involved in the treatment of breast cancer patients at any stage of their disease. Newly diagnosed patients are often treated with a combination of surgery, radiotherapy, chemotherapy and hormone treatments. As a result of this, patients frequently require physiotherapy intervention. Following breast surgery, patients can experience problems with pain, limited shoulder movement and lymphoedema. Radiotherapy to breast tissue can cause soft tissue fibrosis, resulting in movement limitation and lymphoedema. Chemotherapy and hormone therapy can lead to changes in menopausal status and general debility. Physiotherapists' knowledge of anatomy and normal movement makes them ideally suited to treating this group of patients.

Progressive breast disease can result in bone, brain, lung or liver metastases. Patients can present with a variety of symptoms affecting their mobility and respiratory function, and may benefit from assessment and treatment by a physiotherapist. Again, they may undergo a combination of treatments as they enter the palliative phase of their disease, and the physiotherapist should take a holistic approach towards the patient.

PHYSIOTHERAPY AND BREAST SURGERY

Referral criteria

Not every patient undergoing breast surgery will need to be seen by a physiotherapist, as more minor surgery is unlikely to cause problems. Appropriate referrals include:

- Axillary intervention, i.e. axillary lymph node dissection, axillary sampling and sentinel lymph node biopsy;

Breast Cancer Nursing Care and Management, Second Edition, Edited by Victoria Harmer
© 2011 by Blackwell Publishing Ltd.

- Mastectomy, i.e. simple, modified radical and subcutaneous;
- Reconstructive surgery, i.e. myocutaneous flap repair and tissue expander.

Inappropriate referrals include:

- Lumpectomy, wide local excision without axillary dissection;
- Wire localisation and excision biopsy;
- Implant exchanges;
- Mastopexy.

Patients are usually seen by the physiotherapist from the first post-operative day, although pre-operative assessment would be useful in some cases, e.g. patients with pre-existing mobility or shoulder problems. This may be difficult, however, due to limited access to patients pre-operatively and limited resources in staffing levels. Seeing patients at pre-admission clinics would be ideal, as this would allow the physiotherapist an opportunity to assess the patient's pre-operative range of shoulder movement and to discuss any history of joint problems and their current level of function. This might necessitate early referral to other members of the multidisciplinary team if there are issues relating to safe discharge planning following surgery.

It appears to be well documented that impaired shoulder function is frequently seen after breast cancer surgery, and there is a role for active physiotherapy intervention (Wingate, 1989; Box, 2002; Lauridsen, 2005). When surgery is combined with radiotherapy, the risk of shoulder dysfunction increases (Ryttov, 1983; Isaksson, 2000), but there is less literature to support the benefits of physiotherapy in the prevention and treatment of this problem.

This chapter is based on the current practice of the physiotherapy service at the Royal Marsden Hospital in London and Surrey, and the exercise regimes were devised in conjunction with the consultant breast surgeons. The exercise regimes are not evidence-based, as there is little research on this subject, and the timing of post-operative exercises remains controversial with regard to the risk of seroma formation (Shamley, 2005). This will be discussed in further detail later in this chapter.

AIMS OF PHYSIOTHERAPY FOLLOWING BREAST SURGERY

Post-operative physiotherapy should seek to:

- Minimise pain;
- Increase shoulder range of movement;
- Maintain soft tissue extensibility;
- Return the patient to her/his pre-operative level of function;
- Regain muscle strength.

Arm exercise regime

The arm exercise regime should be as follows:

- Set A (Fig. 6.1) – from day 1, short-lever exercises (to minimise the stress placed on the surgical incision during the movement);

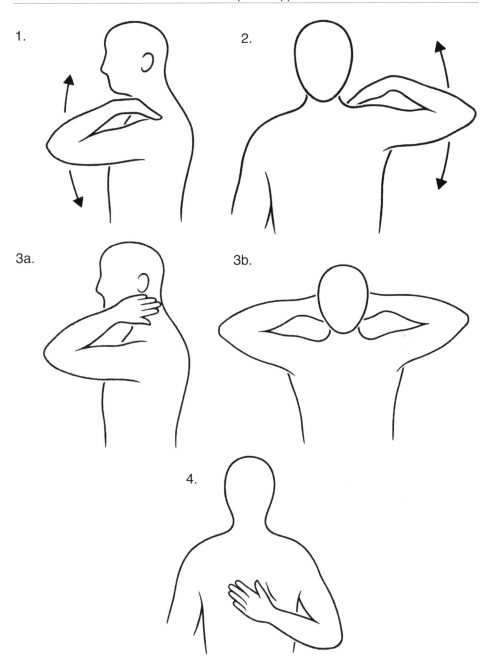

1.

2.

3a.

3b.

4.

Fig. 6.1   Set A arm exercises.

- Set B (Fig. 6.2) – from 1 week, long lever exercises (to increase shoulder range of movement);
- Set C (Fig. 6.3) – following removal of sutures/clips or at 10–14 days if sutures are dissolvable, end-of-range sustained stretches in supine position (to stretch the soft tissues around the shoulder and chest wall).

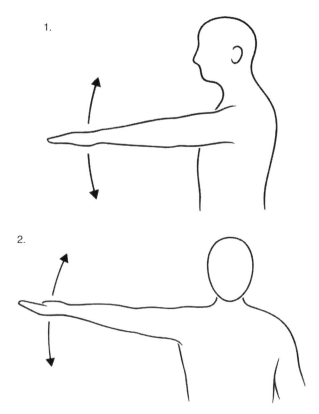

Fig. 6.2   Set B arm exercises.

These exercises should be performed within a pain-free range.

First post-operative day

Assessment

The physiotherapist's initial assessment of the patient will include a review of respiratory status, the number and position of drainage tubes, their wound dressing and analgesia. Questioning of the patient will establish hand dominance, any previous history of shoulder problems, occupational and leisure activities, and level of pain control. An explanation of the effects of the surgery will introduce the need for an exercise regime.

Exercises

Patients are taught Set A exercises and are encouraged to perform these three times a day within their limits of comfort. These movements are similar to functional use of the arm, such as using the affected arm for eating and drinking, washing the face and brushing hair. It is useful at this stage to correct their posture, as patients can easily adopt a position where the shoulder on the affected side is elevated and protracted in response to pain. They can also develop poor patterns of movement to minimise discomfort and should be encouraged to move their affected arm as normally as possible.

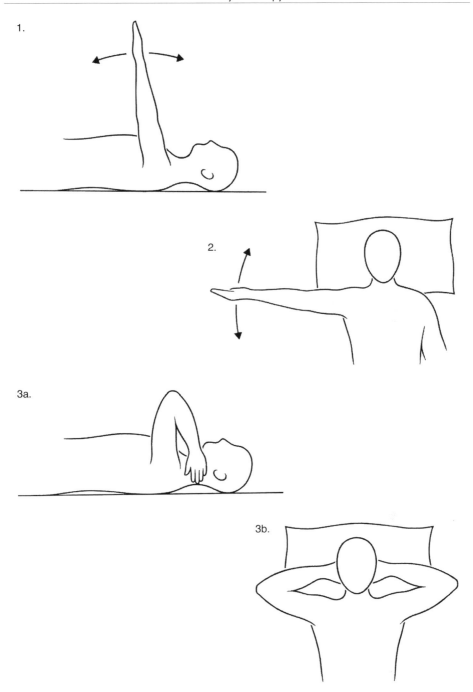

Fig. 6.3   Set C arm exercises.

General advice

Patients are provided with written information regarding the general use of their arm following breast surgery.

- Lifting and housework – for the first 4–6 weeks following their operation patients are advised to lift only light objects with their affected arm. They are also encouraged to use their unaffected arm for heavy or repetitive tasks such as vacuum cleaning, ironing and window cleaning.
- Driving – patients are advised not to drive until after the first outpatient appointment following their operation. They should only resume driving once they feel confident to do so, and should start with short distances. Car insurance should be checked in case there is a clause with regard to driving and the time lapsed post-anaesthetic. If they have also undergone abdominal surgery, it is sensible to wait 6 weeks before driving again.
- Sport and leisure activities – swimming may begin once good shoulder movement is regained and the operation scar has healed (usually after 4–6 weeks). If patients are undergoing radiotherapy by then, they will need to check with their radiographer that swimming will not damage fragile skin. Most other sporting activities can be restarted within 2 months of surgery.

Discuss complications

Patients are informed of the particular complications that are usually associated with axillary intervention, e.g. altered sensation, seroma formation, cording and lymphoedema. These will be discussed later in the chapter.

Pre-discharge

Patients will usually stay in hospital until their drains are removed, although some will be discharged earlier with drains still in situ. Prior to discharge, their range of shoulder movement is checked, and most patients should be able to elevate their affected arm to about 90 degrees.

Set B exercises are taught, and patients are encouraged to progress their range of movement within comfortable limits after 1 week.

Set C exercises are demonstrated to them, and the physiotherapist will discuss the importance of these stretches. Many patients will go on to have adjuvant radiotherapy as part of their treatment. For radiotherapy, patients are required to lie supine with both arms elevated and externally rotated above their head. The Set C exercises will help them achieve and maintain this position.

The physiotherapist may arrange to see patients at their first outpatient appointment if there are concerns regarding their movement, level of pain or ability to perform the exercises. Physiotherapy contact details are given to every patient, and they are encouraged to contact the physiotherapy service or attend a 'drop-in clinic' run by the service if they are concerned about their movement or exercises.

First outpatient appointment

Patients attend for their first outpatient appointment with their surgical team at about 7–10 days after their surgery. At this appointment, their wound is reviewed, and any difficulties with regaining movement may be noted, necessitating a referral to physiotherapy.

Early assessment of shoulder range, level of pain, postural changes and signs of developing cording by the physiotherapist will decide if a patient requires ongoing treatment.

RECONSTRUCTIVE SURGERY

Women may have reconstructive surgery at the time of their cancer surgery, or this may be delayed to a later date.

Latissimus dorsi flap reconstruction

Following latissimus dorsi flap reconstruction, patients are instructed in the set A, B and C exercises, although progress may be slower, and it may take longer for them to resume their normal activities. Within the first few days of surgery, the Set A exercises may need to be modified and shoulder girdle movements encouraged. Particular attention should be paid to posture, and patients should be instructed to avoid forced adduction and extension of the affected arm, such as pushing themselves up and down the bed.

Seroma formation on the scar at the back is a frequent problem and may require repeated aspiration. Additional thoracic expansion and scapular mobility exercises will help to stretch posterior scars.

Lower-abdominal tissue reconstruction

Lower-abdominal tissue reconstruction includes transverse rectus abdominis myocutaneous flap (TRAM), deep inferior epigastric perforator flap (DIEP) and superior inferior epigastric artery flap (SIEA).

The large abdominal wound increases the potential for respiratory complications in the early post-operative stage, and the physiotherapist will assess respiratory function and advise on breathing exercises and supported cough techniques. Set A exercises are started within the patient's level of comfort and pelvic tilting after 3–4 days, once the patient is more mobile and pain is controlled. Progression to Sets B and C are recommended as per the usual protocol. Back-care and lifting techniques are discussed to minimise strain on the abdominal wound. Progressive core abdominal strengthening exercises and stretches are advised from 6 weeks onwards.

Patients are advised to delay driving until 6 weeks after their operation.

RADIOTHERAPY CLASS

A multi-professional information class is available to any patient undergoing radiotherapy to their breast and/or axilla. This class is run jointly by the physiotherapist, lymphoedema nurse specialist and therapy radiographer. Patients are invited to attend this one-off session during their radiotherapy treatment.

The aim of the class is to increase patients' awareness of the potential long-term effects of radiotherapy relating to shoulder movement and lymphoedema (Hammick *et al.*, 1996).

Information includes a description of how soft tissues over the chest wall may be tightened by the fibrosing effect of radiotherapy, and emphasis is placed on the importance of continuing to stretch these structures indefinitely. A review of the lymphatic system, together with prophylactic lymphoedema advice, helps to consolidate the patient's knowledge of this subject. Post-radiotherapy skin changes and care are also discussed.

COMPLICATIONS FOLLOWING SURGERY

Cording

Cording is frequently seen in patients who have had axillary surgery, and can start to form about 1 week post-operatively. In an unpublished MSc study (Williams, 1994), 83% of patients had cording after axillary surgery. A subsequent study by Leidenius (2003) found that 74% of patients experienced movement limitation as a result of this, and Lauridsen found that 57% of patients had axillary 'strings' at 7 weeks post-operatively (Lauridsen, 2005).

Cording is seen as a tight band-like structure of varying thickness arising from the axilla and stretching down the inner aspect of the upper arm when the arm is stretched (Fig. 6.4). In some cases, thinner string-like cords can be felt at the inner aspect of the elbow, or even wrist. Cording may limit arm movement when stretched, and can vary between feeling tight to very painful. Some patients also feel tightness over the front of the ribs below the breast, and cording can, more rarely, be present here.

Although a result of axillary surgery, it is not known which tissue is involved. Researchers at the University of Washington in Seattle first referred to this phenomenon as axillary web syndrome (Moskovitz, 2001) and suggested that it is a result of interruption of the axillary lymphatics during node dissection and is a variant of Mondor disease. Other hypotheses suggest that it may be thickened lymph or blood vessels, or fibrosis in the fascial planes caused by scarring. Both Moskovitz and Leidenius believe the condition is self-limiting, resolving within 2–3 months without long-term sequelae.

We believe resolution of cording is enhanced by stretching exercises and normal range of movement (ROM) is usually regained within 3 months if no other complications are involved. Those women who have had reconstruction of the breast mound may find that recovery takes longer. When done regularly, the exercises outlined above should restore ROM, but a physiotherapist can treat the cords using soft tissue mobilisations to speed up

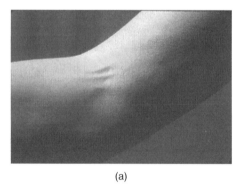
(a)

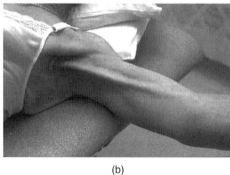
(b)

Fig. 6.4 A patient with cording at the elbow and in the axilla after axillary node surgery. Reprinted with permission of the Royal Marsden Hospital.

recovery. Physiotherapy treatment of axillary web syndrome has been described by Kepics, a physiotherapist specialising in the treatment of breast cancer and lymphoedema (Kepics, 2004).

Patients are encouraged to use the arm as normally as possible, but are advised not to lift or carry heavy objects for 4–6 weeks. They are also advised to avoid prolonged periods of repetitive activity or static muscle contraction with the affected arm such as ironing, driving and computer use. If pain persists or movement remains limited after this time, the patient should be referred to a chartered physiotherapist for assessment and treatment.

Seroma

Seroma formation after axillary surgery is considered the most common complication (Schulz *et al.*, 1997). Controversy surrounds the issue of whether early mobilisation of the shoulder is linked to seroma formation. Some research (e.g. Rodier *et al.*, 1987) suggests early exercise in order to avoid shoulder stiffness caused by scar tissue formation. Early exercise is also thought to encourage normal lymphatic, arterial and venous circulation (Miller, 1998) in a limb predisposed to lymphoedema. Schultz *et al.* (1997) advocate avoidance of early exercise in order to minimise complications with seroma. Even those studies that delayed exercise allowed normal activities of the affected limb immediately post-operatively, and did not restrict shoulder movement completely. The difficulty in assessing the research is the large number of variables, which could influence outcome; for instance, type and extent of surgery, age of patient, surgeon involved, number of nodes removed, number of days with drain, number of positive nodes, level of pain, patient's normal activity levels etc. A systematic review of the literature by Shamley in 2005 supported delaying exercises immediately post-operatively to reduce seroma formation. However, the effect of doing this on early- and long-term shoulder movement remains unclear, and future studies are needed in this area. As discussed earlier in this chapter, the exercises that we advocate mimic normal arm movement, and patients are instructed to follow the recommended number of repetitions as a maximum guideline.

Axillary seroma can be uncomfortable, and the resulting limitation of ROM at the shoulder will not be altered by exercise. Often the fluid can be aspirated, and the exercises resumed. Some patients present with seroma of the anterior chest wall, or under the scar of the latissimus dorsi flap on the posterior thorax. Both these can limit shoulder movement. If patients present with seroma, they are advised to continue set A exercises within the limit of their discomfort, and are reviewed by the doctor for possible aspiration of fluid. Unfortunately, once removed, the fluid can re-accumulate over a few days, and the procedure may need to be repeated several times before the seroma settles.

Altered posture

Resuming normal posture after breast surgery is vital. Patients frequently assume a protracted shoulder position to protect the anterior scar. Many will hold their arm slightly abducted from their side due to skin sensitivity on the inner arm, further enhancing this altered posture. This results in some muscles being stretched while others are shortened. Even after a few days of shortening, the pectoral muscles are over-worked and painful while the scapula muscles are stretched and weakened. Shoulder impingement can occur as the shoulder joint is being worked out of alignment, and this will cause pain on elevating the arm. Later, neck problems and headaches can result from the weight of the head moving forward and the neck losing its normal curvature with a slight increase in thoracic kyphosis. Further muscle imbalance in the upper body and alterations to normal scapulohumeral rhythm can also occur.

From the beginning, simply lying flat on the floor and pushing both shoulders back and down onto the floor will help stretch out the anterior scar and relax the pectoral muscles. This is especially important in those women who have elected to have immediate reconstruction (with or without implant), as the pectoral muscles are more likely to be tight and sore.

Altered movement patterns can be identified and corrected by a chartered physiotherapist. After days or weeks of poor positioning, myofascial trigger points can be found within the affected muscles, exacerbating the pain cycle. A trigger point is defined as a 'hyperirritable locus within a taut band of muscle, located in the muscular tissue and/or its associated fascia. The spot is painful on compression and can evoke characteristic referred pain and autonomic phenomena' (Travell and Simons, 1992). The main culprits tend to be the pectoral muscles, latissimus dorsi, upper trapezius and infraspinatus. These muscles can be responsible for referring pain into the shoulder or arm, and can limit movement of the shoulder. The more complications there are to do with wound healing or pain, the more likely it is that trigger points will be found in these areas. Release of the tension here can ease pain and regain the patient 20–30 degrees more movement in one treatment session.

Sensitivity of the scar

Some women are reluctant to look at the scar, and touching it can be a very emotional issue, not just because of changes in body image, but for fear of damaging the wound or, if they have had a reconstruction, moving the implant. Once the scar has healed and infection is not a risk, it is useful to encourage touch and gentle massage of the area, especially if it is very sensitive or tight. Superolateral movement of the soft tissues across the chest wall is necessary for the arm to move into full elevation, and tethering of post-operative scarring and exudate in the soft tissues will impair movement and cause discomfort. It is useful to encourage the patient to massage the scar gently so that it becomes more supple, and it helps the patient to re-acquaint her/himself with the numb and 'odd feeling' chest wall. Very sensitive scarring can be gradually desensitised in this way, although this would not be advocated during radiotherapy treatment when the skin is more fragile. Once healed, if soft tissue stiffness remains that is painful and limits movement, myofascial release techniques used by a chartered physiotherapist can be useful to lengthen tissues and enable them to move more freely over the chest wall as the arm moves into flexion or abduction.

Nerve damage

Three nerves are at risk of damage during axillary surgery. The most commonly disturbed is the intercostobrachial nerve. Division or damage of this nerve causes numbness of the medial arm from the axilla to the elbow. If it has only been bruised (neuropraxia), patients may complain of an uncomfortable tenderness that keeps them from putting the arm by their side, and they may even present standing with their hand on their hip so that the skin is not disturbed. Some people cannot even bear the feeling of clothing on the skin but, over a period of weeks or months, this feeling should gradually fade.

The long thoracic nerve supplies the serratus anterior muscle. When this is damaged, there will be poor control of the scapula, and it will wing out from the chest wall along its medial border. This results in limited strength and ROM of the arm, and a decrease in stability of the shoulder girdle. The thoracodorsal nerve supplies the latissimus dorsi muscle. If the thoracodorsal nerve is damaged, obvious deformity does not result, but there is weakness of medial rotation and adduction of the arm. In either case, referral should be made to a physiotherapist to provide advice on strengthening of the muscle as the nerve regains function, and on how to avoid further soft tissue damage if weakness is permanent. Needless to say, damage of these two nerves is rare but, if it does arise, it is normally a neuropraxia, which will resolve within weeks or months.

Wound problems

Delayed wound healing in the axilla or on the chest wall due to haematoma or infection will usually cause restriction in arm movement because of pain. Exercises should be kept to a minimum during this phase, using the limb in the pain-free range only. Strong stretches over a troublesome wound must be avoided, or healing may be further delayed. Once healing has occurred, movement may be limited due to fibrosis of scar tissue, but exercises can be resumed as pain allows under the guidance of a chartered physiotherapist. The therapist will need to ascertain which, if any, structures are causing the pain and why. She/he will also need to assess which structures around the chest wall and shoulder are tight, in order to give the right treatment and advice.

Radiotherapy side-effects

Those patients who need radiotherapy as an adjunct to treatment are more likely to notice problems with the ipsilateral arm (Bentzen and Dische, 2000; Isaksson and Feuk, 2000). Radiotherapy damages the soft tissues within the field of treatment and, in the short term, can cause acute inflammatory changes, such as redness, sensitivity and desquamation of the skin. Strong stretches of the shoulder will be uncomfortable, and massage of the skin is not recommended until healing has taken place. Later, skin changes include pigmentation and telangiectasis. Subcutaneous fibrosis of soft tissues is commonly seen by the end of treatment, and can continue to form gradually years after treatment (Ryttov et al., 1983; Kurtz, 1995). Subcutaneous fibrosis can cause a fibrous band of tissue at the anterior axillary fold from the anterior chest wall, along the band of pectoral muscle.

A study in 2003, looking into the current management of radiation-induced fibrosis, suggested that active physiotherapy should be encouraged (O'Sullivan and Levin, 2003). The physiotherapist will instruct the patient to continue putting the shoulder through a full range of movement, stretching out once a day when full movement is regained, just to ensure that stiffness does not recur. Our experience at the Royal Marsden Hospital suggests that patients tend to forget to continue stretches and, as normal daily routines do not put the shoulder through full range of movement, stiffness goes unnoticed until it starts producing arm symptoms later on. Patients sometimes come back to clinic perhaps 1 year after radiotherapy has finished, complaining of symptoms either directly or indirectly related to their breast cancer surgery and radiotherapy, with or without any signs of lymphoedema. It is worthwhile highlighting the need to continue stretches indefinitely after radiotherapy, as research suggests that fibrosis may be a lifelong risk (Jung et al., 2001).

Brachial plexus lesions due to radiotherapy are much less common with modern radio-therapy techniques. Patients who were treated with higher doses and larger fields in the past, however, may develop a progressive weakness in the ipsilateral arm if the radiotherapy field encompassed the nerves lying under the supraclavicular fossa. This can cause profound weakness and atrophy of the arm and, both physically and psychologically, the effects can be devastating. Brachial plexus damage is irreversible, but assessment by a chartered physiotherapist, and occupational therapist, can be helpful to provide advice on symptom control and maximising function. Active exercise and gentle stretches may help to prevent tightening and stiffening of the joints and soft tissues involved. Splinting of the hand and wrist may be appropriate to protect the joints and minimise pain. No amount of exercise will regain lost muscle power, owing to the damage being to the nerve supply, not to the muscle itself. Ill-advised exercise can lead to an increase in symptoms and is best avoided.

Other side-effects worth bearing in mind for the physiotherapist treating this patient group are radiation-induced malignancy, pulmonary fibrosis and lymphoedema of the arm (Wallgren, 1992). Lethargy is a commonly experienced effect, which can limit the patient's capacity for exercise and slow her/his progress with rehabilitation. Lethargy is normally experienced towards the end of treatment and over the next month after treatment has finished. It is often helpful to spend time explaining in detail the effects of the treatment and the rationale for stretches, and to tailor the exercise plan to the individual's ability at the time.

Lymphoedema

Lymphoedema can be a big concern to women who have undergone lymph node removal and/or radiotherapy to lymphatic structures, but sensible precautions will limit the risk of it occurring, and it is usually possible to treat the limb and prevent it from becoming a significant problem. Clinical nurse specialists or physiotherapists should be notified of hand, arm or trunk swelling early on, and gentle exercises and advice on activities and control of the condition will be given. In some cases, elastic support sleeves and gloves or manual lymph drainage can help. Interestingly, although traditionally, women with axillary dissections, with or without radiotherapy, are warned to avoid strenuous and prolonged upper-limb activity in order to decrease the risk of lymphoedema, a study by Harris and Niesen-Vertommen (2000) suggested that this is unsubstantiated by research, and places unnecessary limits on a woman's activities. Harris' study shows it may be relatively safe to exercise vigorously and not develop arm swelling. A pilot study by Kilbreath *et al.* (2006) also challenges the belief that vigorous arm exercise will cause lymphoedema, and a further research proposal plans to look at whether an intensive resistance exercise programme will actually prevent swelling in the upper limb. Positive results will help to enhance quality of life for those people wishing to return to more strenuous recreational activities.

Heavy lymphoedematous arms are uncomfortable and difficult to carry, causing changes in posture at the shoulder girdle, back and neck. Shoulder, elbow and hand joints can become tight, causing more discomfort. Physiotherapy can be useful in maintaining function of the limb, and easing secondary neck, back or other joint pain.

The lymphoedema chapter in this book will explain in more detail the causes of and treatments for the problem.

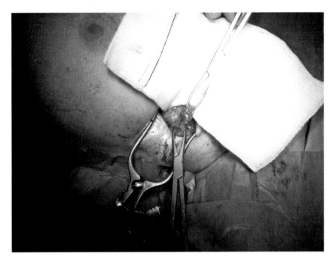

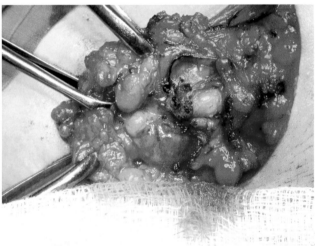

Plates 1 and 2 Intra-operative photographs illustrating the sentinel node as it stains with blue dye. This dye is injected around the breast cancer prior to surgery to allow the surgeon to identify the sentinel node. Reprinted with kind permission of Mr D.J. Hadjiminas, Consultant Breast Surgeon, Imperial College Healthcare NHS Trust.

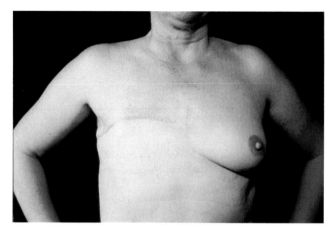

Plate 3 Appearance after a total mastectomy.

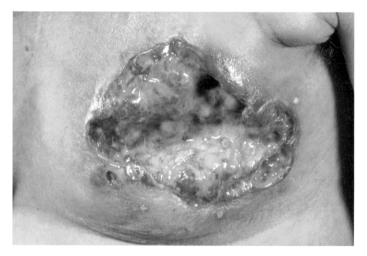

Plate 4 Appearance of a fungating breast wound.

Muscle weakness

Weakness can be caused by surgery for breast cancer for several reasons:

- Pain can inhibit strong muscle contraction (Guymer, 1997). Pain also means that women avoid using the painful body part, and the muscles weaken progressively from under-use.
- Pain can also elicit raised tone in the muscle concerned, or it can irradiate to the surrounding muscles (Guymer, 1997).
- Muscle action can be limited by nerve damage, as discussed above.
- Muscles on excessive stretch are working at a mechanical disadvantage and can be weakened. For example, the submuscular implants placed underneath the pectoralis major put the muscle on stretch, and make it harder to contract.
- TRAM flaps harvested from the rectus abdominis muscle, both pedicled and free flaps, cause weakness of the abdominal wall. This can lead to abdominal herniation, and decreased trunk stability when the patient is faced with functional activities.

Recent innovations in plastic surgery have meant that more surgeons are performing the DIEP flap in reconstructions rather than taking rectus abdominis muscle in a TRAM flap to rebuild the breast mound. It is hoped this will decrease the risk of abdominal herniation and muscle weakness, which can predispose to trunk instability and low back pain. Futter *et al.* (2000) found that, while no muscle was removed in the DIEP flaps, there was still a strength deficit, although not as marked compared to the TRAM flap. Blondeel *et al.* (1997) found that not only was there a deficit in trunk flexion strength following the TRAM flap surgery, but that the oblique muscle function was also impaired, weakening rotation. The abdominal muscles work not only concentrically to flex the trunk, but also work eccentrically and statically to stabilise the lumbar spine, the pelvis and the rib cage, allowing the limbs to move freely. Futter *et al.* found that those women expressing difficulty carrying out activities such as lifting heavy objects or shopping, vacuuming, moving furniture etc. were those who demonstrated weak trunk muscles post-operatively. This means that the TRAM flaps can cause weakness in the abdominal muscles, and also impair normal daily functional activities. Therefore, patients undergoing this type of surgery should be referred to a physiotherapist to be taught appropriate strengthening exercises and back care advice before going home, and may need to be seen on an outpatient basis once discharged.

Pain

Once the initial surgical pain has faded, patients can present with pain for a number of reasons – for example, nerve damage, swelling and altered movement patterns due to stiffness, etc. Many women interpret their pain as disease recurrence, and it is often necessary to reassure them that their discomfort is an unfortunate side-effect of necessary treatment, rather than a sign of returning cancer. If there is any possibility that metastases are present, the doctors concerned should be consulted, and manual physiotherapy techniques to the area abandoned until investigations prove otherwise.

Physiotherapists can help relieve pain caused by muscle spasm, postural changes, joint stiffness, altered biomechanics, scar tissue, cording, or weakness by assessing the probable cause, and using various mobilising and soft tissue techniques. Electrotherapy is contraindicated over any area that may contain cancerous cells, although transcutaneous electrical nerve stimulation (TENS) machines (small portable electrical nerve stimulators) may be useful in some cases to help with pain relief (Forster and Palastanga, 1981). TENS is a non-invasive means of exciting sensory nerves to stimulate the body's specific natural pain relief mechanisms, the pain-gate mechanism and the endogenous opiod system. A recent Cochrane review found insufficient evidence as to whether TENS should be used in the treatment of cancer-related pain and called for further research in this area (Robb et al., 2008).

It is estimated that around a quarter of women go on to develop post-mastectomy pain syndrome (PMPS) (Wallace et al., 1996; Smith et al., 1999). One study (Tasmuth et al., 1996) found that 1 year after surgery, 80% of women had treatment-related symptoms. PMPS symptoms range from infrequent mild problems to pain that constantly disturbs daily activities and sleep. PMPS is a poorly recognised and poorly treated chronic pain condition following breast surgery, where women complain of tight, burning, constricting pain, and loss of sensation in the anterior chest wall, axilla and posterior aspect of the upper arm in the distribution of the intercostobrachial nerve (Granek et al., 1984). They may also demonstrate loss of movement and arm weakness with postural changes. Wallace et al. (1996) found a higher incidence of PMPS with patients who had mastectomy and reconstruction. Smith et al. (1999) found that the main contributing factors to PMPS in their group of patients were surgery and age. Heavier and taller patients in this study seemed more likely to develop pain, and those reporting PMPS were more likely to have had chemotherapy, post-operative radiotherapy and tamoxifen. Tasmuth et al. (1996) found a correlation between anxiety levels and depression with PMPS.

A study of long-term follow-up of patients with PMPS found that 52% still had symptoms at a mean of 9 years since surgery (Macdonald et al., 2005). Causes of PMPS remain uncertain, although work by Gottrup et al. (2000) suggests a neurological central sensitisation of pain mechanisms similar to that seen in other neuropathic pain patients. Neuropathic pain has been shown to be effectively treated by drugs acting on the nervous system, such as amitriptyline (Kalso et al., 1996) and gabapentin (Mao and Chen, 2000). Owing to the complexity of the problem, it may be best treated using a multidisciplinary approach, using pharmacological and physical modalities such as analgesia, physiotherapy, massage, exercise, acupuncture, TENS, and psychological help, e.g. cognitive behavioural strategies to cope with chronic pain. Robb and Newham (personal communication, 2002) showed that a combination of physiotherapy and psychology interventions helped patients to recognise the many factors contributing to their pain, and that it improved their ability to cope with these factors.

PMPS is a condition that is more prevalent than previously thought and is still underdiagnosed and poorly understood. Further research is needed to improve our understanding of its aetiology and treatment. A wide range of treatment modalities may help, and more research is needed to examine the effects of holistic approaches to treatment.

CHEMOTHERAPY AND HORMONE THERAPY

Primary chemotherapy for early-stage breast cancer may result in neutropenic episodes requiring hospital admission. The patient may present with a respiratory infection and difficulty expectorating. Appropriate chest physiotherapy techniques may be of benefit. General muscle weakness and loss of mobility may also be a symptom in this group of patients, and a graduated exercise programme will encourage a return to normal function.

Menopausal symptoms as a result of chemotherapy and hormone therapy can cause hot flushes and night sweats, leading to disturbed sleep patterns, tiredness, fatigue, low mood, anxiety and depression. Physiotherapists may be involved with teaching relaxation and breathing techniques to help patients cope with these symptoms.

Bone, joint and muscle aches are a frequent side-effect of hormonal treatments, and physiotherapists may be asked to provide advice on gentle exercise regimes to ease the symptoms of stiffness and fatigue.

Increased survival rates following breast cancer treatments have resulted in a 5-year survival rate of over 80% (Cancer Research UK, 2005). For many patients, this involves living with the ongoing effects of their treatments such as reduced levels of physical fitness and quality of life. There is evidence to suggest that exercise is beneficial for cardiorespiratory function, muscle and bone strength, mobility, fatigue and improving quality of life in breast cancer patients and survivors (McNeely *et al.*, 2006; Stevinson *et al.*, 2004). Fatigue is a well-recognised side-effect of cancer treatments, and a Cochrane review found that physical exercise helped to reduce fatigue both during and after treatment (Cramp and Daniel, 2008). However, at present, there is not sufficient evidence as to what type of exercise should be taken, or its intensity.

A recent study has indicated a 50% risk-reduction in mortality in patients who are regularly active in comparison to those with a sedentary lifestyle (Holmes *et al.*, 2005). Mutrie *et al.* (2007) looked at the benefit of supervised group exercise for patients during treatment for early breast cancer. Their results showed functional and psychological benefits following the 12-week programme and at the 6-month follow-up. They concluded that patients should be encouraged to exercise and that 'policy makers should consider the inclusion of exercise opportunities in cancer rehabilitation services.' Physiotherapists may become increasingly involved in setting up outpatient exercise programmes for patients both during and after their treatments. Patients frequently express concern about returning to sporting activities and prefer guidance from health professionals before doing so.

PHYSIOTHERAPY AND METASTATIC DISEASE

When considering the patient with metastatic breast disease, the physiotherapist rarely works in isolation and liaises closely with occupational therapists, social workers, community liaison nurses, lymphoedema nurses, doctors and other members of the multidisciplinary team. Good communication within the team and with the patient and her/his family is vital to ensure that everyone is working towards the patient's goals. This may mean helping the patient continue to care for their family at home, or to adjust to the terminal phase of the disease and finding the most appropriate setting for them.

Breast cancer metastasises primarily to bone, lung, liver and brain. Patients may present with a multitude of problems, i.e. pain, fractures, spinal cord compression, hypercalcaemia, chest infections, dyspnoea, pleural effusions, lymphangitis, abdominal ascites, hemiplegia, ataxia etc. Physiotherapy assessment and treatment can begin once the patient is medically stable.

Bone metastases

Depending on the site of bony involvement, patients will usually present with pain and limited mobility. Some patients will require an orthopaedic assessment. Once the patient is adequately pain controlled and there is minimal risk of pathological fracture according to the doctors, the physiotherapist will assess the range of movement of the affected joints, look for signs of muscle wasting and weakness and, where appropriate, analyse the patient's gait pattern.

Treatment may involve teaching the patient maintenance and strengthening exercises and possibly providing a walking aid to encourage a more normal gait. Gait re-education is important to facilitate the patient's return to their normal functional independence. Daily physiotherapy sessions may be appropriate in the initial stages of the patient's treatment, and the physiotherapist will then monitor progress. Prior to any discharge planning, the physiotherapist will review the patient's function, i.e. can she/he transfer independently from a lying to a sitting position, from sitting to standing, maintain a safe standing balance, walk with or without a walking aid and climb stairs?

Pathological fractures

Bony metastases that have resulted in pathological fracture may require orthopaedic in-tervention, depending on the fracture site. Upper-limb fractures are not always surgically stabilised and may require some form of arm support, for example a polysling. Exercises are begun under the guidance of the physiotherapist, and particular attention is paid to functional activities.

Lower-limb fractures are often surgically fixated, allowing the patient to weight-bear again. It is important to encourage early exercises of the affected and unaffected limbs to maintain muscle strength. The patient should be provided with the appropriate walking aid as soon as possible and encouraged to resume weight-bearing as pain and stability of the fracture site allow. The physiotherapist will assess and re-educate her/his gait pattern, and teach the patient how to manage stairs and other functional activities with a walking aid if appropriate.

Spinal cord compression

Spinal cord compression is an oncological emergency, and immediate medical attention is vital to limit the amount of permanent neurological damage. Spinal cord compression is caused by invasion of the epidural space with involvement of the spinal cord or nerve roots at any level, and is characterised by sensory and/or motor impairment and pain. It may also be accompanied by bladder and bowel symptoms (Lindsay and Bone, 1997). Radiotherapy is the treatment of choice, although surgical intervention may be useful to decompress the nerves or cord or to stabilise bony collapse. In the acute phase, a physiotherapist may be involved in assessing respiratory status if the respiratory system is compromised. Once the lesion is known to be stable, further assessment by physiotherapists and occupational therapists will determine the extent of the patient's functional deficit and potential for rehabilitation, which may be restorative or palliative. The goal of therapy is maximum independence and quality of life, whether the patient is walking or restricted to a wheelchair. New NICE guidelines regarding the management of patients with spinal cord compression are due to be published in the near future.

Hypercalcaemia

Patients with bony metastatic disease may develop hypercalcaemia where there is a rise in serum calcium levels. The main symptoms include confusion, nausea, vomiting and lethargy. Following medical intervention, patients may be referred to the physiotherapist to increase their general mobility prior to discharge home.

Lung metastases

Respiratory infections and progressive breathlessness are common features of lung involvement. As a result, the patient's general mobility may become limited, which can lead to a decrease in their exercise tolerance and function.

Chest physiotherapy techniques may be appropriate for patients who have a productive chest infection, with difficulty expectorating sputum. The physiotherapist should be cautious, however, if there is evidence of metastatic rib disease, as some techniques may cause fracture. Advice on positioning, relaxation and breathing control may be useful adjuncts for these patients. The physiotherapist will encourage the patient to increase her/his mobility gradually, and will advise on pacing. The provision of a walking aid may help to increase stability and conserve energy.

Pleural effusions and lymphangitis

Both pleural effusions and lymphangitis require medical intervention. Advice on positioning of the patient may be useful.

Liver metastases

Physiotherapists may be involved with patients suffering from abdominal ascites and/or lower-limb lymphoedema. Appropriate walking aids may be provided, and strategies taught for moving in bed or transferring from bed to chair. Positioning may help with shortness of breath resulting from abdominal swelling, which compromises diaphragmatic excursion.

Brain metastases

Brain metastases can cause a variety of impairments such as movement, speech, cognitive or visual problems. Physiotherapists, occupational therapists, and speech and language therapists work together in assessing these deficits, providing support for patients and their families. Hemiplegic patients present with limb weakness, alteration in muscle tone, and varying degrees of difficulty in functional movement of upper and/or lower limbs. Ataxic patients have difficulty in coordinating movement and have impaired balance reactions. Physiotherapy can help normalise tone, improve mobility and provide strategies for maximising function.

Pain

Pain caused directly by the disease is usually well controlled by drugs, but some pain can be relieved by the physiotherapist, particularly if it is positional, muscular, caused by stiffness, or due to abnormal posture or movement. Some patients may find TENS beneficial and use this in conjunction with pharmacological interventions. TENS is a small, portable electrical nerve stimulator, which can be purchased, although it is recommended to try one out before buying one, as some people do not find them beneficial.

CONCLUSION

Physiotherapists may be involved with breast cancer patients from diagnosis through to terminal stages of their disease. They may be involved in treating problems caused by the cancer itself or its treatment, most especially surgery and radiotherapy. An increase in survivorship means that many patients are living with long-term implications of their treatments, and physiotherapists are becoming more involved with helping patients regain health and deal with issues of fatigue. Recurrence of breast cancer may present in a variety of ways, and all health professionals must be vigilant. If recurrence is suspected, the patient must be referred back to the oncologist or surgeon for appropriate treatment. Physiotherapists are often actively involved in providing symptom control and palliative care. This may be in a hospital, hospice or in the patient's home.

REFERENCES

Bentzen SM and Dische S (2000) Morbidity related to axillary irradiation in the treatment of breast cancer. *Acta Oncologica* (39)3: 337–347.

Blondeel Ph N, Boeckx W, Vanderstraeten G *et al.* (1997) The fate of the abdominal muscles after free TRAM flap surgery. *British Journal of Plastic Surgery* 50: 315–321.

Box R, Reul-Hirche H, Bullock-Saxton J and Furnival C (2002) Shoulder movement after breast cancer surgery: results of a randomised controlled study of postoperative physiotherapy. *Breast Cancer Research and Treatment* 75: 35–50.

Cancer Research UK. Breast cancer survival statistics 2005: info.cancerresearchuk.org/cancerstats/ types/breast/survival.

Cramp F and Daniel J (2008) Exercise for the management of cancer-related fatigue in adults. *Cochrane Database of Systematic Reviews* 2.

Forster A and Palastanga N (1981) *Clayton's Electrotherapy: Theory and Practice* 9th edn. Amsterdam: Bailliere Tindall.

Futter C, Webster M, Hagen S and Mitchell S (2000) A retrospective comparison of abdominal muscle strength following breast reconstruction with a free TRAM or DIEP flap. *British Journal of Plastic Surgery* 53: 578–583.

Gottrup H, Andersen J, Arendt-Neilson L and Jensen T (2000) Psychophysical examination in patients with post-mastectomy pain. *Pain* (87) 275–284.

Granek I, Ashikari R and Foley K (1984) *The Post-Mastectomy Pain Syndrome: Clinical and Anatomical Correlates.* New York: Memorial Sloan-Kettering Cancer Centre.

Guymer A (1997) The neuromuscular facilitation of movement. In: Wells, Frampton, Bowsher (Eds) *Pain Management by Physiotherapy*, 2nd edn. Oxford: Butterworth Heinemann.

Hammick M, Howard E, Macleod H and Smith J (1996) A multidisciplinary symptom control class for breast cancer patients. *British Journal of Therapy and Rehabilitation* 3(6): 333–336.

Harris S and Niesen-Vertommen S (2000) Challenging the myth of exercise-induced lympoedema following breast cancer: a series of case reports. *Journal of Surgical Oncology* (74), 95–99.

Holmes M, Chen W, Feskanich D, Kroenke T and Colditz G (2005) Physical activity and survival after breast cancer diagnosis. *Journal of the American Medical Association* 293: 2479–86.

Isaksson G and Feuk B (2000) Morbidity from axillary treatment in breast cancer. *Acta Oncologica* (39)3: 335–336.

Jung H, Beck-Bornholdt H, Svoboda V *et al.* (2001) Quantification of late complications after radiation therapy. *Radiotherapy Oncology* (61) 233–246.

Kalso E, Tasmuth T and Neuvonen P (1996) Amitriptyline effectively relieves neuropathic pain following treatment of breast cancer. *Pain* (64) 293–302.

Kepics J (2004) Physical therapy treatment of axillary web syndrome. *Rehabilitation Oncology* 22: 21–22.

Kilbreath S, Refshauge K, Beith J and Lee M (2006) Resistance and stretching shoulder exercises early following axillary surgery for breast cancer. *Rehabilitation Oncology* 24(2): 9–14.

Kurtz JM (1995). Impact of radiotherapy on breast cosmesis. *The Breast* 4, 163–169.

Lauridsen M, Christiansen P and Hessov I (2005) The effect of physiotherapy on shoulder function in patients surgically treated for breast cancer: A randomised study. *Acta Oncologica* (44): 449–457.

Leidenius M, Leppanen E, Krogerus L and von Smitten K (2003) Motion restriction and axillary web syndrome after sentinel node biopsy and axillary clearance in breast cancer. *American Journal of Surgery* 185(2): 127–130.

Lindsay KW and Bone I (1997) *Neurology and Neurosurgery Illustrated.* Section IV. London: Churchill Livingstone.

Macdonald L, Bruce J, Scott N, Smith W and Chambers W (2005) Long-term follow-up of breast cancer survivors with post-mastectomy pain syndrome. *British Journal of Cancer* 92(2): 225–230.

Mao J and Chen L (2000) Gabapentin in pain management. *Anaesthesia and Analgesia* 91: 680–687.

McNeely M, Campbell K, Rowe B, Klassen T, Mackey J and Courneya K (2006) Effects of exercise on breast cancer patients and survivors: a systematic review and meta-analysis. *Canadian Medical Association Journal* 175: 34–41.

Miller L T (1998) Exercise in the management of breast cancer-related lymphoedema. *Innovations in Breast Cancer Care* 3(4): 101–106.

Moskovitz A, Anderson B, Yeung R, Byrd D, Lawton T and Moe R (2001) Axillary web syndrome after axillary dissection. American Journal of Surgery 181(5): 434–439.

Mutrie N, Campbell A, Whyte F *et al.* (2007) Benefits of supervised group exercise programme for women being treated for early stage breast cancer: pragmatic randomised controlled trial. *British Medical Journal* 334: 517–520B.

O'Sullivan B and Levin W (2003) Late radiation-related fibrosis: pathogenesis, manifestations, and current management. *Seminars in Radiation Oncology* 13(3): 274–289.

Robb K and Newham D (2002) *Non-pharmacological interventions in the management of chronic pain associated with breast cancer treatment.* Personal communication.

Robb K, Bennett M, Johnson M, Simpson K and Oxberry S (2008) Transcutaneous electrical nerve stimulation (TENS) for cancer-related pain in adults. *Cochrane Database of Systematic Reviews* 3.

Rodier JF, Gadonneix P, Dauplat J, Issert B and Giraud B (1987) Influence of the timing of physiotherapy on the lymphatic complications of axillary dissection for breast cancer. *International Surgery* 72: 166–169.

Ryttov N, Blichert-Toft M, Madsen EL and Weber J (1983) Influence of adjuvant irradiation on shoulder joint function after mastectomy for breast carcinoma. *Acta Radiologica Oncology* 22(1): 29–33.

Schultz I, Barholm M and Grondal S (1997) Delayed shoulder exercises in reducing seroma frequency after modified radical mastectomy: a prospective randomized study. *Annals of Surgical Oncology* 4(4): 293–297.

Shamley D, Barker K, Simonite V and Beardshaw A (2005) Delayed versus immediate exercises following surgery for breast cancer: a systematic review. *Breast Cancer Research and Treatment* 90: 263–271.

Smith W, Bourne, D, Squair J, Phillips D and Chambers W (1999). A retrospective cohort study of post mastectomy pain syndrome. *Pain* 83: 91–95.

Stevinson C, Lawlor D and Fox K (2004) Exercise interventions for cancer patients: systematic review of controlled trials. *Cancer Causes and Control* 15: 1035–1056.

Tasmuth T, Von Smitten K and Kalso E (1996) Pain and other symptoms during the first year after radical and conservative surgery for breast cancer. *British Journal of Cancer* 74: 2024–2031.

Travell J and Simons D (1992) Myofascial pain and dysfunction. In: *The Trigger Point Manual.* Philadelphia: Lippincott Williams and Wilkins.

Wallace M, Wallace A, Lee J and Dobke M (1996) Pain after breast surgery: a survey of 282 women. *Pain* 66: 195–205.

Wallgren A (1992) Late effects of radiotherapy in the treatment of breast cancer. *Acta Oncologica* 31(2): 237–242.

Williams C (1994) Pain and upper limb function following breast surgery: an investigation into the effect of physiotherapy. Unpublished MSc study.

Wingate L (1989) Rehabilitation of the mastectomy patient: a randomised, blind, prospective study. *Archives of Physical Medicine and Rehabilitation* 70: 21–24.

7 Breast Reconstruction

Nicola West

INTRODUCTION

> Breasts are exalted as the epitome of all that is feminine and desirable in a woman. They are the basic stock in trade of the adman's art and the romantic novelist's passionate pen. (Faulder, 1982)

It is hardly surprising, therefore, that women undergoing treatment for breast cancer not only have the fear of a potentially life-threatening disease, but also the worry of disfigurement, and possible rejection following the loss of a breast with all its associated psychological and psychosocial problems, especially a dramatic change in body image (Kissane *et al.*, 1998; Kasper, 1995; Harcourt *et al.*, 2003). Indeed around 50% of women undergoing mastectomy and wide local excision suffer high levels of anxiety and depression pre-operatively, and one third suffer from psychological problems up to 1 year post-operatively (Goldberg *et al.*, 1992). Sexual problems occur in approximately 25% of women regardless of the surgery received (Schover, 1991; Young McCaughan, 1996).

The modern management of breast cancer aims to minimise chest wall deformity following all types of surgery. The cosmetic result is now given much more attention without compromising the wellbeing and safety of the patient.

Although mastectomy has been the standard treatment for breast cancer for almost a century, a wide local excision followed by radiotherapy is now the more modern form of treatment, with the same long-term survival (Veronesi *et al.*, 1981; Fisher *et al.*, 1989). Where possible, women are now also given a choice in their treatment. It is worth remembering, however, that of the 44 000 women diagnosed in the country each year, up to 40% will still require a mastectomy (Callaghan *et al.*, 2002). In a small study conducted by Cotton *et al.* (1991) of those women offered a choice, approximately 50% chose mastectomy and 50% chose wide local excision. Morrow *et al.* (1998) reported that more than 50% of women chose mastectomy compared to wide local excision. Not all women, however, welcome this choice of treatment, and find having a choice stressful (Pierce, 1993; Fallowfield *et al.*, 1994). There are also cultural differences in the choice process. Asian cultures, for example, place far less importance on the breast. They value role fulfilment and place

Breast Cancer Nursing Care and Management, Second Edition, Edited by Victoria Harmer
© 2011 by Blackwell Publishing Ltd.

greater value and emphasis on this than on physical characteristics as a sign of femininity and beauty. Roles such as manager and that of mother are far more significant than physical images to one's sense of self (Kagawa Singer *et al.*, 1997). In Japanese culture, the nape of the neck and lightness of the skin are central to the foci of beauty and, in Chinese culture, deportment depicts the essential elements of beauty.

Having a choice of treatment can depend, however, on the patient's view, the expertise and attitude of the surgeon, the position of the tumour in the breast and where a woman receives her treatment. For those women with large tumours, central tumours or multifocal disease, a mastectomy is usually recommended, and breast reconstruction should therefore be an integral part of the patient's overall treatment. The surgeon's priorities, however, are obviously to eradicate the disease and decrease the potential for future recurrence. That said, surgeons are increasingly recognising the importance of patient-centred care and informed consent. The latest guidelines produced by the Association of Breast Surgeons at BASO (2007) reflect this.

BREAST RECONSTRUCTION

Breast reconstruction is a term used to describe a range of surgical procedures with the aim of recreating breast shape. It can also be offered to women who have risk-reducing mastectomies, wide excisions where large amounts of tissue are removed (mini-flap), skin-sparing mastectomy, asymmetry of one breast and, of course, a mastectomy. Women with Poland's Syndrome or congenital absence of a breast may also seek breast reconstruction. It is not contra-indicated in patients who require adjuvant treatment, it is cost effective and it does not compromise further detection of disease (Matala *et al.*, 2000).

The NHS Executive in 1996 recommended that all women undergoing mastectomy should be given the option of breast reconstruction, both immediate and delayed due to the benefits of improving quality of life and cosmetic satisfaction for those facing a mastectomy (Wilkins *et al.*, 2000). However, despite the availability and a consistent increase in demand for breast reconstruction in specialist units in the UK, less than half of the women offered it actually take it up (Watson *et al.*, 1995). Significant variation also exists in the delivery of breast reconstruction in the UK and Ireland (Callaghan *et al.*, 2002).

The age, workload, and personal characteristics of the surgeon are important factors in determining reconstructive practice (Callaghan *et al.*, 2002).Overall, it is estimated that 10–20% of patients eventually take up the offer of breast reconstruction (Handel *et al.*, 1990). This figure is slightly higher in America, where it is taken up by approximately 30% of women undergoing mastectomy (cited in Rowland *et al.*, 1995). Most women who choose mastectomy, opt to wear an external prosthesis which for some can be heavy, embarrassing, uncomfortable and inconvenient (Schain *et al.*, 1985).

The purpose of breast reconstruction is to reconstruct a 'breast mound' in order to produce some symmetry of the size and contour of the lost breast. It has to be acknowledged that a reconstructed breast, however, does not have the function or physiological attributes of a natural breast (Ward, 1981). It should aim to match the remaining breast, thus restoring feelings of attractiveness and wholeness.

Breast-reconstruction techniques and results have improved considerably over the past decade. There has also been an increase in the number of specialist surgeons performing breast reconstruction, and an improvement in the quality of implants with the introduction of textured-surface implants that now come in varying shapes and sizes. This is in contrast to the late 20th Century, when attempts at breast reconstruction resulted in substantial scarring, failed procedures and poor results (Bostwick, 1990).

TYPES OF BREAST RECONSTRUCTION

With any breast-reconstruction technique, various factors have to be taken into consideration. These include; the patient's body shape, size of remaining breast and lost breast, skin condition, health status, patient choice, adjuvant therapy, previous surgery, lifestyle, occupation and, finally, expectations. The two main methods of breast reconstruction are implants and autologous tissue flaps.

Implant surgery

Implant surgery (Fig. 7.1) involves the use of either silicone gel or saline implants. The implants are placed sub-muscularly as opposed to subcutaneously because the cosmetic result is superior. Silicone implants were introduced in the 1960s (Bostwick, 1990) and, since then, major improvements have been achieved with the use of temporary expanders, introduced in the 1970s to gradually stretch the skin. Much of the controversy surrounding the safety of silicone implants has now been resolved, with the conclusion that silicone is safe to use and does not cause further cancer, connective tissue disease or any life-threatening illness. Soya bean oil and trilucent implants, once thought to be safer than silicone implants, were removed from the UK market in 1999 because of their questionable safety with regard to toxic leaks. Polyurethane-covered implants were also removed in 1991 due to concerns around safety (Department of Health, 1999). Implants can obscure breast tissue, making future mammography more difficult. Women having local excisions with implants should therefore inform the radiographer.

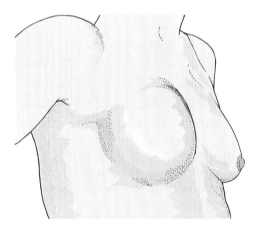

Fig. 7.1   Implant surgery.

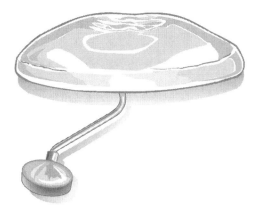

Fig. 7.2   Becker implant.

Tissue expanders

Introduced in the 1970s, tissue expanders (see Fig. 7.2 and Fig. 7.3) may be temporary or permanent, smooth or textured. Expanders are used when there is insufficient skin to cover an implant and its purpose is to gradually create a submuscular space. Expanders are placed under the pectoralis major muscle and gradually expanded every few weeks. Temporary expanders are usually saline and are removed in a second operation, when the desired size has been reached. Permanent expanders, e.g. Becker expanders, are left in place when the volume and desired shape have been achieved. The best results with implants are seen in those women who have small/moderate–sized breasts, have little or no ptosis, have healthy skin that can stretch, and have had no muscle removed during the mastectomy. Tissue expanders are generally not suitable for those women who have undergone radiotherapy, because the skin will not stretch adequately and the complication rates are higher (Jahkola *et al.*, 2003; Vandeweyer and Deraemaecker, 2000). There is now evidence that radiotherapy

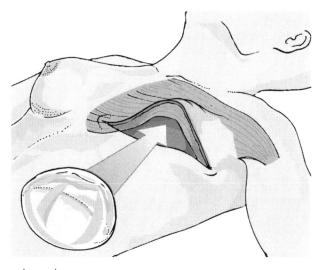

Fig. 7.3   Submuscular implant.

can have detrimental effects on immediate implant-based reconstructions, both in terms of the cosmetic result and the complication rate, especially capsular formation. Capsular formation is three times more likely to occur following immediate reconstruction within a radiotherapy field (Hussein *et al.*, 2004; Behranwala *et al.*, 2006; Gui *et al.*, 2005).

For those women who are particularly keen and suitable for implant/expander–breast reconstruction, however, and who have larger breasts, reduction of the contralateral breast may also be required, in order to produce symmetry.

Both temporary and permanent expanders are inserted under the pectoralis major muscle and expanded gradually through a fill port every few weeks by injecting sterile saline. It is an aseptic technique carried out as an extended role by a clinical nurse specialist, or a doctor. Temporary expanders are usually textured, round or anatomical, and their availability will depend on the hospital and surgeon involved. They are easier and less painful to expand than smooth-surfaced implants. Smooth-surfaced implants tend to cause more capsular contractures than textured implants and are nowadays being replaced by textured ones.

Once inflation has been achieved with a temporary expander and the 'reconstructed' breast is larger than the natural breast, the patient is given some months for the skin to adjust. When the permanent implant is then inserted, this will give a more natural look. The permanent implant is silicone. A second operation is necessary to remove the inflatable implant and insert the permanent one. This method is useful for the patient with insufficient tissue after mastectomy and where the desired shape and size of the breast cannot be achieved with a single-stage procedure.

Permanent expanders

Permanent expanders have a double lumen with an outer shell of silicone gel and a saline-filled inflatable inner chamber. The implant is gradually expanded using sterile saline through a remote port connected to the inflatable chamber. Again, the implant is over-inflated but then deflated after a few months by removing some of the saline through the same fill port, with the aim of matching the contralateral breast. This deflation also attempts to achieve some ptosis. The port may then be removed at a later date under local anaesthetic in day surgery. Patients suitable for this method are those women who have small/moderate–sized breasts, and who desire a simple reconstruction, have mild ptosis and realise that it may not perfectly match the opposite breast.

Fixed-volume implants

Where a woman has sufficient skin and is small-breasted, a satisfactory result may be achieved in theatre with a fixed-volume implant that is permanent. These are used for women who desire a simple, quick reconstruction.

Round versus anatomical devices

The first implants introduced were round, but it was soon recognised that not all breasts are round, and these early round smooth-surfaced implants showed little promise. The idea, in the 1990s, to produce implants with different base widths, heights and projections on textured surfaces, therefore led to major improvements.

The advantages of any implant breast reconstruction compared to 'flap' surgery, is that it is less invasive and relatively simple to do. Patients have a quicker recovery with minimal

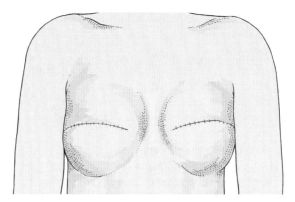

Fig. 7.4   Bilateral mastectomy with implants.

scarring, and the skin colour and texture is better (Beasley and Ballard, 1990) (Fig. 7.4 and Fig. 7.5).

The disadvantages of implant surgery are that women may need surgery to the contralateral breast to achieve symmetry, the implant may need replacing at some time, infection may occur and implant leakage or contracture formation are also potential complications, as is expander valve dysfunction. Some discomfort is experienced after inflation and, in the long term, a patient may be displeased with the final result.

There is still some debate as to the lifespan of implants. The general consensus is that an implant may need replacing at between 10 and 25 years, but views on this vary, and there is no evidence to support these figures. Implants are generally removed if there is a problem.

Summary of potential implant complications

Potential implant complications can be summarised as follows:

- Infection;
- Capsular contractures;

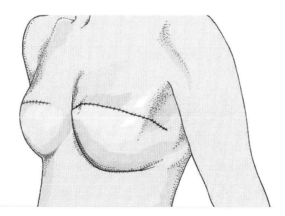

Fig. 7.5   Bilateral mastectomy with implants.

- Deflation – especially with a saline-only implant;
- Haematoma;
- Expander valve dysfunction.

It is not necessarily a medical problem if an implant shows signs of wear and tear, ruptures, or the gel leaks into the fibrous capsule. If the gel moves outside the shell and capsule, however, it can form a series of lumps, causing local tenderness which may mimic cancer. Implants are only generally removed at the patient's request, when a capsular contracture forms or when aesthetic considerations predominate.

Capsular contracture, which is generally a later complication of breast-implant surgery, is caused by fibrous tissue forming a band or capsule around the implant. As the fibrous tissue contracts, it may become more uncomfortable, cause hardness in the breast and change the shape of the breast reconstruction. Surgery may be required to break or remove the capsule and replace the implant. Capsular formation following radiotherapy can be as high as 39% (Gui *et al.*, 2005). However, as 60% of patients do not develop capsular contractures after radiotherapy; this could still be a viable option in selected cases. Evidence suggests that it remains an acceptable technique to patients (Cordeiro *et al.*, 2004; Bronz and Bronz, 2002).

Dickson *et al.* (1987) reported increased capsular contracture in patients who had received post-operative radiotherapy with an implant. In addition, Krueger *et al.* (2001), Jahkola *et al.* (2003), Ringberg *et al.* (1999) and Tallet *et al.* (2003) all found an increased expander implant failure in patients who received radiotherapy compared to non-irradiated patients. There have also been reports of implant failure leading to removal in patients undergoing radiotherapy (Barreau-Pouhaer *et al.*, 1992). It is generally seen that those patients subjected to adjuvant chemotherapy or radiotherapy have worse cosmetic results with breast reconstruction than those not subjected to it (Von Smitten and Sundell, 1992). Radiotherapy to an implant or an expander is sometimes possible however, following immediate breast reconstruction when healing has occurred and inflation is complete, but the overall cosmetic result will be compromised. Those women having flap surgery and requiring radiotherapy generally have a better cosmetic result, less capsular contracture and the radiotherapy is well tolerated (Senkus-Konefka *et al.*, 2004). However, other adverse reactions such as ischaemic events, fat necrosis and volume loss can occur (Alderman *et al.*, 2002; Zimmerman *et al.*, 1998; Kroll *et al.*, 1994).

- Length of operation: 1–2 hours;
- Hospital stay: 4–7 days;
- Convalescence/recovery time: 4–6 weeks.

Pre-operative marking-up by the surgeon is essential. Breast-width measurement is more important than volume measurement. Implants feel firmer than the natural breast, remain upright whilst lying down and feel a little cooler than the rest of body temperature. The implant usually has little movement (see Fig. 7.1).

AUTOLOGOUS TISSUE RECONSTRUCTION

Autologous tissue reconstruction involves taking muscle and subcutaneous tissue, plus or minus skin from a donor site, and transferring it to the breast site. The donor site is either

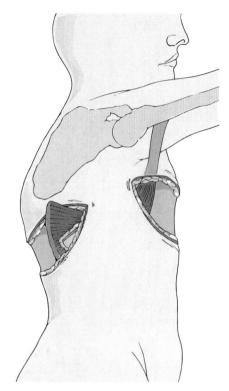

Fig. 7.6   Latissimus dorsi flap reconstruction, side view.

the tissue of the lower abdominal wall, based on the rectus abdominus muscle, or the back muscle (latissimus dorsi). Occasionally, the gluteus maximus muscle can be used.

Pedicled latissimus dorsi flap

The latissimus doris muscle is a fan-shaped muscle that extends over the back from the lower six thoracic spines and thoracolumbar fascia to the humerus (see Fig. 7.6 and Fig. 7.7). A recent survey of breast units in the UK showed that this is the most common type of reconstruction offered to women (Callaghan, 2002).

With this type of reconstruction, the latissimus dorsi muscle from the back, with its overlying skin and blood supply, is dissected and rotated under the arm and placed on the front of the chest wall, where the diseased breast has been removed. Depending on the size of the contralateral breast, a woman usually requires an implant to go under the muscle and skin. The woman has either a horizontal scar on her back or, with a more recent technique, a vertical scar hidden when the arm is placed by the patient's side. This type of reconstruction is recommended when a woman is larger breasted, where there is inadequate skin or muscle on the chest wall or damaged skin from radiotherapy, when there has been a failed attempt at tissue expansion or when the patient chooses it. It is not usually recommended for women who are very slim or who require their latissimus dorsi muscle, for example rock climbers or tennis players.

A latissimus dorsi skin flap can also be used to close a wound following mastectomy where there is insufficient skin, for example following radical surgery for a large tumour.

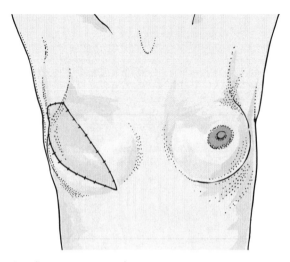

Fig. 7.7   Latissimus dorsi flap reconstruction, front view.

The latissimus dorsi muscle alone can be used when there is sufficient skin; for example, after a wide local excision but not enough volume. This is known as a mini-flap. Women with ductal carcinoma in situ and who are very keen on breast conservation but would lose most of the breast tissue following a wide excision, benefit from a mini-flap. Some surgeons perform the mini-flap at a second operation when they are sure that excision margins are clear and have been examined. Other surgeons perform this at the same time as removing the initial cancer. The latissimus dorsi muscle can also be used with a skin-sparing mastectomy, where the skin and nipple are preserved and where the deficit needs filling with the muscle only and an implant.

The advantages of a latissiumus dorsi reconstruction include its safety and the fact that it gives a good contour, is reliable and dependable and gives a more natural looking breast with some ptosis. It also has a good blood supply. In order to prevent the potential problems of a longer operation and possibly a longer recovery, women often choose this reconstruction instead of a transverse rectus abdominis musculocutaneous flap reconstruction.

The disadvantages include some shoulder impairment, scars either on the back or vertically on the side and the fact that women still require an implant in many cases. Potential complications with this type of breast reconstruction include: seroma formation on the back, infection, flap necrosis and capsular contracture, although contracture rates are lower when the latissimus dorsi muscle is used than when an implant is used alone (Vasconez *et al.*, 1991).

- Length of operation: 3–5 hours;
- Hospital stay: 5–10 days;
- Convalescence/recovery time: 2–3 months.

Transverse rectus abdominis musculocutaneous flap

The rectus abdominis muscle is a long flat muscle that runs from the fifth, sixth and seventh ribs to the pubis. The transverse rectus abdominis musculocutaneous flap (TRAM) was developed in the early 1980s. Women who benefit from this type of surgery include larger-breasted women with ptotic breasts. Women who choose this type of reconstruction are usually averse to the implant method of breast reconstruction and have enough abdominal tissue to remove. The TRAM reconstruction can give a more natural feel and look to the breast than other methods, and women often think that, because it is their own tissue and muscle, it is more natural. Also, the skin from the abdomen provides a better colour and texture match than the latissimus dorsi flap. The TRAM flap can either be performed using a pedicle or as a free flap.

Pedicled TRAM flap

The pedicled TRAM flap is performed by removing an area of skin and fat from the abdomen with its blood supply, rotating the abdominal muscle and passing it through a subcutaneous tunnel onto the chest wall, where it is constructed into a breast shape. Women often feel that the tram flap operation also gives them a tummy tuck by removing excess fat from their abdomen. Women who are heavy smokers, have diabetes, are generally unfit or have had an extensive abdominal operation in the past are not suitable candidates for this operation. It is a long operation to perform, and is thus classed as major surgery (approximately 5–6 hours), and the blood supply is impaired if the patient is a heavy smoker which compromises healing and the survival of the flap. The recovery from this operation is longer than both the implant and latissimus dorsi operation. Flap failure and donor-site morbidity are higher with the TRAM method of reconstruction than the pedicled latissimus dorsi. Occasionally, an implant is also required with a TRAM flap reconstruction.

The disadvantages of the pedicled TRAM flap reconstruction include a longer recovery, horizontal scars on the abdomen, and abdominal muscle weakness, and therefore potential for hernia formation and fat necrosis where ischaemia to the flap occurs, and which can be very painful. Women who have had flap breast reconstruction sometimes have a normal or reduced sensation of the breast, especially if the skin envelope has been preserved. Flap surgery also tends to move with the patient on mobility and is generally softer than an implant. When a woman's weight changes, the TRAM flap can also change in size (Vasconez et al., 1991) (see Fig. 7.8, Fig. 7.9 and Fig. 7.10).

Free TRAM flap

The free TRAM flap is tissue and muscle cut completely free from the abdomen, with its own blood supply, and moved to the breast area where it is reconnected to vessels in the axilla using microsurgical techniques. This technique can be used for unilateral or bilateral breast reconstruction. In addition, it relies on the more robust deep inferior epigastric vessels and has less fat necrosis and less risk of ischaemia and partial flap loss than the pedicled TRAM flap. It carries a larger volume of skin and fat than the conventional tram flap, so it is most suitable for larger-breasted women. Patients who are obese, smoke, have diabetes, peripheral vascular disease, autoimmune disease and cardiovascular disease are not good choices of patients to undergo this procedure. Its downfall is the amount of theatre time required, the fact that it is difficult to perform and the possibility of total flap loss, which is in the region of 5–6% (Arnez et al., 1991). Free flaps avoid the bulge in the epigastrum from tunnelling of the pedicled flap. The free TRAM flap technique is now less commonly employed (see Fig. 7.11, Fig. 7.12 and Fig. 7.13).

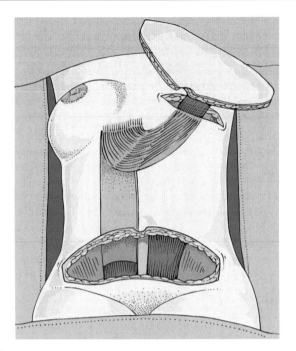

Fig. 7.8 TRAM flap.

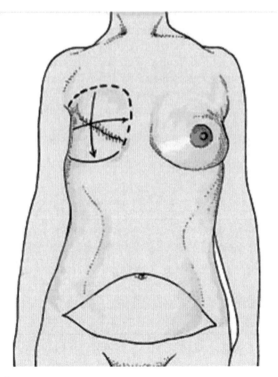

Fig. 7.9 The TRAM flap reconstruction.

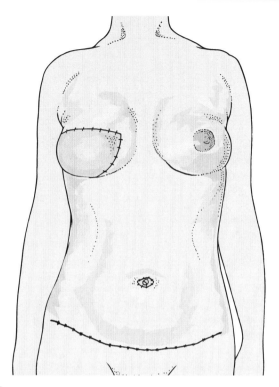

Fig. 7.10   TRAM flap.

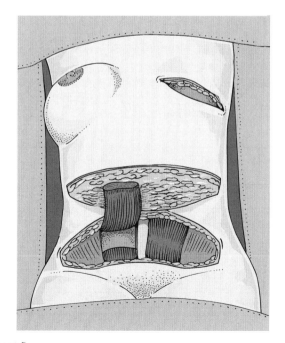

Fig. 7.11   Free TRAM flap.

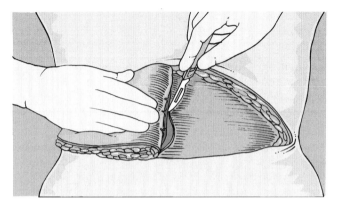

Fig. 7.12 Free TRAM flap incision.

TRAM reconstruction

- Length of operation: approximately 6–10 hours;
- Hospital stay: 7–12 days;
- Convalescence/recovery time: 2–9 months.

Diep flap (perforator flap)

The Diep flap (perforator flap) is the latest innovation and is similar to the TRAM but it utilises the abdominal fat and tissue only. The deep inferior epigastric artery and veins are disconnected from their anatomical source, and the vessels are then connected to the internal

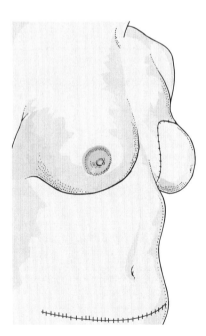

Fig. 7.13 Free TRAM flap.

mammary artery. This technique involves microvascular surgery which spares the muscle, resulting in minimal disruption to the rectus muscle. Hernias and bulges are therefore avoided and, for the patient, there is less pain and a reduced hospital stay. In addition, there is no need to close the abdomen with a tight synthetic mesh as with the TRAM flap. This is ideal for the young athletic patient for whom an intact abdominal wall is important, and also those wanting bilateral breast reconstruction, as preserving the rectus abdomini muscle significantly decreases donor site morbidity (Vasconez *et al.*, 1991).

Inferior gluteus maximus musculocutaneous flap reconstruction

Inferior gluteus maximus musculocutaneous flap reconstruction is one of the most favourable free flaps because the patient has a breast reconstruction and a buttock reduction and lift. The main advantage of this flap is that an extremely large flap can be based on the vessel and muscle. The main disadvantage is the position of the patient on the operating table because the patient needs to be on her side when the flap needs to be harvested. It involves microsurgery to restore the blood supply of the flap. In addition, the posterior cutaneous nerve of the thigh has to be sacrificed, which results in a small area of sensory loss on the posterior thigh. This technique is rarely performed by breast surgeons and is more popular with plastic surgeons.

Although infrequent, complications from any type of breast reconstruction include seroma formation, infection, pain, flap loss and fat necosis, capsular contracture with an implant, asymmetry, rupture and leaking, hypertrophic scars and a weakness at any of the donor sites. Many of the women undergoing breast reconstruction will need some form of extra minor surgery to rectify small surgical problems and obtain better symmetry (Vasconez, 1991).

SKIN-SPARING MASTECTOMY

Skin-sparing mastectomy was introduced in 1991 by Toth and Lappert. This technique removes the breast, nipple–areola complex and the tumour. Local recurrence rates are not increased, but complication rates can be higher. Its advantages include preserving the native skin and inframammary fold, lessening the chance of performing surgery on the contralateral breast and reducing the size of the mastectomy scar. The peri-areola incisions are also inconspicuous. An implant plus or minus a flap using the latissimus dorsi muscle is used to fill the deficit.

Peyser *et al.* (2000) reported this technique to be oncologically safe and to involve minimal scars, but emphasised that it needs to be performed by trained surgeons in oncoplastic techniques.

RISK-REDUCING MASTECTOMIES

It is easier to create symmetric breasts if both breasts need to be reconstructed. This type of surgery is ideal for implants or expanders because symmetry can be achieved. All of the breast tissue with skin and nipple is usually taken to ensure safe removal and reduce the risk of breast cancer recurring. It cannot be guaranteed, however, that all of the breast tissue has been removed.

NIPPLE–AREOLA RECONSTRUCTION

Most operations for a mastectomy involve removing both the areola and nipple in order to successfully remove all the disease. A new nipple, however, can be created on the reconstructed breast, giving some symmetry in an attempt to achieve a more natural look (Fig. 7.14). This is usually performed at a later date to the breast reconstruction, in order to allow the reconstruction to settle into its final shape and to allow time for healing. Some women, however, do not want another operation and decide to wear a silicone stick on nipple which can be custom-made (to match the shape and colour of their existing nipple) or ready made. There are two methods of nipple reconstruction. The skate flap and the C-V flap, although these techniques are rarely performed.

With both methods, a layer of skin and fat on the reconstructed breast is shifted to the centre of the future nipple–areola area and formed into a nipple. More recently, the nipple projection is made with local skin flaps from the breast. A new nipple can also be created by taking part of the nipple from the remaining natural breast. This can also be done to create the areola, but it is only performed if the patient has large nipples and if breast cancer has been ruled out. Cosmetically, a superior result can be achieved in terms of size, colour and texture. For many patients, the nipple can flatten and fade over time, and women need to be informed this may happen. It can be tattooed using a pigmented dye which is now the more common and preferred option.

Healing of the reconstructed nipple can take many months. There is usually no sensation in the reconstructed nipple and it doesn't function as a natural one. Some women may experience phantom nipple sensations which will eventually disappear.

Although, with any breast reconstruction, the aim is to achieve as natural a look as possible for the woman, it does not look exactly the same. It may look flatter, firmer, higher or lower that the natural breast. The reconstructed breast can change shape over time especially following flap surgery, when the muscle can atrophy and the breast can become smaller. Therefore surgery to the contralateral breast is often required. This can be carried out at the same time as the initial reconstruction but, more often, it is advised as a delayed procedure. Contralateral surgery can be a reduction mammoplasty, a mastopexy or an augmentation (Vasconez, 1991).

REDUCTION MAMMOPLASTY

When a woman's remaining breast is large, she may wish to have it reduced to match the reconstructed breast. A reduction mammoplasty may also make it easier to perform the breast reconstruction on the treated side. The incision used for a breast reduction resembles an upside down T. If only a moderate amount of tissue requires removal, smaller, shorter scars can result. The final result is a scar around the nipple, which is lifted and repositioned. A vertical scar down the middle of the breast and, in some cases, a small scar in the inframammary fold is also possible. For larger amounts of tissue to be removed, the nipple

(a) Nipple reconstruction 1

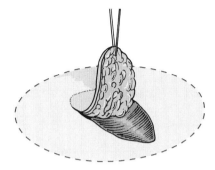

(b) Nipple reconstruction 2

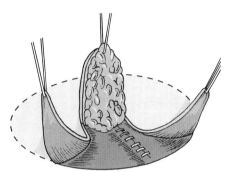

(c) Nipple reconstruction 3

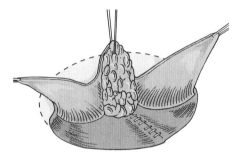

(d) Nipple reconstruction 4

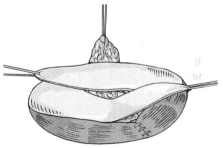

(e) Nipple reconstruction 5

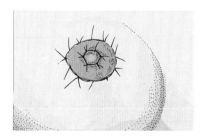

Fig. 7.14   Nipple reconstruction.

will need to be used as a free flap and repositioned, but the rate of nipple loss is higher with this latter surgery.

MASTOPEXY (LIFT)

If the remaining breast is of a reasonable size but sags because of excess skin, a mastopexy may improve the situation. With this technique, the surgeon moves the nipple–aerola complex upwards to a new position on the breast and removes the skin below the nipple and above the lower breast crease.

The incisions are similar to a breast reduction, but may be shorter. If the breasts are not too ptotic, an incision around the aerola and down to the inframammary fold may be all that is necessary.

BREAST AUGMENTATION

If a woman's remaining breast is small and flattened, an option after mastectomy and breast reconstruction is to consider having the remaining breast enlarged. The reconstructed breast can then be created to resemble the larger breast, especially if an expander has been used. The incision is usually made under the breast, around the areola or, occasionally, through the lower axilla. An implant is then inserted behind the existing breast tissue or muscle.

Finally, women differ in their satisfaction with the breast reconstruction's end result, and so expectations of this are especially important to identify. For this reason, all women considering undergoing breast reconstruction should receive appropriate in-depth counselling and should see the surgeon, the specialist nurse and possibly a patient volunteer. Photographs should be seen of realistic results, and all the patient's information needs should be addressed.

TIMING OF BREAST RECONSTRUCTION

Breast reconstruction can be carried out at the same time as a mastectomy (immediate breast reconstruction, IBR) or as a delayed procedure (delayed breast reconstruction, DBR). If reconstruction is to be carried out as a DBR, it must be delayed for at least 3–6 months to allow adequate recovery, but views on this vary. Evidence to date on the correct timing of breast reconstruction is inconclusive and inconsistent. The National Institute of Clinical Excellence currently advocates immediate reconstruction to be superior in terms of psychological advantages and cost effectiveness (NICE, 2002). From the patient's point of view, having everything done at the same time seems sensible. One of the worries of surgeons in the past was that IBR may delay the administration of adjuvant therapies e.g. chemotherapy; however, this does not seem to be the case and does not increase the time to treatments (Allweis *et al.*, 2002). This observation is supported by Malata *et al.* (2000) who found that IBR is safe, acceptable and there is no evidence that it has untoward oncological consequences.

Pre-1980, however, most breast reconstructions were carried out in a separate operation so that any treatment necessary could be completed and there would be greater healing of the mastectomy scar. For many surgeons, delaying a breast reconstruction gave a woman time to grieve and to accept the loss (Winder and Winder, 1985).

Various arguments have been put forward supporting both IBR and DBR. Generally, the main reason for offering women IBR is to spare them the psychological and psychosocial problems associated with breast loss (Maguire *et al.*, 1978; Fallowfield *et al.*, 1986) as well as being more cost effective. This is especially relevant in the current financial climate where all aspects of breast cancer treatment have to be cost effective. Furthermore IBR, compared to DBR, not only offers the benefits of being more cost effective, but some women have a quicker recovery and there is less inconvenience for the patient, as there is no need for a separate admission (Bremner-Smith *et al.*, 1996). In addition, women who have had IBR have reported less distress at the time of the mastectomy and less of a fear about cancer (Rosenqvist *et al.*, 1996). Other authors have also reported that post-operative psychological morbidity is lower in those who have IBR (Stevens *et al.*, 1984; Singletary, 1996), although the evidence is not compelling. Some authors, however, argue that IBR gives a lower score of satisfaction amongst patients (Wellisch *et al.*, 1985). In addition, those women undergoing IBR have no experience of living without a breast, so a comparison cannot be made.

Initially, the basic premise was that women need to have experience of a mastectomy in order to benefit from breast reconstruction, despite the fact that there is lack of sound research evidence to support any of the initial theories. There is also a general feeling that delayed DBR may produce psychological trauma and morbidity (Scott *et al.*, 2001), but again the evidence to support this is limited. Most of the studies on breast reconstruction are retrospective and assess decisions after they have been made, failing to portray actual feelings at the time. Furthermore, many of the studies on breast reconstruction are not random controlled trials and do not compare like with like. Breast reconstruction can be a traumatic and upsetting experience whether immediate or delayed for some women (Ward, 1981; Fentiman, 1990), but can be a positive and rewarding outcome for others.

PSYCHOLOGICAL BENEFITS OF BREAST RECONSTRUCTION

> We restore, repair and make whole those parts, which nature has given but which fortune has taken away, not so much that they may delight the eye but that they may buoy up the spirit, and help the mind of the afflicted (Tagliacozzo and De Curtorum [1597] in Walsh Spencer, 1986, page 131).

After critically reviewing the literature, there is an obvious lack of conclusive evidence on the psychological aspects of breast reconstruction (Harcourt and Rumsey, 2001). This is mainly due to the number of inappropriate randomised controlled prospective studies. Most studies to date are retrospective.

According to the literature, the main reasons for undertaking breast reconstruction include practical reasons, for example the ability to wear certain clothing and to go swimming improves confidence and self-esteem, takes the emphasis off the cancer and allows women to be less sexually inhibited. Reasons against breast reconstruction include fear of scars and pain, and worries that it may not meet expectations and that it is not essential for one's wellbeing, together with the possibility of an unclear future (Schain, 1991), and these facts remain consistent. It is also well documented that women undergoing breast-conserving surgery report a significantly more positive body image than women who have either mastectomy with or without reconstruction (Mock, 1993). Furthermore, Al Ghazal *et al.* (2000) found that patients undergoing breast-conserving surgery had less psychological morbidity and greatest satisfaction than patients undergoing mastectomy with reconstruction. However, other quality of life issues, for example anxiety and depression, have been reported to be worse for women undergoing breast-conserving surgery or breast reconstruction (Nissen *et al.*, 2001). The greatest mood disturbance and poorest wellbeing was actually reported in the mastectomy-with-reconstruction group (Nissen *et al.*, 2001). In addition, Gilboa and co-workers in 1990 reported higher levels of anxiety and depression in the younger patient requiring adjuvant treatment despite having undergone breast reconstruction.

Although some studies have reported psychological benefits and less psychological disturbance to patients undergoing breast reconstruction (Dean *et al.*, 1983; Berry *et al.*, 1998), results concentrate mainly on satisfaction rates and techniques. Many other authors have reported no significant difference between women who undergo breast reconstruction and those who do not in terms of body image, depression, anxiety, social support and self-esteem (Owens *et al.*, 1988; Reaby and Hort, 1995; Holly and Kennedy, 1998).

Psychological assessment is also very difficult because of the complexity of the issues involved as there is, for example, no gold standard assessment for body image so researchers develop their own tools. Despite the inconclusive evidence, however, there is a general view that women who undergo breast reconstruction have good psychological functioning and adaptation (Anderson and Kaczmarek, 1996).

There is also a general belief that women who do not undergo breast reconstruction will not cope with their mastectomy. In 1991, McKenna *et al.* wrote: 'not electing for breast reconstruction may add to the cost of medical and psychiatric follow up' (page 1182), suggesting that breast reconstruction is essential for all women to prevent psychological problems. This reinforces the fact that many clinicians may not fully understand the patient and the complexity of the decision process.

In 1983, Morris wrote: 'there is still much ignorance of what women feel and many assumptions are made on their behalf by clinicians treating them' (page 1725).

NURSING CARE

Pre-operative care

Pre-operative care is the most important time for the patient and the nurse specialist to address all of the information needs and make an assessment of the patient. Women with breast cancer should have access to a specialist nurse in breast care who has received adequate training in the area and works as part of a multidisciplinary team. This is in line with both national and local guidelines. There is also no doubt that women facing decisions about their treatment for breast cancer need support, and this has been widely acknowledged (Fallowfield *et al.*, 1994). Furthermore, there is now strong evidence that the clinical nurse specialist has a significant impact on psychological outcome (McCardle *et al.*, 1996). It is also felt that breast-care nurse specialists should extend their support to include care of the woman undergoing breast reconstruction (Harcourt *et al.*, 2003).

The decisions that women and their partners have to make often run far beyond the type of surgery they want to undergo at initial diagnosis. They have to make decisions on issues which include surgery, adjuvant treatment (e.g. chemotherapy, hormone therapy and radiotherapy), clinical trials and breast reconstruction. Nurses caring for women with breast cancer include ward nurses, clinic nurses, district nurses and practice nurses, and so a sound knowledge in breast care is also imperative for all the above to ensure continuity for the patient.

The decision of breast reconstruction is an extremely difficult one to make for some women, especially when a woman has just been diagnosed, is feeling vulnerable and is not taking in all the information the professionals are imparting. Clifford (1979) found that a quarter of patients used denial or avoidance when working through the decision process regarding breast reconstruction. Excellent communications skills, as well as a sound knowledge in breast reconstruction, are paramount when caring for such women and their families. Women considering breast reconstruction may not always be those who have just been given the initial diagnosis of breast cancer. They may be women who have just been told that the conservative treatment they have undergone has been unsuccessful. They may also be women who have developed a recurrence or been referred from another hospital. The psychology therefore for these groups of women is extremely diverse, and individual assessment is critical.

When a woman is diagnosed with breast cancer, this is not always the best time to discuss the surgical options, especially in a busy clinic. Most clinical nurse specialists make appointments to see the woman and her family either in their home, which ensures privacy, or in a separate private counselling room. All nurses working with the patient can assess the individual's understanding of the meaning of the diagnosis of breast cancer. The anxiety levels, fears and feelings about having a mastectomy with, or without breast reconstruction, can also be determined. Basic communication skills of listening, gentle probing and reflection can assess what the most important issues are for the woman. The clinical nurse specialist is in an ideal position to build a good rapport with the patient and family due to their autonomy, availability, experience, advanced clinical decision making and expertise. A woman's individual femininity, sexuality and body image are especially important to ascertain because these issues can ultimately affect the decision that she finally makes on breast reconstruction. However, the nurse specialist can only identify these issues when a sound relationship has been established with trust and when a woman feels that confidentiality will be maintained.

Nurses often feel inadequate when faced with issues of sexuality and feel that they do not possess the skills to assess these sensitive issues. However, much can be assessed by what the patient says and by her actions without any strong enquiry coming from the nurse. Often women think they want breast reconstruction but, after talking to the specialist nurse and surgeon, seeing relevant photographs and speaking to other women, they decide against it. Body image and sexuality are important issues in the decision of breast reconstruction but are not, however, the only factors that influence a woman's decision. Other issues surrounding the decision process include: the support network within the family, occupation and financial issues, dependants, amount of information available and the likely adjuvant treatment required. There, is however, little research evidence on the factors that enable women to decide on breast reconstruction and their coping abilities around this decision period (Harcourt and Rumsey, 2004).

The surgeon would have already ascertained and physically assessed the patient's suitability for breast reconstruction before it is offered. In order to make such a huge decision, a woman needs adequate information, given clearly and in stages, both verbally and written.

She also needs time to make her decision. Clifford (1979) reported that several women felt that not enough time had been given to them to decide. Often, women benefit from talking to someone who has undergone the procedure, and also seeing photographic results. This is in addition to the specialist nurse's consultation. Women and their families can consider the pros and cons of the procedures involved, with all the potential problems. Some women are well informed about breast reconstruction, others know very little. The woman who does not want to discuss breast reconstruction or wants minimal input from any nurse, including the clinical nurse specialist, has to be respected; the nurse can only offer her support and a contact number should the woman change her mind.

Once the surgeon and the patient have discussed briefly the breast-reconstruction options, there is usually one option of breast reconstruction that appeals to a woman. For example, the TRAM reconstruction is popular because it usually doesn't involve an implant and gives a 'tummy tuck' at the same time. However, for some women, because of their shape, size, health status and previous circumstances (e.g. radiotherapy), only one option may be suitable. This makes it easier for the nurse specialist to discuss the issues with the patient. When a woman, however, has the option of all three methods of breast reconstruction and is unsure, she will need more information, more time and additional support to enable her to decide on the right option.

Some women have unrealistic expectations of the final result, and the pre-operative time is very important for discussing all the issues. It has been found that specific pre-operative counselling for breast reconstruction does not increase the likelihood that a woman will choose breast reconstruction but, rather, has more to do with a woman's own desires than the need for access to education (Finlayson *et al.*, 2001). Nevertheless, quality information, time to make an informed decision and careful patient selection is paramount. Pre-operative counselling not only enables the woman to consider all the issues but allows the nurse specialist to make a thorough psychological assessment of the patient.

Continuous education and support are very important for women who accept and refuse breast reconstruction. Those who refuse may want to reconsider, change their mind, or have a DBR.

If surgery needs to be performed on the contralateral breast, photographs can also be seen of this surgery. Again a volunteer can be provided if the woman so wishes, and the procedure needs to be fully discussed. In addition to the education and information given by the nurse specialist and nurses caring for the woman, information booklets provided locally or by cancer organisations like Breast Cancer Care and CancerBacup can be given, although some of the photographs shown can raise women's expectations and are not realistic. For many women, the role of the nurse specialist extends beyond the initial pre-operative assessment, to full recovery. Although policies vary between regions, a contact number is usually given even if the clinical nurse specialist cannot visit in the community. Women who refuse to accept breast reconstruction need to feel just as supported. The relationship with the primary health-care team is also very important. Support may be given from the district nurses, GP and possibly practice nurses.

When the patient is admitted to the hospital, the ward nurses care her for, so it is imperative that good communication exists between the nurse specialist and the ward team, ensuring continuity of care. Pre-operative marking-up is essential, especially for nipple reconstruction, and it is a good idea for patients to wear a prosthetic nipple for a few weeks pre-surgery to enable accurate placement of the new nipple. On admission, the patient will have an anaesthetic assessment and a general history will be taken.

Post-operatively

Following surgery, the ward nurses take the usual observations for blood pressure, temperature, pulse, pain and any post-operative complications, for example bleeding. The breast reconstruction should also be monitored, especially 'flap' surgery, for colour, temperature and swelling. If the flap is not a healthy pink colour but is dark and cold to the touch, this needs to be reported, as venous congestion is indicated. Blanching, which is touching the flap to ensure venous return, can be performed by the nurse. These observations are usually carried out half-hourly until stable. Most women have a PCA in place (patient-controlled analgesia) to stabilise their own pain, especially women undergoing TRAM reconstruction as it can be very uncomfortable. Pain management is extremely important. Women vary in their recovery and progress. An intravenous infusion is also in place until the woman is eating and drinking, and there are always drains in place that require either changing daily, or careful output recording. Removal of drains will depend on the hospital policy and particular surgeon. The drains should be observed for excess blood volume, indicating bleeding, and also for patency to ensure that the drain is draining freely. Drains may reduce the risk of infection and haematoma, although there is no evidence to support this.

Tight dressings or any pressure should not be put on the wounds post-surgery as they may interfere with the circulation, especially flap surgery. For those women with implant surgery, the chest wall may already feel very tight. Women need to be informed that, post-surgery, they will feel this tightness across their chest where the implant has been placed under the muscle and that, when they relax and become more mobile, the tightness will improve. The wound needs to be observed for bleeding or swelling which may indicate a haematoma.

As the patient recovers, the woman becomes more mobile, the drains are removed, the dressings are changed according to surgeon's preference and arm exercises are increased. The physiotherapist, as well as the specialist nurse and ward nurses, normally visits the woman, and arm exercises are encouraged and demonstrated as soon as possible. Women need reassurance that they will not damage anything by moving their arm at the earliest opportunity. Leaflets on arm exercises can also be given. In addition, the arm can be particularly painful after axillary surgery. The wounds must also be observed for signs of infection and tissue necrosis. Any signs of redness, heat, discharge or a rise in temperature need reporting. Infection must be addressed immediately as it may compromise the success of the breast reconstruction. Antibiotics are commenced if infection occurs, but will also be given in theatre prophylactically. The chances that an implant needs removal post-surgery as a result of infection is low, as is the need for more surgery following flap breast reconstruction for necrosis. The clinical nurse specialist will usually visit the patient on the ward, check wounds and support the patient psychologically.

The duration of the hospital stay varies for each woman and for each breast-reconstruction technique and particular hospital. It is now common practice to discharge women home with their drain in place, so this could be as early as 2–4 days. Seroma formation after removal of drains, whether in hospital or at home, is a possibility and common. It occurs in 10–52% of patients (Tadych and Donegan, 1987). The patient is made aware of this and is told that any signs of swelling in the wound need to be reported and reassurance needs to be given that it can be easily aspirated. District nurses are also involved with the patient on discharge which means that patients have the primary healthcare team, the ward and the breast team as sources of contact. Some clinical nurse specialists visit the patient at home post-surgery and can assess for any problems physically or psychologically and refer to the appropriate person. It must be remembered that women are not only coming to terms with their new body image and reconstruction, but they may also have worries concerning the cancer, survival and adjuvant therapy.

Women usually return to the hospital 1 week following surgery for their results and to check their wounds. The breast reconstruction when swelling and bruising have disappeared, and when healing has taken place, can change shape and look very different to its appearance during the initial post-operative period.

Any signs of tissue necrosis (dark hard areas), need to be reported early, and therefore the primary care team, following discharge, are invaluable. Any discoloration of skin, discharge, protrusion of an implant from a mastectomy wound or any signs that a wound is not healing, should be reported. An earlier outpatient appointment may be necessary. The clinical nurse specialist usually makes contact post-surgery and becomes aware of any complications. Advice on bras is given by the nurse specialist and also by the ward nurses. Initially, a soft bra is advised with a more supportive bra when the wounds have healed. Wearing a bra is very individual, and there is no evidence that wearing one immediately affects the breast reconstruction. It is, however, more comfortable for the larger-breasted patient. Patients who want to wear under-wired bras, once healed, are able to do so. Information, support and psychological care are usually continued after discharge until the patient and nurse feel it can be given less frequently. The patient should always have a contact number. For those patients assessed by the clinical nurse specialist to be in need of more expert intervention, referrals to counsellors, psychologists or psychiatrists can be made.

CONCLUSION

Breast reconstruction is not essential for everyone in order to improve psychological well-being, but access to breast reconstruction should be available to all women. Although there have been major improvements in surgical techniques and availability, breast reconstruction is not accepted by the majority of women facing breast surgery. Generally those who do accept the procedure are younger patients, whose appearance is a high priority. Satisfaction rates are generally very high. Those not suitable seem to self-select themselves out of the process after adequate counselling by the clinical nurse specialist and surgeon.

To date, there is clearly little conclusive research evidence surrounding the psychological benefits of breast reconstruction and, in particular, little is known of the decision process and the enabling or disabling factors influencing women at the time (Harcourt and Rumsey, 2004). This, in itself, presents the clinical nurse specialist and nurses involved with such patients with a major nursing challenge, because they are at the forefront of care. To date, the key psychological influences include body image, personality, sexuality, cancer treatments, fear, expectations, scars and the amount and quality of available information.

Although body image and sexuality are two consistent factors influencing the decision on breast reconstruction, they are not the only ones. Some women with a high body image, for example, refuse breast reconstruction because of many of the other issues involved.

The clinical nurse specialist in breast care has a key role to play, not only caring for the woman with breast cancer but also for those women with breast cancer who are considering breast reconstruction. Her advanced nursing skills and in-depth knowledge, as well as the close relationship and rapport built with the patient, equip her with the necessary resources to do this.

In conclusion, patients considering breast reconstruction need and want information, both written and verbal. This information needs to be given in stages, and it has been suggested that a video would also be helpful. Too much information too soon is not processed, and patients may require continuous support in order to make a final decision. A few consultations may be necessary. Patients value the input of the clinical nurse specialist, and the nurse specialist is in an ideal position to make assessments, physically and psychologically, understanding the whole cancer journey for the patient. This can then be communicated to the multidisciplinary breast team, thereby ensuring individualised intervention and careful patient selection.

Acknowledgement

All illustrations © Nicola West, Cardiff and Vale University Health Board, July 2002.

REFERENCES

Al Ghazal SK, Fallowfield L and Blamey RW (2000) Comparison of psychological aspects and patient satisfaction following breast conserving surgery, simple mastectomy and breast reconstruction. *European Journal of Cancer* 15(36): 1938–1943.

Alderman AK, Wilkins EG, Kim HM and Lowey JC (2002) Complications in post mastectomy breast reconstruction: two-year results of the Michigan Breast Reconstruction Outcome Study. *Plastic Reconstructive Surgery* 109(7): 2265–2274.

Allweis TM, Boisvert ME, Otero SE, Perry DJ, Dubin NH and Priebat DA (2002) Immediate reconstruction after mastectomy for breast cancer does not prolong the time to starting adjuvant chemotherapy. *American Journal of Surgery* 183(3): 218–221.

Anderson R and Kaczmarek B (1996) Psychological well-being of the breast reconstruction patient: A pilot study. *Plastic Surgical Nursing* 16: 185–188.

Arnez ZM, Bajec J, Bardsley AF, Scamp T and Webster MH (1991) Experience with 50 TRAM flap breast reconstructions. *Plastic Reconstruction Surgery* 87: 470–478.

Association of Breast Surgeons at BASO (2007) BAPRAS and the Training Interface Group in Breast Surgery. Oncoplastic breast surgery – a guide to good practice. *European Journal of Surgical Oncology* doi:10.1016/j.ejso.04.014.

Barreau-Pouhaer L, Le MG, Rietjens M, Arrlagada R, Contesso G and Martins R (1992) Risk factors for failure of immediate breast reconstruction with prosthesis after mastectomy for breast cancer. *Cancer* 70: 1145–1151.

Beasley ME and Ballard AR (1990) Immediate breast reconstruction: A comparison of techniques utilizing the pedicled TRAM and tissue expanders. Presented at the Annual Meeting of the American Association of Plastic Surgeons, Hot Springs, VA, USA, 7 May 1990.

Behranwala KA, Dua RS, Ross GM, Ward A, Ahern R and Gui GPH (2006) The influence of radiotherapy on capsule formation and aesthetic outcome after immediate breast reconstruction using biodimensional anatomic expander implants. *J Plastic and Aesthetic Surgery* 59: 1043–1051.

Berry MG, Al-Mufti RA, Jenkinson AD, Denton S, Sullivan M, Vaus A and Carpenter R (1998) An audit of outcome including patient satisfaction with immediate breast reconstruction performed by breast surgeons. *Annals of the Royal College of Surgeons of England* 80: 173.

Bostwick III J (1990) *Plastic and Reconstructive Breast Surgery*, Vol II, St Louis: Quality Medical Publishing.

Bremner-Smith A, Straker V, Abel A and Rainsbury R (1996) Choices and experiences of women offered breast reconstruction. British Association of Surgical Oncologists, Winter Meeting, London: Royal College of Surgeons.

Bronz G and Bronz L (2002) Mamma reconstruction with skin expander and silicone prosthesis. *15 years experience. Aesthetic Plastic Surgery* 26(3): 215–218.

Callaghan CJ, Couto E, Kerin MJ, Rainsbury RM, George WD and Purushotham AD (2002) Breast reconstruction in the UK and Ireland. *British Journal of Surgery* 89: 335–340.

Clifford E (1979) The reconstruction experience: the search for restitution. In: Georgiade, NG (ed.) *Breast Reconstruction following Mastectomy* St Louis: Mosby, pp 22–34.

Cordeiro PG, Pusic AL, Disa JJ, Mccormick B and Vanzee K (2004) Irradiation after immediate tissue expander/implant breast reconstruction: outcomes, complications, aesthetic results, and satisfaction among 156 patients. *Plastic Reconstructive Surgery* 113(3): 877–881.

Cotton T, Locker A, Jackson L *et al.* (1991) A prospective study of patient choice in treatment for primary breast cancer. *European Journal of Surgical Oncology* 17: 115–117.

Dean C, Chetty U and Forrest AP (1983) Effects of immediate breast reconstruction on psychosocial morbidity after mastectomy. *The Lancet* 1: 459–462.

Department of Health (1999) *Withdrawal of Oil Based Breast Implants*. London: HMSO.

Dickson MG, Sharpe DT, Dickson WA, Wilde GP, Brennan TG and Roberts AH (1987) Breast reconstruction by tissue expansion. *Annals of the Royal College of Surgeons of England* 69: 19–21.

Fallowfield LJ, Baum M and Maguire P (1986) Effects of breast conservation on psychological morbidity associated with diagnosis and treatment of early breast cancer. *British Medical Journal* 193: 1331–1333.

Fallowfield LJ, Hall A, Maguire P, Baum M and A'Hern RP (1994) A question of choice: results of a prospective 3-year follow-up study of women with breast cancer. *The Breast* 3: 202–208.

Faulder C (1982) *Breast cancer: a guide to its early detection and treatment*. London: Pan Books.

Fentiman IS (1990) *Detection and treatment of early breast cancer*. London: Martin Dunitz.

Finlayson CA, Macdermott TA and Jyoti Arya MD (2001) Can specific pre-operative counselling increase the likelihood a woman will choose post mastectomy breast reconstruction. *American Journal of Surgery* 182: 649–653.

Fisher B, Redmond C, Poisson R *et al.* (1989) Eight year results of a randomised controlled study comparing total radical mastectomy and lumpectomy with or without radiation in the treatment of breast cancer. *New England Journal of Medicine* 320: 822–828.

Gilboa D, Borenstein A and Floro S (1990) Emotional and psychological adjustment of women to breast reconstruction and detection of sub-groups at risk for psychological morbidity. *Annals of Plastic Surgery* 25: 397–401.

Goldberg IA, Scott RN, Davidson PM *et al.* (1992) Psychological morbidity in the first year after breast surgery. *European Journal of Surgical Oncology* 18: 327–331.

Gui GPH, Behranwala K, Dua RS, Ward A and Ahern R (2005) The impact of radiotherapy on capsule formation and aesthetic outcome after immediate breast reconstruction using biodimensional anatomic expander implants. *Breast Cancer Research and Treatment* 94(1): S37.

Handel N, Silverstein MJ, Waisman E and Waisman JR (1990) Reasons why mastectomy patients do not have breast reconstruction. *Plastic and Reconstructive Surgery* 86(6): 1118–1125.

Harcourt D and Rumsey N (2001) Psychological aspects of breast reconstruction: a review of the literature. *Journal of Advanced Nursing* 4(35): 477–487.

Harcourt D and Rumsey N (2004) Mastectomy patients decision making for or against immediate breast reconstruction *Psycho-Oncology* 13: 106–115.

Harcourt DM, Rumsey NJ, Ambler NR *et al.* (2003) The psychological effect of mastectomy with or without breast reconstruction; a prospective, multicenter study. *Plastic Reconstructive Surgery* 111(3): 1060–1068.

Holly P and Kennedy P (1998) The psychological benefits of immediate breast reconstruction in women who have undergone surgery for breast cancer. *Proceedings of the British Psychological Society* 6: 32.

Hussein M, Salah B, Malyon A and Weiler Mithoff EM (2004) The effect of radiotherapy on the use of immediate breast reconstruction. *European Journal of Surgical Oncology* 30: 490–494.

Jahkola T, Asko-Seljavaara S and Von Smitten K (2003) Immediate breast reconstruction. *Scandanavian Journal of Surgery* 92(4): 249–256.

Kagawa-Singer M, Wellisch DK and Durvasula R (1997) Impact of breast cancer on Asian American and Anglo American Women. *Culture, Medicine and Psychiatry* 21(4): 449–480.

Kasper AS (1995) The social construction of breast loss and reconstruction. *Women's Health* 1(3): 197–219.

Kissane DW, Clarke DM, Ikin J *et al.* (1998) Psychological morbidity and quality of life in Australian women with early stage breast cancer: a cross sectional survey. *Medical Journal of Australia* 169(4): 192–196.

Kroll SS, Schusterman MA, Reece GP, Miller MJ and Smith B (1994) Breast Reconstruction with Myocutaneous flaps in previously irradiated patients. *Plastic Reconstructive Surgery* 93(3): 460–469; discussion 470–471.

Krueger EA, Wilkins EG, Strawderman M *et al.* (2001) Complications and patient satisfaction following expander/implant breast reconstruction with and without radiotherapy. *International Journal of Radiation Oncology Biological Physics* 1, 49(3): 713–721.

Maguire G P, Lee EG and Bevington DT (1978) Psychiatric problems in the first year after mastectomy. *British Medical Journal* 282: 963–965.

Matala CM, McIntosh SA and Purushotham AD (2000) Immediate breast reconstruction after mastectomy for cancer. *British Journal of Surgery* 11(87): 1455–72.

McCardle J, George W, McCardle C *et al.* (1996) Psychological support for patients undergoing breast cancer surgery: A randomised study. *British Medical Journal* 312: 813–817.

McKenna R, Grene T, Hang-Fu L *et al.* (1991) Implications for clinical management in patients with breast cancer. *Cancer* 68 (Suppl.): 1182–83

Mock V (1993) Body image in women treated for breast cancer. *Nursing Research* 42(3): 153–157.

Morris T (1983) Psychosocial aspects of breast cancer: a review. *European Journal of Cancer and Clinical Oncology* 19: 1725–1733.

Morrow M, Bucci C and Rademaker A (1998) Medical contraindications are not a major factor in the utilisation of breast conserving therapy. *Journal of the American College of Surgeons* 186(3): 269–273.

National Institute for Clinical Excellence (2002) *Guidance on Cancer Services: Improving Outcomes in Breast Cancer: Manual Update*. London: National Institute for Clinical Excellence.

Nissen MJ, Swenson KK, Ritz LJ, Farrell JB, Sladek ML and Lally RM (2001) Quality of life after breast carcinoma surgery: a comparison of 3 surgical procedures. *Cancer* 91(7): 1238–1246.

Owens RG, Ashcroft JJ, Slade PD and Leinster SJ (1988) Psychological effects of the offer of breast reconstruction following mastectomy. In: Watson M (ed.) *Psychosocial Oncology* Oxford: Pergamon.

Peyser PM, Abel JA, Straker VF, Hall VL and Rainsbury RM (2000) Ultra conservative skin sparing keyhole mastectomy and immediate breast and areola reconstruction. *Annals Royal College of Surgeons of England* 82: 227–235.

Pierce P (1993) Deciding on breast cancer treatment: a description of decision-making behaviour. *Nursing Research* 42: 22–27.

Reaby LL and Hort LK (1995) Post mastectomy attitudes in women who wear external breast prosthesis compared to those who have undergone breast reconstruction. *Journal of Behavioural Medicine* 18: 55–67.

Ringberg A, Tengrup I, Aspergren K, Palmer B (1999) Immediate Breast Reconstruction after Mastectomy for Cancer *European Journal Surgical Oncology* 25(5): 470–476.

Rosenqvist S, Sandelin K and Wickman M (1996) Patients' psychological and cosmetic experience after immediate breast reconstruction. *European Journal of Surgical Oncology* 22: 262–266.

Rowland J, Dioso J, Holland J C, Chaglassian T and Kinne D (1995) Breast reconstruction after mastectomy. Who accepts it, who refuses! *Plastic and Reconstructive Surgery* 95(5): 812–822.

Schain WS (1991) Breast reconstruction: update of psycho social pragmatic concerns. *Cancer* 68 (Suppl. 5): 1170–1175.

Schain WS, Wellisch DK, Pasnaw RO and Landsverk J (1985) The sooner the better: a study of psychological factors in women undergoing immediate versus delayed breast reconstruction. *American Journal of Psychiatry* 142: 40–47.

Schover LR (1991) The impact of breast cancer on sexuality. Body image and intimate relationships. *Cancer Journal for Clinicians* 41(2): 112–120.

Scott L, Spear MD and Spittler CJ (2001) Breast reconstruction with implants and expanders. *Plastic and Reconstructive Surgery* 107: 177–187.

Senkus-Konefka E, Welnicka-Jasiewicz M, Jasiewicz J, Jassem J (2004) Radiotherapy for breast cancer in patients undergoing reconstruction or augmentation. *Cancer Treatment Reviews*; 30: 671–982.

Singletary SE (1996) Skin sparing mastectomy with immediate breast reconstruction; The MD Anderson Cancer Centre experience. *Annals of Surgical Oncology* 3: 411–416.

Stevens LA, McGrawth M, Druss RG, Kister SJ, Gump FE and Forde K (1984) The psychological impact of immediate breast reconstruction for women with early breast cancer. *Plastic and Reconstructive Surgery* 73: 619–628.

Tadych K and Donegan W L (1987) Post mastectomy seroma and wound drainage. *Surgical, Gynaecology and Obstetrics* 165: 483–487.

Tallet AV, Salem M, Moutardier V *et al.* (2003) Radiotherapy and immediate two-stage breast reconstruction with a tissue expander and implant: complications and esthetic results. *International Journal Radiation Oncology Biological Physics* 57(1) 136–142.

Toth BA, and Lappert P (1991) Modified skin incisions for mastectomy: the need for plastic input in pre-operative planning. *Plastic and Reconstructive Surgery* 87: 1048–1053.

Vandeweyer E, Deraemaecker R. (2000) Radiation therapy after immediate breast reconstruction with implants. *Plastic Reconstructive Surgery* 106: 56–58; discussion 59–60.

Vasconez LO, Lejour M and Gamboa-Bobadilla M (1991) *Atlas of Breast Reconstruction.* New York: Gower Medical Publishing.

Veronesi V, Saccozzi R and Vecchio M (1981) Comparing radical mastectomy with quadrantectomy, axillary dissection and radiotherapy in patients with small cancers of the breast. *New England Journal of Medicine* 305: 6–11.

Von Smitten K and Sundell B (1992) The impact of adjuvant radiotherapy and cytotoxic chemotherapy on the outcome of immediate breast construction by tissue expansion after mastectomy for breast cancer. *European Journal of Surgical of Surgical Oncology* 18: 119–123.

Walsh Spencer K (1986) The significance of the breast to the individual and society. *Plastic Surgical Nursing* 16(3): 131–132.

Ward CM (1981) Breast reconstruction after cancer. Aesthetic triumph or surgical disaster? *British Journal of Plastic Surgery* 34: 124–127.

Watson JD, Sainsbury DRD and Dixon JM (1995) ABC of breast disease: Breast reconstruction after surgery. *British Medical Journal* 6310: 117.

Wellisch DK, Shain WS, Noone RB and Little JW (1985) Psyco social correlates of immediate versus delayed reconstruction of the breast. *Plastic and Reconstructive Surgery* 76: 713–718.

Wilkins EG, Cederna PS, Lowery JC *et al.* (2000) Prospective analysis of psychosocial outcomes in breast reconstruction; One year postoperative results from the Michigan Breast Reconstruction Outcome Study. *Plastic Reconstructive Surgery* 106: 1014–1025.

Winder AE and Winder BD (1985) Patients' counselling: clarifying a woman's choice for breast reconstruction. *Patient Education and Counselling* 7: 65–75.

Young-McCaughan S (1996) Sexual functioning in women with breast cancer after treatment with adjuvant therapy. *Cancer Nursing* 19(4): 308–319.

Zimmerman R, Mark R, Kim A *et al.* (1998) Radiation tolerance of transverse rectus abdominus myocutaneous free flaps used in immediate reconstruction. *American Journal of Clinical Oncology* 21(4): 381–385.

8 Chemotherapy as a Treatment for Breast Cancer

Elaine Lennan (previous contribution by Joan Klein née McCoy)

INTRODUCTION

The term chemotherapy was first coined to describe the use of chemicals or drugs to treat microbial and later neoplastic diseases. After the first promising results of cytotoxic treatment, during studies in the 1940s, there was a tremendous surge of activity to discover new anti-cancer agents in the hope of finding the ideal drug that would eradicate a tumour whilst having no harmful effects on normal tissue (Wagener, 2009). More than 60 years later, this hope is yet to be realised. The search for new cytotoxics has yielded many hundreds of compounds with possible therapeutic applications, but only 40 or so compounds are in common use. Most recently, efforts have turned to targeted therapies rather than the crude attack by cytotoxic agents.

Chemotherapy for breast cancer has become firmly established as one of the major therapeutic modalities. Although introduced much more recently than other treatments, chemotherapy has assumed an increasing importance.

This chapter will explain how chemotherapy works, how it is used and the side effects of treatment, with some basic detail on side-effect management. In addition, in recent years, the development of new approaches to treating breast cancer – particularly the use of monoclonal antibodies – has become standard practice, and its clinical use will be discussed including administration and side effects.

HOW CHEMOTHERAPY WORKS

Cytotoxic drugs are defined as 'cell-killing drugs' and they act against cancer cells in two main ways:

1 Killing dividing cancer cells;
2 Interfering with cell reproduction.

In this way, such drugs eradicate or control cancer cell growth.

Chemotherapy cannot, however, distinguish between normal and malignant cells. This means that when a cytotoxic drug is introduced into the body, it will attack not only dividing

Breast Cancer Nursing Care and Management, Second Edition, Edited by Victoria Harmer
© 2011 by Blackwell Publishing Ltd.

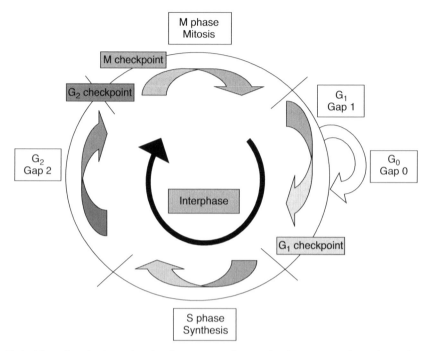

Fig. 8.1 The cell cycle. Reproduced with permission from Gabriel, J. (2007) *The Biology of Cancer*, 2nd edn. Copyright © Wiley-Blackwell.

cancer cells but also normal cells which are proliferating as part of the normal physiological processes of repair and replacement e.g. bone marrow, hair, gastrointestinal tract, skin etc. It is this effect that leads to the well-known common side effects including, neutropenia, nausea and vomiting, stomatitis and alopecia. These side effects will be discussed in more detail later in this chapter.

Knowledge of the way in which normal cells and tumours grow is important in understanding the way in which cancer chemotherapy is used. The cell cycle is shown in Fig. 8.1.

After cell division, each cell enters a growth phase, G_1, which lasts for a variable length of time in different tissues. Cells which are not dividing are said to be in G_0 phase. After G_1, the cells move into the phase of DNA synthesis, the S phase, in which the amount of chromosomal material is doubled. The cell then passes through a pre-mitotic or pre-division phase, G_2, and then into mitosis, M, in which the pairs of chromosomes separate and the cell divides.

The rate of cell division both in normal cells and in human tumours varies considerably from one site or disease to another. The speed at which tumour cells grow also varies depending on the original cell type and, whilst proliferation in a normal cell remains controlled and regulated, the tumour cell proliferation becomes uncontrollable and de-regulated.

CLASSIFICATION OF CYTOTOXIC DRUGS

Cytotoxic drugs can be classified in several ways, e.g. the mode of action and the biochemical group. By mode of action, cytotoxic drugs can be divided into three groups:

1 Cell-cycle phase-specific drugs. Only a limited number of cells will be sensitive to these drugs; they are more powerful in specific phases of the cell cycle, e.g. vinblastine is specific to the M phase.
2 Cell-cycle phase non-specific drugs. These drugs are toxic to cells in the cycle, regardless of the phase, e.g. cyclophosphamide.
3 Cell-cycle non-specific. These drugs act on the cell in or out of the cycle, e.g. BCNU.

Cytotoxic drugs can be classified into six biochemical groups:

1 Alkylating agents. Alkylating agents prevent certain enzymes from carrying out their biological role within the cell, preventing formation of new DNA and inhibiting mitosis. They also form breakages and cross-links with DNA chains. Most alkylating agents are cell-cycle non-specific, destroying resting and dividing cells. Examples of alkylating agents are cyclophosphamide and ifosphamide.
2 Anti-metabolites. The chemical structure of anti-metabolites is similar to some essential metabolites required for synthesis of nucleic acid and protein. These drugs are taken in place of essential components and cause breakdown of synthesis and thus prevent cell division. They are most active in the S phase and are therefore cell-cycle phase-specific. Examples of anti-metabolites are methotrexate and 5-fluorouracil.
3 Vinca alkaloids. These drugs are derived from the periwinkle plant. They prevent spindle formation and mitosis at metaphase by binding tubulin, which is an intracellular protein, required to achieve mitosis. Examples of vinca alkaloids are vinblastine, vinorelbine, vincristine and vindescine.
4 Anti-mitotic antibiotics. Anti-mitotic antibiotics bind directly to the DNA and change its makeup, therefore preventing normal duplication. There are two groups of these drugs:
  (a) Anthracyclines, e.g. doxorubicin and epirubicin.
  (b) Non-anthracycline antibiotics e.g. mitomycin C.
5 Taxanes. Taxanes are derived from yew trees and work by inhibiting mitosis. Examples of taxanes are docetaxel and paclitaxel.
6 Miscellaneous compounds. The action of these drugs is not fully understood and does not conform to other groups. Drugs in the miscellaneous compounds group include cisplatin, carboplatin, etoposide and dacarbazine.

COMBINATION CHEMOTHERAPY

Many cancers are treated with a combination of several drugs. The principles of this are:

- A combination of drugs, with different mechanisms of action, will act on the different phases of the cell, resulting in greater cell death and playing a part in reducing the risk of drug resistance. They may be synergistic, interacting with each other to produce increased activity, which is greater than the effect achieved by giving the same drugs separately.
- A combination of drugs with different toxicities can be given to a maximum tolerated dose without causing unacceptable or irreversible toxicity.

The principles for the choice of drugs to be used in combination chemotherapy are as follows:

- Drugs should be proven to have value in the treatment of the disease.
- Drugs should have different modes of cytotoxic action.
- The dose-limiting toxicities of drugs should be different, so additive toxicity does not limit the dose or intensity of the treatment.

SCHEDULING OF CHEMOTHERAPY TREATMENTS

The interval between treatments is very important. Too short an interval and normal cells do not have sufficient time to recover and repair. Too long an interval and cancer cells have more time to replicate and the tumour may get larger. The exact interval between treatments or cycles varies depending on the drug combination as does the duration of treatment.

A given dose of chemotherapy kills a proportion of cells, not a given number. Because only a proportion of the cells die with a given treatment, repeated doses of chemotherapy must be used to continue to reduce the number of cells.

In an ideal system, each time the dose is repeated, the same proportion of cells, not the same absolute number is killed. The 'log kill graph' (Fig. 8.2) demonstrates this diagrammatically.

Between doses, cell regrowth can occur. When therapy is successful, cell killing is greater than cell regrowth. Drugs should therefore be scheduled in such a way as to produce maximum killing. This will depend on the rate of recovery of the normal tissues which have been most damaged by the drug. These tissues are usually the gut and bone marrow, which regenerate quickly in comparison to most cancer tissue. For this reason, pulsed intermittent therapy, with time for normal tissues to recover, is the usual method of drug administration.

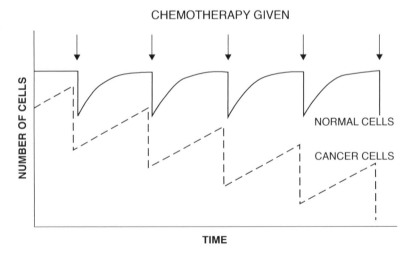

Fig. 8.2 'Log kill graph' – demonstrating the effect of chemotherapy on normal and malignant cells in a tumour which is responding to treatment.

It is also important to note that, in some instances, breast cancer cells can be completely resistant to the cell-killing effects of cytotoxic drugs.

Most recently, educational efforts have been put into understanding dose intensity. There is evidence to suggest that planned dose on time is optimal for patients and results in improved outcomes. This was highlighted as early as 1995 by Bonadonna *et al.* The researchers found that 52% (22/44) of women who received at least 85% of the planned dose of chemotherapy were still alive 20 years later compared with 32% (30/94) of those who received 65–84% of the planned dose, 25% (18/71) of those who received less than 65% and 25% (44/179) of the controls, who received no chemotherapy (Young *et al.*, 2009).

In addition, for those women who received less than 65% of the planned dose, this was equivalent to receiving no treatment at all in terms of survival! It remains important therefore to aim to give the planned dose on time to maintain dose intensity and to prevent suboptimal outcomes.

THE ROLE OF CYTOTOXIC CHEMOTHERAPY IN BREAST CANCER

Chemotherapy has an important part to play in the treatment of breast cancer. The treatment aims to cure some women but, for others who are not going to be cured, it serves to prolong life and to affect or palliate symptoms. Choice of chemotherapy should always be determined by the aim of the treatment, but is clearly influenced by age, performance status, hormone receptor status and stage of disease (National Institute for Health and Clinical Excellence, 2009). Aggressive management of metastatic disease must be carefully considered against the predicted side effects of chemotherapy that would have a significant effect on quality of life. It has become increasingly important to determine and take note of an individual's performance status when deciding fitness for chemotherapy, and is now a recommended pre-treatment assessment. Two examples of the scales used can be seen in Table 8.1. This recommendation follows a recent national audit of deaths within 30 days of receiving chemotherapy, which showed that many patients were noted to have been grade 3 or 4 just prior to their last cycle (National Confidential Enquiry into Patient Outcome and Death [NCEPOD], 2008).

However, the management of metastatic breast cancer has been a major advance in the past decade, with many women now living active and rich lives with active cancer.

Table 8.1 Two scales used for performance status.

Karnofsky scale		Zubrod scale	
Normal – no evidence of disease.	100	Normal activity	0
Able to perform normal activity with only minor symptoms	90		
Normal activity with effort, some symptoms.	80	Symptomatic and ambulatory	
Able to care for self but unable to do normal activities	70	care for self	1
Requires occasional assistance cares for most needs	60	Ambulatory for >50% of time,	
Requires considerable assistance	50	occasional assistance	2
Disabled requires special assistance	40	Ambulatory for <50% of time,	
Severely disabled	30	nursing care needed	3
Very sick, requires active supportive treatment	20	Bedridden	4
Moribund	10		

Current chemotherapy approaches include neoadjuvant chemotherapy, adjuvant chemotherapy, high-dose chemotherapy and palliative chemotherapy.

Neoadjuvant chemotherapy

Chemotherapy may be used as first-line treatment for large or inflammatory breast tumours. The aim of neoadjuvant chemotherapy is usually to shrink the tumour prior to surgery. This may avoid mastectomy and often renders inoperable breast tumours operable (Mansi *et al.*, 1989). Neoadjuvant chemotherapy has been shown to prevent up to 90% of women from undergoing mastectomy (Bonadonna *et al.*, 1990).

Adjuvant chemotherapy

Adjuvant chemotherapy involves the administration of chemotherapy following local treatment for the tumour by surgery or radiotherapy. This means that, at the time of administration of the chemotherapy, the complete tumour has been removed and the chemotherapy is aimed at killing any undetectable or sub-clinical disease. This is sometimes described as the insurance or a belt-and-braces approach. The aim of adjuvant chemotherapy is to reduce the risk of metastatic disease and improve disease-free survival. It is normally used for women who have poor prognostic indicators such as lymph node metastases. However, there has been an increasing trend to give chemotherapy to almost all fit patients with operable breast cancers regardless of lymph node status, as there is increasing evidence of real benefit in disease-free survival.

A recent addition to breast cancer management is the decision-making tool 'Adjuvant! Online'. This tool enables patients with early breast cancer and their oncologists to assess the risks/benefits of adding additional therapy such as chemotherapy and/or hormone therapy after surgery. The information provides an estimate of the risk of negative outcome should further treatment not be used (http://www.adjuvantonline.co.uk).

High-dose chemotherapy

High-dose chemotherapy involves the delivery of high doses of chemotherapy in an attempt to eradicate the cancer, sometimes with stem cell rescue (autologous bone marrow/stem cell transplant). However, to date, the results of clinical trials using high-dose chemotherapy regimens have not been encouraging. Several international studies looking at high-dose treatment for metastatic disease and in the adjuvant setting have shown that there is no appreciable survival benefit over conventional treatment (Berger, 1999).

Palliative chemotherapy

Metastatic breast cancer is currently incurable. Palliative chemotherapy is used to control the disease and also to relieve symptoms associated with cancer spread, i.e. liver pain or dyspnoea. The overall aim of treatment is to improve quality of life, and so the benefits must always out-weigh the side effects.

It is important that patients fully understand the treatment intention in these circumstances, whether at diagnosis or at key changes in the disease management. Nurses fulfil an important role in meeting information needs at all stages and ensuring patients have realistic expectations. In addition, coordination of care is increasingly becoming a key nursing role, requiring full involvement in the multidisciplinary team.

DRUG ADMINISTRATION

Dose calculation

The dose of drug to be administered is generally based on the individual's body surface area (BSA), usually expressed in milligrams per square meter. The patient's BSA is determined by a height and weight nomogram (DuBois *et al.*, 1916). A formula is used to estimate the approximate surface area if the height and weight are known. These are readily available in electronic prescribing systems and drug texts.

Chemotherapy agents for breast cancer are most commonly administered via the intravenous route, though oral drugs are now being routinely used. The intravenous route is the most reliable method of drug delivery, as absorption rates are predictable and administration is the responsibility of the nurse. With oral medicines, the administration responsibility shifts to the individual, and these patients need careful counselling to ensure that they understand the safety aspects of oral administration.

It has long been a recommendation that patients who have undergone breast surgery, particularly those that require axillary lymph node removal, should avoid any injury including venepuncture or cannulation on the affected side. The fear is the development of lymphoedema, due to a reduced capacity to drain the lymphatic fluid. Whilst this recommendation is good practice, it must be weighed up against the need to deliver life-saving drugs and the risks of having a permanent vascular access device. A decision to use the affected side should not be taken lightly and should only be taken with full discussion between the patient, their consultant and the chemotherapy nurse. Further advice regarding the management and prevention of lymphoedema can be found on the website http://www.lymphoedema.org.

CYTOTOXIC DRUGS COMMONLY USED TO TREAT BREAST CANCER

The drugs commonly used to treat breast cancer are detailed in Table 8.2.

PROFESSIONAL ISSUES

The delivery of chemotherapy, as well as the education of the patient and family, is primarily the responsibility of the registered nurse. Only specifically trained nurses working as part of a multidisciplinary oncology team should administer chemotherapy (Calman and Hine, 1995).

Each Hospital Trust involved in the delivery of chemotherapy should have a comprehensive policy detailing all the necessary precautions for the safe handling and administration of cytotoxic drugs.

The Manual of National Cancer Standards (Department of Health, 2001) details the minimum standards a hospital must meet in order to be recognised as delivering the

Table 8.2   Examples of chemotherapeutic agents used to treat breast cancer.

Drug	Route	Delivery	Use	Examples of use in regimens
Doxorubicin	IV bolus	Alone or in combination	Adjuvant or metastatic	AC; FAC
Epirubicin	IV bolus	Alone or in combination	Adjuvant	ECMF; FEC
Cyclophosphamide	IV bolus or oral	Combination	Adjuvant	CMF; FEC
Methotrexate	IV bolus	Combination	Adjuvant	CMF; MMM
Mitomycin C	IV bolus	Combination	Metastatic	MMM
Mitoxantrone	IV bolus	Combination	Metastatic	MMM
5-Fluorouracil (5-FU)	IV bolus	Combination	Adjuvant	CMF
Docetaxel	IV infusion	Alone or in Combination	Adjuvant or metastatic	FEC-T
Paclitaxel	IV infusion	Alone or in Combination	Adjuvant or metastatic	AC-T
Vinorelbine	IV infusion or oral	Alone or in combination	Metastatic	
Capecitabine	Oral	Alone or in Combination	Adjuvant or Metastatic	E Cap
Carboplatin	IV infusion	Combination	Metastatic	Carbo Gem
Gemcitabine	IV infusion	Combination	Metastatic	Carbo Gem

AC: adriamycin and cyclophosphamide; FAC 5: fluorouracil adriamycin and cyclophosphamide; ECMF: epirubicin cyclophosphamide methotrexate 5 fluorouracil; FEC 5: fluorouracil epirubicin cyclophosphamide; CMF cyclophosphamide methotrexate 5 fluorouracil; MMM: mitoxantrone, mitomycin C, methotrexate; FEC-T: 5 fluorouracil epirubicin cyclophosphamide docetaxel; AC-T: adriamycin, cyclophosphamide paclitaxel; E Cap: epirubicin capecitabine; Carbo Gem: carboplatin gemcitabine.

minimum standards of safe practice. Most recently, the national chemotherapy advisory board has produced a policy document to ensure the safety and quality of all chemotherapy services (Department of Health, 2009). Updated peer-review measures will follow shortly.

Information needs

In order to offer informed consent and develop a clear understanding of potential side effects, clear information is required. Indeed, a recent review of all deaths within 30 days following administration of chemotherapy highlighted that, whilst the majority had received information about what do if they developed a side effect, only 19% actually called the helpline (NCEPOD, 2008). There is a clear role for nursing in ensuring that patients are equipped to recognise and act if they develop symptoms related to their chemotherapy. All patients should be given access to a 24-hour helpline, written and verbal information, and the nurse and patient should rehearse actions to be taken based on locality. Indeed, most recently, the National Chemotherapy Advisory Group (NCAG) has recommended a proactive monitoring of patients on chemotherapy, and several studies are currently looking at the benefits of this approach (McKenzie *et al.*, 2008).

COMMON TOXICITIES OF BREAST CANCER CHEMOTHERAPY

The common side effects of toxicities of anti-cancer cytotoxic agents used to treat breast cancer are classified using common toxicity criteria and are generally graded 1–5, with 5 always being death (Food and Drug Administration, 2008). Common toxicity criteria are detailed in Table 8.3.

Table 8.3 Common toxicity criteria.

	1 Mild	2 Moderate	3 Severe	4 Life-threatening
Neutrophils	$<1.5 \times 10^9$/litre	$<1.5–1.0 \times 10^9$/litre	$<1.0–0.5 \times 10^9$/litre	$<0.5 \times 10^9$/litre
Platelets	$<75 \times 10^9$/litre	$<75–50 \times 10^9$/litre	$<50–25 \times 10^9$/litre	$<25 \times 10^9$/litre
Hair loss	Thinning or patchy	Complete	–	–
Nausea	Loss of appetite without alteration in eating habits	Oral intake decreased without significant wt loss dehydration or mal nutrition	Inadequate oral calorific or fluid intake; IV fluids; tube feedings or total parenteral nutrition (TPN) indicated	Life-threatening consequences
Vomiting	One episode in 24 hours	Two to five episodes in 24 hours. IV fluids indicated	>Six episodes in 24 hours. IV fluids indicated or TPN	Life-threatening consequences
Hyperpigmentation	Slight of localise	Marked or generalised	–	–
PPE	Numbness; dysaesthesia/ paraesthesia; tingling; painless swelling or erythema of the hands and/or feet and/or discomfort which does not disrupt the patient's normal activities	Painful erythema and swelling of the hands and/or feet and/or discomfort affecting the patient's activities of daily living (ADLs).	Moist desquamation; ulceration; blistering and severe pain of the hands and/or feet and/or severe discomfort that causes the patient to be unable to work or perform ADLs	–
Nail changes	Discolouration, ridging or pitting	Partial or complete loss of nail(s); pain in nail bed	Interfering with ADLs	
Peripheral neuropathy	Asymptomatic; loss of tendon reflexes or paraesthesia (including tingling) but not interfering with function	Sensory alteration or parasthesia (including tingling) interfering with function but not interfering with ADLs	Sensory alteration or parasthesia interfering with ADLs	Disabling

(Continued)

Table 8.3 (Continued)

	1 Mild	2 Moderate	3 Severe	4 Life-threatening
Stomatitis	Erythema of the mucosa	Patchy ulcerations or pseudomembranes	Confluent ulcerations or pseudomembranes bleeding with minor trauma	Tissue necrosis significant spontaneous bleeding; life-threatening consequences
Diarrhoea	Increase of <4 stools per day over baseline; mild increase in ostomy output compared to baseline	Increase of 4–6 stools per day over baseline; IV fluids indicated; moderate increase in ostomy output compared to baseline; not interfering with ADLs	Increase of >7 stools per day over baseline; incontinence; IV fluids; hospitalisation; severe increase in ostomy output compared to baseline; interfering with ADLs	Life-threatening consequences, i.e. haemo-dynamic collapse
Constipation	Occasional or intermittent symptoms; occasional use of stool softeners, laxatives, dietary modification or enema	Persistent symptoms with regular use of laxatives or enemas indicated	Symptoms interfering with ADLs; manual evacuation required	Life-threatening consequences, i.e. obstruction; toxic megacolon

Bone marrow depression (myelosuppression)

Myelosuppression is not only the most common dose-limiting side effect of chemotherapy, but is also potentially the most life-threatening (Maxwell *et al.*, 1992). All haematopoietic cells divide rapidly and are therefore vulnerable to chemotherapy.

Neutropenia

Neutrophils are the most important of the blood cells to be affected by chemotherapy. Neutropenia, a condition of an abnormally low number of neutrophils, typically develops 8–12 days post-chemotherapy, with full recovery 21–28 days post-treatment.

Most patients receiving chemotherapy for breast cancer will be given their treatment as an outpatient and will only need admission to hospital if they develop a fever. The presence of fever makes this situation an oncological emergency requiring immediate attention.

A patient with fever and presumed neutropenia must attend the hospital immediately for assessment. Urgent intravenous antibiotic therapy will almost certainly be required, and the patient will need close observation of vital signs, observing for septic shock. Indeed, recent guidelines recommend a door-to- needle time for antibiotics of 1 hour (NCAG, 2009). Left untreated, a fever in a neutropenia patient will lead to septic shock, which will most likely be fatal. In this situation, the health professional receiving the patient for assessment should not hesitate to prescribe and administer broad-spectrum antibiotics.

Whilst neutropenia is predictable, neutropenic sepsis needs good management strategies that begin with good patient education and vigilance. Patients at home should be advised to monitor themselves for fever, sore throat, dysuria or productive cough. If a patient has any sign of infection, they should be advised to contact the hospital chemotherapy unit immediately. Rehearsals about what to do, should this situation arise, are a clear recommendation of national policy (NCAG, 2009).

In some cases, it may be necessary for the patient to be prescribed a Granuloycte Colony Stimulating Factor (GCSF) to promote the production of neutrophils produced by the bone marrow. This is used to prevent or recover low blood counts and may contribute to the reduction of febrile episodes during neutropenia (Aappro *et al.*, 2006).

Anaemia

Anaemia is common and generally worsens the more treatment is given. However, most patients can function and manage with low haemoglobin levels, and generally transfusions are only given if patients are symptomatic or are compromised in any way. Each hospital will have local guidelines as to when to transfuse. Similar to the growth factors available to recover neutrophils, a substance called erthropoetin is available to stimulate red cell production. However, this is not available to mainstream practice (British National Formulary [BNF], 2009).

Thrombocytopenia

Similarly, thrombocytopenia is common, but dropping to levels requiring intervention is uncommon. Again, local guidelines determine management. Low platelets may, however, cause a delay in treatment until levels return to normal.

Chemotherapy services will have comprehensive guidance available for the care of a myelosuppressed patient. This is a treatment-related complication, not cancer related. The NCEPOD report into deaths within 30 days of receiving anti-cancer treatment has revealed neutropenic sepsis to be a major cause for concern (NCEPOD, 2008). It is advisable that these patients should be cared for on wards where the nursing staff have experience of managing post-chemotherapy complications.

Alopecia

The myth that all chemotherapy causes alopecia is wrong although, for some, it is the most noticeable and often the most distressing side effect. Although not a life-threatening event, loss of hair has a profound social and psychological impact on individuals and their acceptance of treatment. Some may even refuse potentially curative treatment for fear of this effect (Freedman, 1994).

Cancer chemotherapy agents affect actively growing hairs. Since actively growing hair is the most rapidly proliferating cell population in the human body, alopecia is a common toxicity manifestation of these drugs. The extent of hair loss ranges from thinning of scalp hair to total body hair loss. With an average of 85% of scalp hair follicles in the active growing phase at any one time, the most common location for hair loss is the scalp.

Unlike natural hair loss, chemotherapy-induced alopecia occurs rapidly and usually starts 2–3 weeks following a dose of chemotherapy. It is most apparent after 1–2 months. Hair loss is diffuse and usually asymptomatic; however, some patients have described scalp discomfort 1–2 days prior to and during hair shedding.

Alopecia is temporary and reversible. After discontinuation of the drugs, regrowth is visible within 6–8 weeks. As hair grows back, alterations in hair pigment (lighter or darker), texture (finer or coarser) and hair type (straight or curly) may be evident.

Prevention of alopecia

Since the 1960s, considerable efforts have been directed at reducing the incidence and severity of alopecia using scalp hypothermia or scalp cooling (Dean *et al.*, 1983). The rationale is that it causes vasoconstriction of the superficial scalp veins, temporarily preventing drug uptake, and it also reduces cellular uptake of drugs that are temperature-dependent such as doxorubicin. There are several types of scalp-cooling systems available in the UK, e.g. Penguin and Paxman, all working on the above basic principles, but employed slightly differently.

Hair contributes greatly to body image. Consequently, the loss of hair can have a devastating emotional impact on a patient. In the absence or failure of hair-preserving techniques, more emphasis needs to be placed on the psychological support of the patient and on creative measures to preserve self-image. Advice on the use of scarves and hats may also help patients to cope with hair loss; an information booklet is available from the cancer charity BACUP, entitled Coping with Hair Loss. This booklet is available free of charge to patients and their relatives. (http://www.cancerbacup.org.uk).

One UK charity, 'Look Good feel Better', offers free consultation to patients on applying makeup and on skin care for patients with cancer (http://www.lookgoodfeelbetter.co.uk).

This service aims to improve self-esteem and confidence for women with cancer. Similarly, a recent endeavour by Trevor Sorbie, celebrity hairdresser, has seen the launch of a charity called 'My New Hair'. This charity aims to support women who require a wig by offering product support and training hairdressers up and down the country in the skill of wig-cutting. This helps individualise an 'off the shelf' wig. In addition, advice about ongoing care of the wig and products for new hair growth can be found on the website www.mynewhair.org.

It is often helpful for patients to prepare for probable alopecia by obtaining a wig before it becomes absolutely necessary. This will reduce the anxiety associated with uncertain timing of hair loss and makes it easier for a hair stylist to match colour and style. Wigs are not free of charge unless the individual is on low income. For those on a low income, most hospitals provide wigs free of charge, being paid for by a charitable fund. Details of funding can be found on the Department of Health website (http://www.dh.gov.uk).

Nausea and vomiting

Nausea and vomiting associated with cancer chemotherapy can be classified as anticipatory, acute and delayed.

Anticipatory nausea and vomiting occurs in approximately 25% of patients (Aappro, 1991), and this occurs before chemotherapy is administered. It is difficult to control and is associated with worsening acute nausea and vomiting (Goodman, 1997). Triggers for anticipatory nausea and vomiting include previous unsuccessful control of emesis, smells, sight of chemotherapy nurse, hospitals etc.

The administration of lorazepam prior to treatment has been found to relieve anticipatory effects, but should be used with great caution due to its sedative effects (Malik *et al.*, 1995). Lorazepam used in this setting manipulates its amnesic effect and allows the patient to forget the sensation of nausea (BNF, 2009).

Acute nausea and vomiting occurs from a few minutes to 1–2 hours after treatment, usually resolving within 24 hours. This is generally associated with the emetogenicity of the drugs administered and can be counteracted with the administration of appropriate anti-emetics prior to administration.

Delayed nausea and vomiting persists or develops 24 hours after chemotherapy administration. Oral Granisetron or Ondansetron (5HT3 antagonists) have been found to control delayed nausea and vomiting for up to 72 hours post-chemotherapy.

Management of nausea and vomiting

Management of nausea and vomiting should begin with obtaining an in-depth emetic history and developing a prevention action plan with anti-emetics. Characteristics that affect the occurrence of nausea and vomiting include susceptibility to motion sickness, poor previous emetic control and being young. Individuals with a heavy alcohol intake seem to have a decreased occurrence of nausea and vomiting (Goodman, 1997; Aapro, 1991).

Anti-emetics interrupt the stimulation of the vomiting centre in the brain. The choice of anti-emetic drugs should be made according to the emetic potential of the chemotherapy drugs. Anti-emetic protocols direct the health-care professional to prescribe the most effective anti-nausea drugs. Each chemotherapy unit will have a detailed anti-emetic protocol, and organisations such as the American Society of Clinical Oncologists (ASCO) the will have guidance (ASCO, 2006;,). Anti-emetic drugs commonly used with chemotherapy include:

- Granisetron
- Domperidone
- Ondansetron
- Cyclizine
- Dexamethasone
- Metoclopramide
- Lorazepam
- Aprepitant.

As part of patient education, it is important to inform patients about the potential side effects of anti-emetic therapy. For example, dexamethasone (steroid) can cause hyperactivity, sleeplessness and weight gain; Granisetron/Ondansetron can cause constipation and headaches.

As well as the provision of pharmacological agents, there is general advice regarding management of nausea and vomiting. This includes eating little and often, avoiding strong smells, and an understanding it is safe to abstain from food intake for 24 hours as long as fluid intake is good

Non-pharmacological interventions have also been used, including acupressure and acupuncture, with some effect (Dibble *et al.*, 2000; Molassiotis 2007; Ezzo *et al.*, 2006).

Skin and nails

Several chemotherapy drugs are associated with altered skin pigmentation. This is a purely cosmetic reaction, and the aetiology is poorly understood. It is unclear why some drugs are associated with widespread alteration of pigmentation and others are confined to darkening specific areas, e.g. nails and tongue. Hyperpigmentation occurs more commonly in dark-skinned individuals.

Hyperpigmentation associated with cyclophosphamide can be diffuse or confined to the palms, soles, nails or gums. With 5-FU, hyperpigmentation occurs most readily in sun-exposed areas. Patients may also experience hyperpigmented streaks overlying veins that have been used repeatedly for infusions of 5-FU. This generally occurs without any clinical evidence of cutaneous inflammation or phlebitis.Cyclophosphamide, doxorubicin and 5-FU have been associated with hyperpigmentation of the oral mucosa and tongue, especially in Afro-Caribbeans. Doxorubicin and 5-FU may also cause skin darkening over the knuckles.

Hyperpigmentation generally subsides once treatment is finished.

A specific skin reaction to capecitabine is known as plantar palmer erythema or PPE. The patient first experiences tingling and/or numbness of the palms and soles that evolves into painful, symmetric, and well-demarcated swelling and red plaques. This is followed by peeling of the skin and resolution of the symptoms. The occurrence of PPE may result in discontinuation of capecitabine until resolved and then subsequent dose-reduction. The use of pyridoxine is also commonly used in the treatment of PPE, along with good skin care.

Changes in toe and fingernails are commonly seen in patients receiving chemotherapy. Pigmentation is seen most commonly and occurs more regularly and intensely in Afro-Caribbeans than in whites. The pigment is deposited at the base of the nail, causing dark lines that correspond with the times the drug was administered. This reaction occurs most commonly with cyclophosphamide, doxorubicin and docetaxel.

Beau's lines (transverse white lines or grooves in the nail) indicate a reduction or cessation in nail growth in response to cytotoxic chemotherapy.

After treatment, the nails will resume a normal growth pattern, and the evidence of any damage will grow out.

More severe nail toxicity is seen in taxane therapy. This can be a simple erythema or may result in desquamation of the nails. The incidence is more common in weekly regimens than in 3-weekly regimens, but can have a devastating psychological effect on the patient. Cold gloves, using the same technology as head cooling, has been tried in this situation but, whilst effective, the tolerability of the glove has been poor (Scotté *et al.*, 2005).

It is important that nurses are aware of these effects as they are all too often overlooked. Although these effects do not make the patient unwell, it can be a very frightening time. The alteration in skin and nail pigmentation will add to a patient's altering self-image. Nail varnish can be used to disguise pigmented nails, and patients may find value in seeking makeup and skin-care advice from the charity 'Look Good Feel Better'.

Weight gain

Weight gain is a troublesome side effect of chemotherapy, and is due to increased calorie intake and reduced activity owing to fatigue (Grindel *et al.*, 1989). Significant correlations exist between weight gain and subjective feelings of unhappiness and worry. Factors contributing to weight gain include use of steroids, taste changes, increased appetite, depression, psychological distress and mild nausea that is relieved by eating (Grindel *et al.*, 1989; Knobf 1986; Knobf *et al.*, 1983). It is not unusual for some women to gain as much as 6 kg (1 stone) in weight.

The potential problem of significant weight gain should be discussed with patients prior to commencing treatment, as most patients assume they will lose weight during treatment. Weight gain can add to poor self-image and self-esteem.

Peripheral neuropathy

Peripheral neuropathy can be caused by several drugs, but those drugs used in breast cancer that are most likely to cause peripheral neuropathy include, vinorelbine, carboplatin and, the most likely, the taxanes, i.e. docetaxel and paclitaxel.

The symptoms of peripheral neuropathy vary depending on which nerves are affected, but the most commonly affected are the hands, feet and lower legs. This is because the longer a nerve is, the more vulnerable it is to injury. Symptoms may be initially mild, but progress with further treatment, and so patients need careful assessment at each visit. As there is no treatment for the peripheral neuropathy itself, the treatment would be to stop the causative agent, i.e. the chemotherapy. This is a difficult choice for many, and one in which the nurse has a clear supportive role. The management of peripheral neuropathy involves the use of analgesics, massage and TENs machine, as well as learning techniques to prevent injury. Several neuroprotective agents, including thiols, neurotrophic factors and antioxidants, are considered promising for their ability to prevent neurotoxicity resulting from taxanes exposure. However, further confirmatory trials are warranted on this important clinical topic (Argyriou *et al.*, 2008).

Fatigue

Fatigue is a common subjective complaint associated with adjuvant therapy, and symptoms such as total body tiredness, forgetfulness (often patients describe a 'chemo head') and wanting to rest increase over time throughout therapy (Knobf *et al.*, 1983). Patients should be advised to take regular breaks throughout the day as necessary and to try to plan activities as much as possible.

Stomatitis

The oral mucosa, with its rapid proliferation rate, is a prime target for complications secondary to cancer chemotherapy. In addition to infective complications, a severely compromised oral mucosa can have significant effects on ingestion, resulting in weight loss or nutritional imbalance, communication difficulties, psychological morbidity and pain-control issues.

Oral complications resulting from treatment can be acute or chronic.

- Acute – mucosal inflammation; ulceration; infections including herpes simplex and candida;
- Chronic – taste alteration; xerostomia (salivary gland dysfunction causing a dry mouth).

Treatment of drug-induced stomatitis is essentially palliative, involving topical anaesthetics, analgesics, coating agents and cleansing mouthwashes. Time will resolve each episode of mucositis, usually in relation to rising blood counts.

Infections need to be treated with the appropriate agents, e.g. candida should be treated with anti-fungal preparations. These include topical treatment with mouthwash/lozenge or systemic treatment with fluconazole.

Herpes simplex can be treated topically with acyclovir cream or systemically with intravenous or oral preparations of acyclovir. This will be dependent on the severity of the infection and whether or not the patient is neutropenic.

It is the nurse's role to provide education on good oral hygiene. There is evidence to suggest that the performance of good oral care may be of greater significant benefit in reducing the effects of chemotherapy than the actual agents used.

Patients should be advised to clean their teeth or dentures twice per day with a soft toothbrush, and the brush should be rinsed well after use. A mouthwash should be used.

In an attempt to relieve xerostomia, patients can be advised to chew sugarless gum, suck a hard sour sweet or use regular mouth-rinses with iced water to promote saliva production. It may be necessary to employ a saliva substitute. Patients should be advised that irritants such as tobacco, alcohol and caffeine should be avoided as they dry and irritate the mucous membranes.

Chemotherapy drugs cause direct injury to taste bud cells, resulting in taste changes that vary widely. Common changes include an increased threshold for sweet taste, a decreased threshold for bitter taste and complaints of a metallic taste. Some agents, like cyclophosphamide, can be tasted whilst being injected.

Unless patients are specifically questioned, taste alterations are seldom reported.

Bowel disturbances

Diarrhoea

Just as the mouth can been affected by chemotherapy, so can the rest of the gut. Any chemotherapy can cause diarrhoea but, specifically in 5-FU and capecitabine therapy, it is commonly seen. It is particularly important to note diarrhoea in association with capecitabine therapy, as the ability to prevent further diarrhoea is possible by stopping the tablets. Diarrhoea can be relatively severe, but can usually be controlled with medicines. If the bowels are opening four to five times a day, an anti-diarrhoeal should be commenced, and the individual should contact the hospital for further advice. Prolonged inflammation of the bowel at best is debilitating and, in a worst-case scenario, can lead to perforation and death.

Constipation

Constipation is often caused by a multitude of factors such as loss of appetite, anti-emetic therapy, inactivity, analgesia and chemotherapy agents. However, one particular drug used in breast cancer, vinorelbine, can cause marked constipation owing to a slowing down of the nerves that stimulate the bowel. Aperients should be encouraged in this case, and advice sort if they are ineffective.

Fertility

Infertility and sterility after chemotherapy have been noted since the early 1970s, with reports of amenorrhoea after single agent or combination therapy. The likelihood that chemotherapy will affect a patient's fertility depends on gender, age and the specific drugs (Lamb, 1995).

Chemotherapy can produce significant effects upon patient fertility. These affects are dependent on a number of factors:

- Radical versus adjuvant chemotherapy. Radical chemotherapy regimens generally are more likely to have impacts upon fertility than single-agent regimens.
- Dose-dependent effects. In principle, increased doses are likely to have more profound effects on fertility than lower doses.
- Drug-dependent effects. Different agents have a markedly different impact, having more profound effects on fertility than adjuvant chemotherapy.
- Single-agent versus combination chemotherapy. Increasing complexities of chemotherapy upon fertility can be seen, with some chemo-therapeutic agents sparing fertility whilst others are extremely toxic in this regard.
- Age-dependent affects. In the female in particular, age has a profound affect on chemotherapy toxicity. Women administered chemotherapy under the age of 40 years have a much higher chance of regaining the normal ovarian cycle, whilst the majority of women aged over 40 years administered toxic chemotherapy will be rendered

menopausal by their treatment. Presumably, part of the reason for this observation is the fact that the natural attrition rate of oocyte sees a large drop in oocyte numbers over the age of 40 years, and this corresponds with decreased live birth rates in fertility patients over the age of 40 years (Larson-Disney, 2007).

Many pre-menopausal women who receive chemotherapy for breast cancer will experience ovarian failure and early menopause. In contrast to males, the age of women is an important predictor of treatment-induced sterility. The probability of premature menopause occurring and being permanent increases for women as they near the age of 40 years (Chapman, 1982; Royal College of Physicians *et al.*, 2007).

For most women, menses cease during therapy or become erratic over 2–3 years and amenorrhoea occurs. Levels of follicle stimulating hormone (FSH) increase gradually and remain elevated for 2–5 years. FSH levels >30 ng/litre are generally considered diagnostic for ovarian failure. Estradiol and testosterone levels decrease by 60%, which may account for the reports of lessened sexual desire and arousability (Goodman, 1996).

Pre-menopausal women who receive chemotherapy should be clearly informed of their risk for temporary or permanent ovarian failure. Excellent information is now available regarding this subject (Royal College of Physicians *et al.*, 2007). Menopausal symptoms that commonly occur include hot flushes, night sweats, vaginal dryness and irregular menses. Patients will need support and advice on how to manage these symptoms.

Two options are now possible for pre-menopausal women who wish to preserve their reproductive ability. These are fertility preservation or embryo storage.

Fertility preservation

Hormone protection by suppressing ovaries

Drugs have been utilised during chemotherapy to suppress ovarian cycling and induce a temporary medical menopause. The action is not clearly understood. The Option Trial (Ovarian Protection Trial in Oestrogen Non-Responsive Pre-menopausal Breast Cancer Patients Receiving Adjuvant or Neo-Adjuvant Chemotherapy) is examining this topic.

Embryo storage it is an established technique which has been available since the mid-1980s. IVF offers a success rate of approximately 25% per cycle. It involves a stimulated ovarian cycle using fertility drugs which result in high oestrogen levels. This will raise some concerns in the breast cancer setting but has been used.

Embryo storage is ideal for an adult woman in a stable relationship in the breast cancer setting.

Oocyte storage

Oocyte storage is suitable for adults and for older teenagers who do not have a current partner. Success rates are low at present, with perhaps only 5% success rates achievable per cycle. Less than 100 pregnancies have been documented worldwide using this technique. The technique involves stimulation of mature eggs, harvesting of these eggs and then freezing them, which is technically very difficult. It also requires a delay in chemotherapy treatment whilst eggs are harvested, which might not be acceptable for some patients.

Oocyte storage is very much experimental at the present time. Laparoscopy is required to undertake a biopsy of an ovary or to remove the whole ovary for storage.

Ovarian tissue storage: preservation

Fewer than 15 patients worldwide have had their thawed ovarian tissue re-implanted. Two pregnancies have been reported (Donnes and Dolmans, 2004; Meirow *et al.*, 2005; Royal College of Physicians *et al.*, 2007).

Patients, surviving cancer, who are considering starting a family are generally advised to wait at least 2 years from the completion of therapy, although this advice is currently being challenged. The main reason for waiting is that most recurrences of cancer occur within 2 years (Shrover, 1991). Although the evidence is from small case and epidemiological studies, pregnancy after breast cancer does not seem to have an adverse effect on cancer recurrence irrespective of endocrine status, and some now recommend awaiting 6 months post-treatment be sure the chemotherapy is fully excreted before getting pregnant (Ives 2007; Kromen *et al.*, 2009).

Contraception

Although many patients experience reproductive dysfunction during chemotherapy, information should still be given around contraception. A woman may still be fertile during treatment even if her menstrual cycle is irregular. The combined oral contraceptive pill is not currently recommended in patients with breast cancer, so alternatives will need to be explored with the patient and her partner.

In general, most chemotherapy drugs are excreted from the body within 72 hours of administration. Patients need to be advised to use condoms and to avoid oral sex during this period as it is possible that the vaginal secretions contain chemotherapy metabolites.

Accurate information can make a significant difference in the patient's ability to deal with sexual concerns regarding chemotherapy.

RECENT DEVELOPMENTS IN BREAST CANCER MANAGEMENT

Targeted therapies: monoclonal antibodies

Trastuzumab (Herceptin) is a monoclonal antibody that binds to the HER2 (Human Epidermal Growth Factor Receptor 2) cell-surface receptor, which is over-expressed in some breast cancer patients. It is now used in the adjuvant and metastatic setting.

HER2 is a protein product of a specific gene with cancer-causing potential. Under normal conditions, two copies of the HER2 gene in a cell produce small amounts of a protein product on a cell surface called the HER2 growth factor cell-surface receptor, which appears to play a role in transmitting growth signals and controlling normal cell growth and division (Piccart *et al.*, 2005).

Researchers have discovered that sometimes the HER2 gene is amplified, resulting in multiple copies in a single cell. It is not yet known what factors trigger this genetic event. This, in turn, triggers HER2 over-expression. The over-production of HER2 receptors seems to stimulate some cells to divide, multiply and grow at a faster rate than normal cells, thus contributing to the occurrence and progression of cancer. Slamon *et al.* (1989) demonstrated that HER2 is amplified or over-expressed in as many as 20–30% of breast cancer patients.

The significance of over-expression of HER2 in breast tissue is that these patients are at greater risk of aggressive disease. These markers are directly related to a poor overall prognosis, with faster relapse and shorter survival time at all stages of breast cancer development (Slamon et al., 1989). When compared to women whose tumours do not over-express HER2, these women's cancer may spread to other parts of the body at a faster rate, progress more rapidly after standard treatment including chemotherapy, and affect long-term survival. However, the success of trastuzumab in targeting HER2 has challenged the idea of more aggressive disease. Having a target to attack has possibly changed this thinking, but the early trials are yet to report.

Trastuzumab works by binding to the HER2 cell-surface receptors, blocking their action. Unlike cytotoxic chemotherapy, trastuzumab does not have a significant effect on normal healthy cells as it is a targeted therapy attracted to the HER2 receptor. The presence of trastuzumab stimulates the body's own natural defences (killer cells and macrophages) to help destroy the tumour cells.

Trastuzumab can be administered in several ways. As an adjuvant treatment, it is given every 3 weeks for 1 year, usually beginning after completion of adjuvant chemotherapy, although there is increasing use in the neoadjuvant setting and during the adjuvant chemotherapy. Studies are ongoing to determine whether this 1-year treatment period can be reduced. In the metastatic setting, it is given weekly or 3-weekly for life. Controversies exist regarding the notion of continuing beyond progression. A loading-dose is required for the first cycle (8 mg/kg) administered over 90 minutes, and subsequent doses (6 mg/kg) are administered over 30 minutes. Any adverse reactions are generally manageable. Patients can receive this treatment in the outpatient setting or at home, thus minimising disruption to their lifestyle (Cobleigh et al., 1999).

The major difference between chemotherapy and trastuzumab is the side-effect profile. Trastuzumab does have side effects including transient infusion-associated fevers, chills and pain. These are experienced with the initial infusion in around 40% of patients (Baselga et al., 1996; Cobleigh et al., 1999) but do not usually occur during subsequent infusions.

Although these adverse effects can be managed effectively, the experience can be very frightening for the patient and the nurse. It is therefore imperative that oncology nurses caring for patients receiving trastuzumab are confident in the management of adverse effects, and that emergency drugs and equipment are readily available for the treatment of anaphylaxis. Close observation of the patient is essential during the infusion. Adverse effects can be managed using an analgesic/antipyretic such as paracetamol, or anti-histamine such as chlorphrenamine.

These adverse effects are caused by the body's natural response to a foreign agent but are usually mild as trastuzumab is a humanised antibody. As trastuzumab is a protein produced by living cells, the body accepts the agent more readily and usually adapts to it after the first infusion.

The most concerning adverse side effect reported with trastuzumab is cardiac dysfunction (Stebbing et al., 2000). Cardiac dysfunction has been reported in approximately 5% of patients treated with trastuzumab alone (Cobleigh et al., 1999), and in 13% of patients receiving trastuzumab in combination with chemotherapy (Slamon et al., 1989). However, a later study by Pegram et al. (1999) suggests that it is a much greater problem, with a 28% incidence when administered with concomitant anthracycline chemotherapy, drugs that are also known to cause cardiac dysfunction. Extensive use of trastuzumab has now established that it is a safe drug to use providing ongoing monitoring is maintained. This includes 3-monthly echocardiograms in the adjuvant setting and as required, or yearly, in the metastatic setting. Guidelines are available to assist in decision-making of when to stop or when to continue based on ejection fraction rates. The most recent is the UK National Cancer Institute Guideline (Jones *et al.*, 2009). Key recommendations from this group include a monitoring schedule that assesses baseline and on-treatment cardiac function, strategies for cardiac medication and simplified rules for ceasing and restarting trastuzumab therapy (Jones *et al.*, 2009). Cardiac dysfunction is generally considered reversible on ceasing trastuzumab therapy.

Other monoclonal antibodies

Two other monoclonal antibodies are currently under investigation in the treatment of breast cancer – pertuzumab and bevacizumab.

Pertuzumab

Pertuzumab (Omnitarg), a monoclonal antibody binding to a different receptor than trastuzumab, is under early clinical evaluation. Pertuzumab has been developed for breast cancer patients, whether over-expressing or not. Several clinical trials are currently under-way (http://www.ncri.Gov)

Bevacizumab

Bevacizumab (Avastin) uses a different approach in preventing cell growth by specifically targeting its blood supply. Angiogenesis is the growth of a new vasculature that feeds the tumour (Tortora and Grabowski, 2003). Recent research has targeted killing this blood supply in order to cause cell death (Verheul *et al.*, 2005). Bevacizumab is a monoclonal antibody directed against vascular endothelial growth factor-A, and is being evaluated in the adjuvant and metastatic setting for its antiangiogenic properties, and is showing promising results (Bernard-Marty *et al.*, 2006). The major concern for this line of research was that, if the blood vasculature was destroyed, whether the concurrent chemotherapy would get to the tumour. However, this concern appears unfounded, as it is now known the blood supply developed by the tumour is deranged and the regular blood supply remains untouched and continues to deliver the standard chemotherapy treatment to the cell. Most recently, some concern has been expressed regarding the use of bevacizumab in the adjuvant setting, and whether it could biologically prime the cells for metastatic growth in the future (Miles, 2009). This remains unproven at present.

Lapatinib

Lapatinib (Tykerb) is used in the metastatic setting. It has a novel mode of action, working intracellularly to inhibit both ErbB1 and ErbB2 receptors that are associated with cell proliferation and processes involved in tumour metastasis when stimulated.

Lapatinib is the first oral intracellular small-molecule dual-targeted therapy licensed for use in combination with capecitabine for the treatment of patients with advanced or metastatic breast cancer whose tumours over-express ErbB2 (HER2). It is not currently widely used as studies are ongoing. However, the first trial using combinations of capecitabine and lapatinib was halted early due to overwhelming better outcomes in the combination arm (Geyer *et al.*, 2006). Further trials are examining the potential of this new drug, including the potential to combine lapatinib and trastuzumab together.

CONCLUSION

Currently, there are comprehensive national guidelines for the treatment and management of breast cancer, but it remains important that a patient's treatment should, as far as possible, be tailored to the individual. The current emphasis is on multidisciplinary decision-making and treatment planning involving breast care nurses, surgeons, oncologists, histopathologists and oncology nurses, to name but a few. This is breaking down historical barriers and is a positive step towards the delivery of seamless care.

Many patients with metastatic breast cancer now live full and independent lives with active disease for 10–15 years. This is a great success and a real turnaround from the debilitating death sentence that metastatic disease carried only a few years earlier. There is a great deal of scope for nursing creativity in supporting patients throughout the longevity of their cancer treatment experiences and ultimately their survivorship.

REFERENCES

Aapro M, Tjan-Heijnen VC, Walewski J, Weber DC and Zielinski C (2006) European Organisation for Research and Treatment of Cancer (EORTC) Granulocyte Colony-Stimulating Factor (G-CSF) Guidelines Working Party. *European Journal of Cancer* 42(15): 2433–2453.

Aapro MS (1991) Controlling emesis related to cancer therapy. *European Journal of Cancer* 27: 356–353.

American Society of Clinical Oncologists (ASCO) (2006) *Scientific Proceedings Atlanta*, Georgia, 3 June 2006.

Argyriou A, Koltzenburg M, Polychronopoulos P, Papapetropoulos K and Kalfonus H (2008) Peripheral nerve damage associated with administration of taxanes in patients with cancer. *Critical Review Oncology Haematology* 66(3): 218–228.

Baselga J, Tripathy D, Mendelsohn J *et al.* (1996) Phase II study of weekly intravenous recombinant humanised anti-p185 HER-2 monoclonal antibody in patients with HER-2/neu-overexpressing metastatic breast cancer. *Journal of Clinical Oncology* 14(3): 737–744.

Berger A (1999) High dose chemotherapy offers little benefit in breast cancer. *British Medical Journal* 318: 1440.

Bernard-Marty C, Lebrun F, Awada A and Piccart MJ (2006) Monoclonal antibody-based targeted therapy in breast cancer. *Current Status and Future Direction Drugs* 66(12): 1577–1591.

Bonadonna G, Valagussa P, Moliterni A *et al.* (1995) Adjuvant cyclophosphamide, methotrexate, and fluorouracil in node positive breast cancer: the results of 20 years of follow-up. *New England Journal of Medicine* 332(14): 901–906.

Bonadonna G, Veronesi U, Brambilla C *et al.* (1990) Primary chemotherapy to avoid mastectomy in tumours with diameters of three centimetres or more. *National Cancer Institute* 82: 1539–1545.

British National Formulary (2009) *British National Formulary* 58 (September). Available: http://www.bnf.org.

Calman K and Hine D (1995) *A Policy for Commissioning Cancer Services. A Report by the Expert Advisory Group on Cancer to the Chief Medical officers of England and Wales*. London: Department of Health.

Chapman RM (1982) Effect of cytotoxic therapy on sexuality and gonadal function. *Seminars in Oncology* 9: 84–94.

Cobleigh M, Vogel C, Tripathy D *et al.* (1999) Multinational study of the efficacy and safety of humanized anti-HER-2 monoclonal antibody in women who have HER-2 overexpressing metastatic breast cancer that has progressed after chemotherapy for metastatic disease. *Journal of Clinical Oncology* 17(9): 2639–2648.

Dean JC, Griffiths KS, Cetas TC *et al.* (1983): Scalp hypothermia: a comparison of ice packs and the Kold Kap in the prevention of doxorubicin induced alopecia. *Journal of Clinical Oncology* 1: 33–37.

Department of Health (2001) *Manual of National Cancer Standards*. London: HMSO.

Department of Health (2009) *National Chemotherapy Advisory Board Report. Ensuring Quality and Safety of Chemotherapy Services*. London: HMSO.

Dibble SL, Chapman J, Mack KA and Shih A (2000) Acupressure for nausea: results of a pilot study. *Oncology Nursing Forum* 27(1): 41–47.

Donnez J, Dolmans M, Demylle D *et al.* (2004) Livebirth after orthotopic transplantation of cryopreserved ovarian tissue. *The Lancet* 364(9443): 1405–1410.

DuBois D and DuBois EF (1916) A formula to estimate the approximate surface area if height and weight be known. *Archives of Internal Medicine* 17: 863–871.

Ezzo JM, Richardson MA, Vickers A *et al.* (2006) Acupuncture-point stimulation for chemotherapy-induced nausea or vomiting. *Cochrane Database of Systematic Reviews* Issue 2, Art. No: CD002285.

Food and Drug Administration (2008) *Common Toxicity Criteria for Adverse Events*. Available: http://www.fda.gov.

Freedman TG (1994) Social and cultural dimensions of hair loss in women treated for breast cancer. *Cancer Nursing* 17: 334–341.

Geyer CE, Forster J, Lindquist D *et al.* (2006) Lapatinib plus capecitabine for HER2-positive advanced breast cancer. *New England Journal of Medicine* 355(26): 2733–2734.

Goodman M (1996) Menopausal symptoms. In: Groenwald SL, Frogge MH, Goodman M and Yarbro CH (eds) *Cancer Symptom Management*. Boston: Jones and Bartlett, pp. 77–93.

Goodman M (1997) Risk factors and antiemetic management of chemotherapy induced nausea and vomiting. Oncology Nursing Forum 124(7): Suppl. 20–32.

Grindel CG, Cahill CA and Walker A (1989) Food intake of women with breast cancer during the first six months of chemotherapy. *Oncology Nursing Forum* 16: 401–407.

Ives A, Saunders C, Bulsara M and Semmens J (2007) Pregnancy after breast cancer; population based study. British Medical Journal 334: 194–198.

Jones A, Barlow M, Canney P *et al.* (2009) Management of cardiac health in trastuzumab-treated patients with breast cancer. Updated United Kingdom National Cancer Research Institute recommendations for monitoring. *British Journal of Cancer* 100: 684–692.

Knobf M, Mullen J, Xistris D *et al.* (1983) Weight gain in women with breast cancer receiving adjuvant chemotherapy. *Oncology Nursing Forum* 10: 28–33.

Knobf MT (1986) Physical and psychological distress associated with adjuvant chemotherapy in women with breast cancer. *Journal of Clinical Oncology* 4: 678–684.

Kroman N (2009) Child bearing in pregnancy, *European Journal of Cancer Supplements* 7(2).

Lamb MA (1995) Effects of cancer on the sexuality and fertility of women. *Seminars in Oncology Nursing* 11(2): 120–127.

Larsen-Disney, P (2007) Fertility preservation for cancer. Sussex Cancer Network.

Malik IA, Khan WA, Qazilbash M (1995) Clinical efficacy of oral lorazepam in prophylaxis of anticipatory, acute and delayed nausea induced by high doses of cisplatin. *American Journal of Clinical Oncology* 18: 170–175.

Mansi JL, Smith IE, Walsh G *et al.* (1989) Primary medical therapy for operable breast cancer. *European Journal of Cancer and Clinical Oncology* 25(11): 1623–1627.

Maxwell MB and Maher KE (1992) Chemotherapy induced myelosuppression. *Seminars in Oncology Nursing* 8: 113–123.

McKenzie H, Cox K, Hayes L *et al.* (2008) Chemotherapy outpatients unplanned presentations to hospital. *Proceedings of National Conference of the Clinical Oncology Society Australia*. Sydney, 18–20 November 2008.

Meirow D and Schiff E (2005) Appraisal of chemotherapy effects on reproductive outcome according to animal studies and clinical data. *International Cancer Institute Mongram* 34: 21–25.

Miles D (2009) Anti angiogenic drugs-quo vadis. *European Journal of Cancer Supplements* 7(2).

Molassiotis A, Helin AM, Dabbour R and Hummerston S (2007) The effects of P6 pressure in the prophylaxis of chemotherapy-related nausea and vomiting in breast cancer patients *Complementary Therapies in Medicine* 15: 3–12

Multinational Association of Supportive Care in Cancer (MASCC) (2008) Anti emetics guidelines. Available: http://www.ascc.org.

National Chemotherapy Advisory Group (2009) *Chemotherapy services in England: Ensuring Quality and Safety*. Available: http://www.dh.gov.uk/en/Publicationsandstatistics/Publications/DH_104500.

National Institute for Health and Clinical Excellence (2009) *Advanced Breast Cancer: Diagnosis and Treatment. NICE Clinical Guideline*. London: National Collaborating Centre.

NCEPOD (2008) *For Better, for Worse? A Review of the Care of Patients who Died within 30 Days of Receiving Systemic Anti-Cancer Therapy*. London: National Confidential Enquiry into Patient Outcome and Death (NCEPOD).

Pegram M, Hsu S, Lewis G *et al.* (1999) Inhibitory effects of combinations of HER-2/neu antibody and chemotherapeutic agents used for treatment of human breast cancers. *Oncogene* 18(13): 2241–2251.

Piccart-Gebhart MJ, Procter M, Leyland-Jones B *et al.* (2005) Trastuzumab after adjuvant chemotherapy in HER2-positive breast cancer. *New England Journal of Medicine* 353: 1659–1672.

Royal College of Physicians, Royal College of Radiologists, Royal College of Obstetricians and Gynaecologists (2007) *The Effects of Cancer Treatment on Reproductive Functions*. London: Royal College of Physicians.

Scotté F, Tourani JM, Banu E *et al.* (2005) Multicenter study of a frozen glove to prevent docetaxel-induced onycholysis and cutaneous toxicity of the hand. *Journal of Clinical Oncology* 23(19): 4424.

Shrover L (1991) *Sexuality and Fertility after Cancer*. New York: John Wiley and Sons.

Slamon D, Godolphin W, Jones LA *et al.* (1989) Studies of the HER-2/neu centre for proto-oncogene in human breast cancer. *Science* 244: 707–712.

Stebbing J, Copson E and O'Reilly S (2000) Herceptin (trastuzumab) in advanced breast cancer. *Cancer Treatment Reviews* 26(4): 287–290.

Tortora G and Graboski S (2003) *Principles of Anatomy and Physiology*. Hoboken: John Wiley and Sons.

Verheul, Henk MW, Pinedo and Herbert M (2005) Inhibition of angiogenesis in cancer patients *Expert Opinion on Emerging Drugs* 10(2): 403–412.

Wagener P (2009) *The History of Oncology* Houston: Springer.

Young A, Crowe, M, Lennan E *et al.* (2009) Delivery of chemotherapy at planned dose and on time. *Cancer Nursing Practice* 8(5): 16–19.

9 Radiotherapy as a Treatment for Breast Cancer

Karen Burnet

INTRODUCTION

Comprehensive treatment for breast cancer can include surgery, hormone therapy, chemotherapy, the biological therapies and radiotherapy (RT). This chapter will concentrate on the treatment modality of RT with particular reference to what RT is, when it is used and how it can affect the patient. Nursing care for the patient undergoing RT involves many skills, from a basic knowledge of radiation physics to understanding what physical effects radiation can have on the patient. The inclusion of RT in a patient's treatment programme needs careful explanation and preparation to make the unknown and often misunderstood less of an ordeal to that patient. Since I originally wrote this chapter in 2002, there have been many advances in the delivery and provision of RT owing to robust research projects and improved audit and quality assurance. These initiatives have all contributed to better treatment with RT, and I confidently predict that research will continue to shape the way radiation is given to the patient with breast cancer. RT can be a confusing and difficult treatment to understand, and this chapter aims to separate the facts from the fiction about RT for those who care for patients undergoing this treatment.

RADIOTHERAPY

What is radiotherapy?

Simply, radiotherapy is the use of ionising radiation to kill tumour cells.

Historical context

Ionising radiation, X-rays, was discovered by Röntgen in 1895. He produced these rays by heating an electrode in a sealed airless tube, and applying a voltage across it, which accelerated the electrons towards a target plate. Striking the target, the electrons changed their kinetic (movement) energy into X-rays. The term 'X' was used because, at the time, the nature of these rays was not understood. Röntgen quickly recognised the potential for medical diagnosis and an early X-ray exists of his wife's hand, showing how well bones could be visualised with this type of radiation. The first treatment of a cancer using X-rays took place the following year, in 1896.

Breast Cancer Nursing Care and Management, Second Edition, Edited by Victoria Harmer
© 2011 by Blackwell Publishing Ltd.

Also in 1896, Becquerel further described and quantified radioactivity, and his name is given to the modern SI (Système International) unit of its measurement (Bq). Shortly after, Marie and Pierre Curie extracted radium from pitchblende, a radioactive material containing uranium oxides, contributing further to the understanding of radiation. Their name was given to the first unit of radioactivity (Ci).

Both X-rays (produced by electrons hitting a target) and gamma (γ) rays (produced by the decay of the nucleus of a radioactive atom) are identical forms of electromagnetic radiation. Of all the electromagnetic wave spectrum, which includes light waves, infrared and radio waves, only X-rays and gamma rays have the right amount of energy to produce the ionisation of atoms which takes place when radiation passes through living tissue. These are the main sources of therapeutic radiation used today.

RT today

In the past, patients in the UK with breast cancer requiring RT were treated using ^{60}cobalt machines. Today, these machines have mostly been replaced by the superior linear accelerators, or 'Linacs', which produce X-rays. Linacs are capable of accelerating electrons almost to the speed of light, before they hit a target to produce X-rays. Some Linacs are equipped to allow use of the electron beam (beta particle radiation) itself to treat the patient. Linacs are able to produce a more defined beam, with higher energy than ^{60}cobalt machines, and can achieve greater depth doses through tissue.

Radiation dose is measured as the amount of energy that is absorbed by tissue and is measured in the SI unit termed the gray, usually abbreviated to Gy. One gray is equal to 1 joule of energy absorbed per kilogram of tissue treated. Sometimes doses are expressed in centigray (cGy), 1/100th of a gray.

The penetrating power of high-energy X-rays and gamma rays means that, inevitably, some normal tissues will be irradiated as well as the tumour, which can be problematic. With electrons, the radiation stops after a short distance in tissue, the depth of penetration depending on the energy of the beam. This is useful for giving a 'boost' of radiation to the site of the tumour (tumour bed) which has clearly been proven to reduce the rate of local recurrence in the treatment of breast cancer (Bartelink *et al.*, 2001). Also, clinicians have learned to use the natural falling off from the source of the radiation (the inverse square law –more about this later in the chapter) to reduce the radiation dose to the deeper structures of the chest wall, that is the ribs, lung and heart. Avoiding these organs at risk (OARS) by the careful planning and delivery of radiation has been a great challenge to radiotherapists and radiation physicists over the years and has shaped the necessary advances in the treatment planning and delivery of RT.

How does RT kill cancer cells?

Radiation kills cancer cells by:

- A direct hit, when the radiation damages DNA (deoxyribonucleic acid) directly; or
- An indirect hit, when the radiation produces free radicals in water adjacent to the DNA, which then damage the DNA.

The important cell-killing effect of RT on DNA is the double-strand break, a complete break in the DNA molecule which is contained within the cell nucleus and is responsible for the

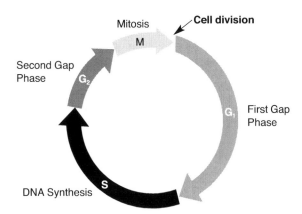

Fig. 9.1   The cell cycle. With thanks to Dr Norman Kirkby, Faculty of Engineering and Physical Sciences, University of Surrey.

function of that particular cell. Although cells can repair some of these breaks, residual breaks lead to cell death, the desired effect against the tumour. If a cell is unable to repair these breaks, it will die when it tries to divide. Fig. 9.1 shows a pictorial representation of the cell cycle and division.

The damaging effects of radiation are less marked in cells that are hypoxic (i.e. have a limited oxygen supply), which is an important consideration when treating large, inoperable breast cancers that are not well vascularised and are therefore not well oxygenated. There are also differences in radiation sensitivity in different phases of the cell cycle, but it is difficult to exploit this clinically (Hall and Cox, 1994).

Cell death is proportional to the amount of radiation given, the more radiation given the greater the number of cells killed. Unfortunately, as mentioned before, the surrounding normal tissues will also receive a dose of radiation. If very high doses of radiation are used, normal tissues may be permanently damaged, which could be very dangerous to the patient (Souhami and Tobias, 1995). The limiting of normal tissue damage is achieved by the biological strategy of dividing the course up into a number of smaller treatments, called 'fractions', and by the physical strategy of careful planning to limit the amount of normal tissue treated. The challenge for the radiotherapist is to give enough RT to achieve optimal local control and survival of the patient, whilst avoiding normal tissue damage and ensuring a good cosmetic outcome.

When is RT used for the treatment of breast cancer?

Breast irradiation is a major part of the RT workload in the UK, and it is estimated that breast irradiation uses about 30% of all RT resources. The UK Department of Health's 2007 Cancer Reform Strategy estimates that an 80% increase in service capacity will be needed by 2016, emphasising the need for optimal treatment regimens, more investment in RT machinery, the development of more efficient RT techniques and defining when RT is *not* needed for the treatment of breast cancer as well as when it is (Hilley *et al.*, 2008). RT has an established and important role in the treatment of breast cancer in several clinical settings.

As a treatment for early breast cancer

Surgery for the treatment of breast cancer has become less radical over the past 30 years with the introduction of wide local excision of the tumour (see Chapter 5) and the use of primary chemotherapy to reduce the size of the tumour (see Chapter 8). If wide local excision has been used, RT is given to complete the treatment of the breast, as an added insurance against local recurrence. The breast surgeon will try to remove the entire breast tumour, but there is always the risk that at a microscopic level some cancer cells will have been left behind, or that a separate focus of cancer has been missed. It has been clearly shown that mastectomy can safely be replaced by wide local excision and RT (Fisher *et al.*, 2002). There is also strong evidence that RT contributes to the systemic control of the disease by improving overall survival of the patient as well as preventing local relapse in the treated breast (Overgaard *et al.*, 1997; Coles *et al.*, 2005a).

RT may be given after a mastectomy if the tumour was close to the chest wall or was large in volume. Patients who have a high number of lymph nodes involved with the tumour (Gebski *et al.*, 2006), or who have received primary chemotherapy to shrink the breast tumour, or in whom the tumour cannot be completely surgically excised, will also be offered RT.

As a treatment for a locally advanced breast cancer

Patients who present with a large, inoperable tumour may receive RT as a primary treatment to shrink the tumour. The response of the tumour to RT will be carefully assessed, and the plan of treatment may change if the tumour shrinks down enough to make surgery possible.

As a treatment for metastatic breast cancer

RT has a very large part to play in the palliation and control of metastatic breast cancer and is generally well tolerated. When used on its own or in conjunction with other treatment modalities, RT can do much to enhance the quality of life of the patient. RT given for the treatment of metastatic disease is described in greater detail later in this chapter.

How is RT given to the patient with breast cancer?

If the patient needs to be treated with RT, she will be advised of the best method of RT for her. External beam radiation remains the most common treatment.

External beam RT (or teletherapy)

External beam RT is given using a Linac. The treatment is given in divided doses, known as fractions, on a daily or every-other-day basis to the breast, chest wall and sometimes to associated lymph nodes. It is recommended that treatment begins about 1 month after chemotherapy has finished, or 1 month to 6 weeks after the surgery if no chemotherapy is given.

Most breast treatment plans in the UK are made in a single two-dimensional (2D) plane which, when translated into the three-dimensional RT treatment, can lead to variations in radiation dose across the breast. In many centres across the UK, greater accuracy of planning is achieved using 3D planning of the breast, incorporating information on the 3D shape of the breast and the chest wall, for example using a computerised tomography (CT) scan (Yarnold 2002;Coles *et al.*, 2005b).

Brachytherapy

Brachytherapy is the use of radioactive material placed within, or near to, the area of the tumour. In the past, empty catheters were placed into the breast by a radiotherapist whilst the patient was anaesthetised. Two systems are used to deliver the radiation. One option was for the iridium wires to be inserted into the catheters manually by the radiotherapist (manual afterloading). The amount of radioactivity was usually low, and the implants would take several days to deliver the required dose of radiation. For the safety of staff and other patients, the woman was nursed in a lead-lined room and behind lead shields to minimise exposure to others. The radioactive implants remained in place until the calculated dose of radiation had been given (usually a few days) and would be removed by a radiotherapist along with the inert tubes. This method is largely being phased out because of the patient's required duration of stay and the safety issues to both staff and patients.

The second, and more widely employed, method is using iridium wire, which has a higher level of activity, afterloaded into the inert catheters by a remote-controlled machine. These treatments take a matter of minutes, but have to be repeated in a daily, fractionated way. Using this remote afterloading machine, the radioactive sources are withdrawn mechanically if the nurse or doctor wishes to enter the room, so there is no exposure to staff.

Intra-operative RT

Although not used in the UK at present, the delivery of intra-operative RT, during the wide local excision procedure, using a portable electron beam device, has become an exciting and innovative way of delivering RT to the breast. This technique has the advantage of focusing RT to a selected part of the breast and avoiding outpatient visits to the RT department for external beam fractions of radiation. However, it can have the disadvantage that the definitive resection margins around the tumour are not known when the radiation is delivered (Coles *et al.*, 2005b).

Although not used in the UK yet, Veronesi *et al.* (2001) have considerable experience of using electron intra-operative therapy or ELIOT and describe the process and outcome in 86 women. A single fraction of 3–9 MeV electrons is delivered using a perspex applicator, the chest wall is shielded and the skin of the breast is pulled out of the radiation field, thus reducing considerably the skin dose (Veronesi *et al.*, 2001). The long-term side effects appear favourable (Orrechia *et al.*, 2006).

Targeted intra-operative radiotherapy (Targit) is currently being evaluated at various RT units across the UK, the USA, Australia and Europe. Targit uses a portable 50-kV photon beam emitting device that has been designed to deliver RT to the tumour bed in a single treatment. This RT machine has a spherical applicator (a little like a lollypop), which delivers RT directly into the wide local excision cavity at the time of surgery, thus negating the need for external beam RT. These methods capitalise on the phenomena of the RT energy falling off from the source (the inverse square law), and so the surrounding normal tissues do not get radiation scatter, making it a relatively safe treatment to deliver (2006).

Another method of delivering partial breast brachytherapy is the MammoSite balloon breast brachytherapy catheter. This can be placed into the tumour cavity, either at the time of the surgery, or afterwards under local anaesthetic. The balloon is inflated with saline and a contrast medium and connected to a brachytherapy source which then delivers the required dose of RT (Keisch *et al.*, 2003). There has been some concern about the conformance of the balloon to the tumour cavity in some patients, and several patients had to have the balloon removed, and the RT source removed. Research continues to evaluate this technique of delivering whole and partial breast irradiation, as this method offers an alternative to women being treated for small, low-risk breast cancers (Coles *et al.*, 2005b).

Planning RT

The patient's initial visit to the RT department will involve an accurate plan being made of where the RT is to be given. The first part of this process is to position the patient in a way that is comfortable and also reproducible. The patient's arm is usually moved up (abducted) so it is clear of the breast area. In most centres, the patient is asked to hold onto a fixed point, often attached to the treatment couch, and sometimes a pole, to keep her arm in the same position from day to day. Imaging is taken to check the positioning of the patient. This can be X-rays or a CT. The RT plan is based on images taken from the CT or an X-ray machine linked to an image intensifier called a 'simulator', and an outline of the shape of the patient's chest. A CT scan will add 3D information, such as the thickness of the chest wall and the position of underlying lung and heart.

Marks are made on the patient's skin that will later be used to ensure that the treatment beam is accurately directed at the precise area required, avoiding as much as possible the delicate structures of the lung, the left anterior ascending coronary artery and the heart. These lines are of semi-permanent pen. Additional permanent 'tattoos' are also made, from a small drop of indian ink introduced under the skin with a small-bore needle. These pin-prick tattoos provide a permanent record of the location of the RT on the patient. The procedure is quick and painless, but the need for these marks introduces yet another assault on the patient's body image that can be very difficult. The necessity for these tattoos needs to be explained to the patient with care and sensitivity ahead of the simulator appointment so that she is prepared.

During planning, the patient will be asked to keep quite still, with her arm up. A good range of arm movement is essential after axillary surgery and, if this has not been achieved, the patient should be referred back to the physiotherapist for more individualised arm exercises. She will remain supine during her treatment. Clear communication is of paramount importance as this will usually be the first time a patient is introduced to the RT department. Being surrounded by large and complicated machinery can be very daunting, and then having to keep still for such a long period of time can make some patients very anxious.

Rarely, when treating with external beam RT, partial volumes of the breast may be irradiated if the patient had a very low-grade invasive breast cancer or ductal carcinoma in situ (DCIS). If the patient has undergone a wide local excision of her tumour, the whole breast will be treated, and sometimes, a 'boost' of radiation to the tumour bed is given. The location of the boost is defined by using the surgical scar as a guide. For patients who need RT to the chest wall following a mastectomy, the chest wall is the target, and a boost is not usually required. Some primary breast tumours which have not been removed are visible to the naked eye, or their dimensions can be defined with mammogram, ultrasound and occasionally magnetic resonance (MR). If the patient has received primary chemotherapy, a titanium clip is sometimes inserted into the breast at the time of the diagnostic biopsy, or the definitive surgery to locate the tumour site for the radiotherapist. Depending on the surgical clearance of the axilla and the lymph node involvement, the axillary lymph nodes and supraclavicular nodes may also be treated. There has been some discussion about the treatment of the axilla with RT because of the rare but serious complication of brachial nerve damage or plexopathy (Maher, 1995; Bates and Evans, 1995) and an increased risk of lymphoedema. There is no consensus as to whether or not the axilla should be routinely treated, although standardisation of what areas of the breast and loco-regional nodes are to be irradiated is under consideration. It is clear that irradiation of the axillary nodes can increase the risk of lymphoedema, particularly if a number of axillary lymph nodes have been dissected (Hayes *et al.*, 2008).

For each patient, the volume of tissue to be irradiated is assessed by the radiotherapist and the therapy radiographer. For treatment to the breast, it is usual to use two directions of radiation beam or fields, striking the breast tangentially, from opposite directions, so that the beams intersect within the breast. This gives the most radiation to the tumour or the tumour bed whilst sparing the skin and normal tissues as much as possible. Since the chest wall is curved, and radiation travels in straight lines, it is inevitable that the ribs and a small amount of the lung are treated. When treating the left side, where the heart lies just below the chest wall, it is especially important to minimise radiation dose to the heart. If the woman has undergone a wide local excision, a boost of RT may be given to the site of the tumour or the tumour bed after the whole breast has been treated. Treating the tumour bed will usually be by a single small-electron beam which can be produced from most Linacs. The radiation physics department will be involved with all treatment plans. Fig. 9.2 shows a breast treatment plan. Note the different isodoses, or concentrations of radiation, throughout the breast shown by the separate contours. This plan shows how effectively the normal tissues can be spared by accurate and careful planning.

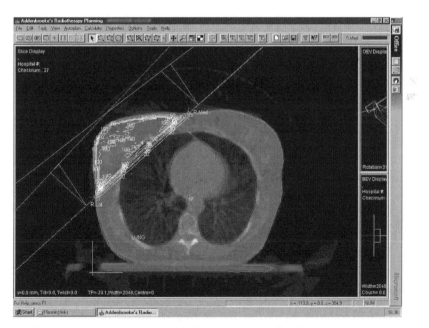

Fig. 9.2   A breast treatment plan. Printed with kind permission of Nikki Twyman, Radiation Physicist, Addenbrooke's NHS Trust.

Intensity-modulated RT

It has long been recognised that treating the breast with radiation is challenging. The breast is a three-dimensional structure, and the effect of surgery, the close relation of the breast to the heart (in left-sided tumours) and the lung all need to be taken into account when planning and delivering RT. In addition, the energy levels across a radiation field fluctuate, which further complicates the treatment levels across the breast and can lead to variation in dose or dose inhomogeneity. To compensate for this variation and to improve dose homogeneity, the technique intensity modulated RT or IMRT has been used. One way to achieve IMRT is to use a multi-leaf collimator (MLC). The MLC is a mechanism of metal leaves that is able to give extra RT to the areas of the breast that need the boost and less to areas that do not need the additional RT.

Other methods of achieving IMRT include inverse planned (by computer) and forward planned (by planner) RT and three-dimensional planning using computed tomography (CT) and MR imaging. All these methods aim to improve dose accuracy and reduce normal tissue toxicity (Coles *et al.* 2005b).

Delivering RT treatment

Once simulated, the patient is expected to adopt the exact position each time she is treated. Laser lines projected from the walls of the Linac room onto the patient are aligned with the tattoos and semi-permanent ink marks to ensure that the positioning is accurate throughout the weeks of treatment.

After the machine is positioned each time the patient is treated, she is left alone in the treatment room. The radiographers do watch the patient on CCTV, but the patient cannot see them. This can be quite frightening for some patients who have been diagnosed with a serious condition and then find themselves isolated whilst they receive the RT – yet another unknown experience. Sometimes music is left on in the treatment room, making the solitude easier, and the radiographers who operate the machinery have an audio link with the patient. Clear explanation of the procedure and the approximate time the patient is left alone can help to relieve her anxiety. For a two-field treatment to the breast alone, the whole treatment lasts only about 10 minutes, including setting-up the patient, so the patient is alone in the room for only 1 or 2 minutes at a time. Fig. 9.3 shows a Linac RT machine.

RT dose

Across the UK, there used to be considerable variation between radiotherapists about the dose and number of fractions of RT that should be given to the patient (Yarnold *et al.*, 1995). Generally, treatment fractions were given at 2.0 gray per day in 25 fractions over 5 weeks, or as 2.67 gray per day in 15 fractions over 3 weeks. A national trial, called START, (UK Standardisation of Breast RT) has studied and recently reported that a radiation schedule delivering 40 Gy in 15 fractions seems to offer equivalent rates of regional control and late adverse effects as the regime of 50 Gy in 25 fractions (Bentzen *et al.*, 2008). As there is a great pressure on radiotherapists to treat patients as soon as they optimally can, then the hypofractionation regimen using 40 Gy in 15 fractions may be the way forward (Bentzen *et al.*, 2008).

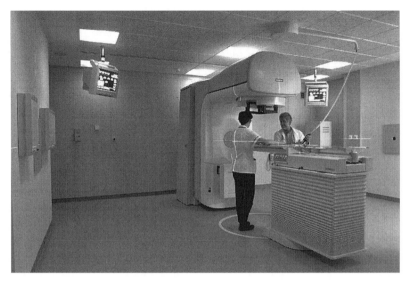

Fig. 9.3   A Linac RT machine. Reproduced with kind permission of the Addenbrooke's NHS Trust Photographic Department.

GENERAL NURSING CARE FOR A PATIENT UNDERGOING RT

Patients who need RT as part of their treatment for breast cancer can have significant concerns about this treatment. They may worry about being badly burned or of being very unwell, thinking that the radiation is a systemic and not a local treatment. Some patients confuse the side effects of chemotherapy with RT and believe that they will lose their hair and be nauseated.

Most people never see a RT machine until they are being treated, so any nursing care should be directed at helping the patient understand the unknown and to support them through their treatment. Sometimes, for patients, attendance at a RT unit can mark the end of the fairly intensive support they will have received during the chemotherapy, and they should be encouraged to call their breast care nurse or treatment radiographer if they are feeling isolated. For many patients who have had adjuvant chemotherapy, RT is not as difficult, but they find that they are still recovering from the physical side effects of their chemotherapy. In reality, RT is painless and quick once the planning has taken place and, for most women, the only acute side effects they experience are fatigue and some skin sensitivity. Other side effects do occur, but these are rare, and the severity of such effects depends on the dose of radiation, the individual's tissue sensitivity and the treatment site. If the patient knows what sort of side effects to expect, and that there are measures to alleviate them, she is usually able to cope much better (Ream and Richardson, 1996). Having to attend for daily or every-other-day RT may cause some problems for a mother or for someone who has a particularly demanding job.

Although most RT centres are working to full capacity, it is often possible for a patient's treatment to be scheduled for early in the morning or later in the day to help her organise her life better, and this should be discussed with the treatment radiographers. Each patient needs to be assessed and cared for as an individual. Patients are seen regularly throughout their treatment by the clinician and the radiographers, so this can be an opportunity to evaluate how things are going as well as assessing the physical effects of the RT. Most patients find that RT is not as bad as they were expecting, and meeting other patients that are going through the same treatment can help the individual cope better with her fears and anxieties.

All patients who receive RT should be assessed before, during and after their treatment. The condition of their skin, risk factors including the technique, volume and dose of RT, chemo-sensitising drugs and the area receiving RT should all be taken into account. Skin-care advice should be given to the patient during their treatment. The patient should be encouraged to use aqueous cream or E45 cream when RT commences to delay the onset of skin erythema. Patients should be encouraged to wash or shower their skin during treatment, although it is important to use tepid water and mild soap, rinsing thoroughly and patting the area with a soft, clean towel. Patients should wear loose-fitting, cotton clothing next to the treated area, and this clothing should be washed using a mild detergent. Bras should be soft but supportive and not underwired. Towards the end of treatment, some women may find that they stop wearing their bra and choose to wear a crop top or a cotton tee shirt. No adhesive tape should be used in the treatment area, and perfumed products such as soap or deodorant should not be used in the treatment area once RT has started. Advice should be given concerning the importance of avoiding swimming in chlorinated water during treatment and also of avoiding extremes of temperature.

Hair follicles and sweat glands are radiosensitive due to their high rate of growth. For this reason, patients who receive axillary RT will lose underarm hair on the treated side and may temporarily stop sweating from that axilla, although the sweat glands usually recover after the treatment. Axillary hair does not normally grow back, which can be seen as an advantage but, if the patient was not expecting this non-regrowth of axillary hair, she may feel concerned.

For women who have undergone a mastectomy, it is recommended that the permanent breast prosthesis is fitted between 4 and 6 weeks after RT, as long as the woman's skin has healed from the RT. For the 'stick-on' type prosthesis, a longer period of time is required to ensure that the skin is completely healed. Careful assessment of the woman's skin will need to be made by the prosthetic fitter, as some women take longer to heal than others.

When receiving RT, the treatment area should not be exposed to full sunlight and, after treatment, the patient should be advised to not expose the treatment area to sunlight until it has completely healed. If, after several months the patient wishes to sunbathe, she should use a high-factor sun cream on the treated area and should not continue to sunbathe if the area becomes red or sore. The skin will stay sensitive to the sun for at least 1 year post-treatment, and caution in future years may need to be taken.

Fatigue and the inability to function as they would wish is very common among patients who have cancer, and this tiredness may be compounded by receiving a course of RT (Poirier, 2007). There may be many practical reasons why RT makes the patient tired.

- Recovering from surgery;
- Receiving concurrent chemotherapy;
- Pain;
- Frequency of visits to the hospital;
- Having to continue parenting or another caring role.

In her research, Faithfull (1998) found that patients attending for RT became very tired. She speculated that this fatigue may be related to the accumulation of metabolites and to cell destruction from tissue damage caused by the radiation. Encouraging the patient to take naps during her treatment can help, and a pre-treatment explanation will help to prepare the woman for this side effect. Some negotiation of treatment times may be possible, although this will depend on the workload of that patient's RT centre.

Early effects of RT to the breast

Skin reactions

The skin is composed of several layers of cells, the normal mature cells which are constantly shed from the skin surface and new cells from the basal layer of the epidermis, which move up to replace the mature cells. This continuous cell renewal explains why skin is radiosensitive. Although the skin is not often the primary target, the RT beams must pass through the skin to treat the underlying breast or chest wall.

Erythema, or a reddening of the skin, may be the only manifestation of mild radiation sensitivity for some women, and may develop 2–3 weeks after RT treatment has started. In some women, if their skin is particularly sensitive, the erythema may progress to itching and dry desquamation, where there is scaly loss of some of the epidermal layer, or moist desquamation, where there is loss of the entire epidermal layer, producing an ulcer. This is more common where skin folds meet, such as the inframammary fold beneath the breast.

The College of Radiographers has produced guidelines on the assessment of skin reactions and how to care for them (Glean *et al.*, 2000). These guidelines suggest that the patient is assessed for her potential to develop skin reactions using an approved assessment tool before RT starts. The guidelines make the point that intrinsic factors may make reactions to RT worse, such as age, infection, and co-existing disease. Extrinsic factors, such as treatment dose, fractionation, adjuvant chemotherapy, site of treatment and energy used, would also affect how patients react to radiation. Even more complicated is the fact that the same amount of radiation given in the same way can cause completely different skin reactions in different women. Skin sensitivity to radiation differs across the population and cannot be routinely tested for at the moment (Burnet *et al.*, 1998). For all these reasons, the patient should be reviewed regularly whilst on treatment. For the individual, assessment is designed to give appropriate care for her individual reaction. For clinical trials, assessment of normal tissue effects is of great importance, and an agreed skin-reaction scoring scale should be used, such as that produced by the Radiation Oncology Group Criteria (RTOG/EORTC) (Cox *et al.*, 1995) or the *Standard Framework/Guide for Patients Receiving RT* (2002).

Specific nursing care for a patient undergoing RT

Skin care

Radiation skin reactions can occur in a large number of patients undergoing RT, and there is little evidence to support a particular skin-care regime (Porock and Kristjanson, 1999). The following general recommendations are based on guidelines from the College of Radiographers (Glean *et al.*, 2000) and on the *Best Practice Statement* from NHS Quality Improvement, Scotland (2010).

Normal tissue reactions are being evaluated in a more scientific way, particularly as new regimens of RT are being developed and trialled. Several scoring systems to assess RT reactions are available. The simplest scoring system is to use a photographic evaluation of the shape of the breast at a given time after the RT. Others include the LENT SOMA system (Late Effects on Normal Tissue, Subjective, Objective, Management and Analytical), RTOG/EORTC or the CTCAE scale (Common Terminology Criteria for Adverse Events).

Dry desquamation can be divided into two categories – faint or dull erythema which can be itchy and uncomfortable, but responds well to aqueous cream and the application of hydrogel sheets, and tender or bright erythema, which responds well to aqueous cream and a limited, prescribed course of hydrocortisone cream 1%. Hydrocortisone cream must be used sparingly and should be discontinued if there is a likelihood of a fungal infection developing or if the skin breaks down.

If moist cell desquamation develops, RT may be interrupted to allow healing, although this is not usually necessary. The moist areas can be dressed using a hydrogel, hydrocolloid or an alginate dressing. If the area becomes infected, a swab should be taken and appropriate antibiotics prescribed. After the RT has been given, healing may be slow but is usually complete and leaves minimal evidence of the acute damage, except for pigmentation or telangiectasia. Telangiectasia is caused by the formation of tiny capillaries in the skin and has no physical consequence apart from the change in appearance of the treated area.

Other immediate problems from radiation may be itchiness of the breast that continues after the RT has finished, and breast lymphoedema, which is being seen much more frequently in lymphoedema clinics. Keeping the skin of the breast well moisturised with aqueous cream can help relieve the itchiness and irritation, as can the use of hydrogel dressings. For breast lymphoedema, referral to a lymphoedema clinic can provide the patient with advice on lymphatic massage or manual lymph drainage (MLD), and the importance of a well-fitted bra is obvious.

Late changes of RT to the breast

The use of modern RT equipment has reduced the incidence of late skin changes to the breast (Sainsbury et al., 2000). These changes can include some thickening or scarring of the breast tissue and some breast shrinkage and telangiectasia.

Despite trying to avoid the lung tissue, some may be treated by radiation. Damage to the lung tissue by radiation or radiation pneumonitis may have two components. Acute inflammation, with cough, can occur during or just after a course of RT, but is uncommon with RT for breast cancer. It is the result of inflammation of the alveolar wall plus an accumulation of exudate in the alveolar air space, similar to pneumonia. Later changes can lead to fibrosis of the lung tissue and thickening of the pleura. Such changes reduce respiratory function in the area treated, but the degree of disability is related to the amount and condition of the remaining lung tissue. It is rarely noticeable by the patient after breast RT, although may be seen on subsequent scans.

Damage to the myocardium and the coronary arteries have been recognised as a serious late change caused by RT to the left side of the chest wall or the left breast (Mangar et al., 2002). With the increased use of anthracycline and taxane chemotherapy, which can damage the myocardium, cardiac tolerance can be further compromised. Clinicians are aware of this problem and now make every effort to individualise treatment planning to reduce the amount of heart tissue that is irradiated in order to minimise cardiac toxicity.

The ribs are often treated by adjuvant RT as they fall within the treatment field. There can be immediate rib tenderness and, over time, the ribs can become more brittle and susceptible to pathological fracture. This is a rare complication.

Swelling of the arm and breast can be caused by RT, due to fibrosis of the lymphatic channels. This risk of lymphoedema is much increased if the patient has undergone surgery to the lymph nodes and then receives RT to the same area. For more detail on care of lymphoedema, see Chapter 11.

Nursing care of patients treated with brachytherapy

The patient is isolated when the radioactive implants are in situ but will be able to have visitors after the daily fraction has been given, and this should be explained to her before she embarks on her treatment. The patient should be prepared for the isolation of a single room by being advised to bring in books and other distractions to help pass the time. A television is usually available in the treatment room. Sensitive emotional support is essential as the patient is not only coping with breast cancer, but also this time away from normal life may provide her with time to reflect on her situation and to ponder her future. When with the patient, the nurse should make a little time to listen to her concerns and be aware that this is an emotional and reflective time for the woman.

Any sign of a wound infection should be reported to the clinician in charge of the patient's care so that antibiotics may be prescribed. Any pain or discomfort should be assessed and treated with appropriate analgesia. Inactivity may cause associated problems of the risk of thrombo-embolic events. The patient should be encouraged to drink plenty of fluids, and she may be given an anti-coagulation therapy and TED (thrombo-embolic deterrent) stockings to wear in order to prevent the formation of deep vein thrombosis.

Safe practice with RT

Significant known hazards are associated with the insertion and removal of radioactive sources and working around radioactive substances, but radiation protection is not within the remit of this chapter. *The Ionising Radiation (Medical Exposure) Regulations* (HMSO, 2000) stipulate regulations on which local radiation protection policies should be written. These regulations apply to patients who are exposed to radiation, and any other individual who might come into contact with radiation as part of health-screening programmes, occupational health surveillance, research or medico-legal procedures (HMSO, 2000). All staff working in areas where there is radiation have a responsibility to themselves, their colleagues and their patients to be aware of these regulations and any other local policies that their hospital trust follows, and should practise strictly according to them.

Safety concerns regarding brachytherapy

For any staff caring for an inpatient with radioactive implants, all be it for a very restricted time, there are three watch words to bear in mind: *time, distance and shielding* (Langmack, 1998). The nursing care of the patient who is receiving brachytherapy should be carefully planned before going into the patients' room so as to avoid the few minutes per day when the fractionated, high-dose rate RT is given. The intensity of the radiation reduces as the distance from the radiation source increases, according to the inverse square law. This means that, if a nurse doubles her distance from the patient, she will reduce her radiation exposure to a quarter. The room in which the patient is cared for is usually lead-lined, and movable lead shields are placed in front of the patient for added staff protection. The area where someone is being treated with RT should be marked very carefully with internationally recognised radiation symbols, and any visitors should also be made aware. The area should be avoided by pregnant woman, women who think they may be pregnant and young children. Other adults will be allowed to visit after the daily fraction has been given.

TREATMENT OF RECURRENT AND METASTATIC BREAST CANCER

RT has a very large part to play in the palliation and control of metastatic breast cancer and is generally well tolerated. When used on its own or in conjunction with other treatment modalities, RT can do much to enhance the quality of life of the patient (Oliver, 1996). External beam RT can be very effective when treating local-regional disease providing that a substantial dose has not been previously given to the chest wall, remaining breast tissue or supraclavicular nodes as part of the original local treatment. RT given to fungating lesions can help to reduce the tumour bulk, reducing the amount of dying tissue and reducing the possibility for infection and odour (Regnard and Tempest, 1998). Painful bone disease can be treated very effectively using standard regimes of 30 Gy in ten fractions, 20 Gy in five fractions or simply a single fraction can reduce pain and promote calcification of the affected area of bone, so preventing unnecessary fractures (Price *et al.*, 1986). If a bone has been stabilised by surgery, RT can re-enforce the bone around the fixation. RT can be given as an emergency treatment for spinal cord metastases and, in conjunction with steroids, can be very effective (White *et al.* 2008). RT may also give considerable relief from pain in other organs, e.g. liver, with a minimum of side effects. Because fewer fractions of RT are given than with a curative dose, there is less risk of skin side effects such as erythema, and dry and moist cell desquamation.

Single brain lesions can be treated very effectively with specialised stereotactic RT given in a single high-dose treatment (known as radiosurgery) which may necessitate an overnight stay for the patient or may be given as an outpatient visit. Steroid pre-medication and continual cover for a few days after should be administered (1996). Adequate treatment of solitary cerebral metastasis is particularly important when a patient's systemic disease is otherwise controlled. Whole-brain prophylactic irradiation is particularly useful when treating the patient with multiple brain metastases.

Generally, RT treatment given in these circumstances is well tolerated and provides an effective treatment without compromising the patients' quality of life too much.

THE FUTURE

As already discussed, RT resources are greatly stretched as the treatments for cancer become more effective and complicated. The pressure on RT departments to treat more patients more quickly is evident, and this is very pertinent to the high number of breast cancer patients who are treated with RT. To optimise RT accuracy, research is being undertaken to refine the way that RT is given.

The targeting of RT to the tumour bed continues to provide a challenge to the clinician and physicist and has certainly improved with the use of clips, CT ultrasound and MR. Research into this particular area will continue.

Dose delivery and accuracy is constantly being evaluated. The use of IMRT planning and the development of newer RT equipment such as the tomotherapy machine will start to have an impact on improving the way RT is given to the patient with breast cancer.

An individual's reaction to radiation may have a genetic basis. If some patients have an intrinsic sensitivity or tolerance to RT, it may be that their RT can be individualised to suit their genetic makeup (Barnett *et al.*, 2009).

CONCLUSION

It is important for nurses to understand that RT is a crucial component of many patients' treatment for breast cancer. It is an ever-developing treatment modality, and its effectiveness continues to be proven. This chapter aims to make clear why and when RT is used and to clarify the needs of the patient undergoing this treatment. Caring for and supporting the patient with breast cancer undergoing RT is exciting and challenging, and it is hoped that this chapter will help to facilitate their care.

REFERENCES

Auchter RM, Lamond JP, Alexander E *et al.* (1996) A multi institutional outcome and prognostic factor analysis of radiosurgery for resectable single brain metastasis. *International Journal of Radiation Oncology, Biology and Physics* 35(1): 27–35.

Barnett GC, West CML, Dunning AM *et al.* (2009) Normal tissue reactions to radiotherapy: towards tailoring treatment dose by genotype. *Nature Reviews Cancer* 1–9.

Bartelink H, Horiot J-C, Poortmans P *et al.* (2001) Recurrence rates after treatment of breast cancer with standard RT with or without additional radiation. *New England Journal of Medicine* 345: 1378–1387.

Bates T and Evans RG (1995) *Report of the Independent Review Commissioned by the Royal College of Radiologists into Brachial Plexus Neuropathy following RT for Breast Cancer.* London: Royal College of Radiologists.

Bentzen SM, Agrawal RK, Aird EG *et al.* (2008) The UK Standardisation of Breast RT (START) Trial B of RT hypofractionation for the treatment of early breast cancer: a randomised trail. *The Lancet* 372(9634): 203–204.

Burnet NG, Johansen J, Turesson I, Nyman J and Peacock JH (1998) Describing patients' normal tissue reactions: concerning the possibility of individualising RT dose prescriptions based on potential predictive assays of normal tissue radiosensitivity. Steering Committee of the BioMed2 European Union Concerted Action Programme on the Development of Predictive Tests of Normal Tissue Response to Radiation Therapy. *International Journal of Cancer* 79: 606–613.

Coles CE, Moody AM, Wilson CB and Burnet NG (2005a) Reduction of RT-induced late complications in early breast cancer: the role of intensity modulated radiation therapy and partial breast irradiation. Part I – normal tissue complications. *Clinical Oncology (Royal College of Radiologists)* 17(1): 16–24.

Coles CE, Moody AM, Wilson CB and Burnet NG (2005b) Reduction of RT-induced late complications in early breast cancer: the role of intensity modulated radiation therapy and partial breast irradiation. Part II – Radiotherapy strategies to reduce radiation-induced late effects *Clinical Oncology (Royal College of Radiologists)* 17(2): 98–110.

Cox J, Stetz J and Pajak T (1995) Toxicity criteria of the radiation therapy oncology group (RTOG) and the European Organisation for Research and Treatment of Cancer (EORTC). *International Journal of Radiation Oncology Biology Physics* 31(5): 1341–1346.

Faithfull S (1998) Fatigue in patients receiving RT. *Professional Nurse* 13(7): 459–461.

Fisher B, Anderson S, Bryant J *et al.* (2002). Twenty year follow up of a randomised trial comparing total mastectomy, lumpectomy and lumpectomy plus irradiation for the treatment of invasive breast cancer. *New England Journal of Medicine* 347: 1233–1241.

Gebski V, Lagleva M, Keech A, Simes J and Langlands AO (2006) Survival effects of post mastectomy adjuvant RT using biologically equivalent doses; a clinical perspective. *Journal of the National Cancer Institute* 98: 26–38.

Glean E, Edwards S, Faithful S *et al.* (2000) Intervention for acute RT induced skin reactions in cancer patients: the development of a clinical guideline recommended for use by the College of Radiographers. *Journal of Radiotherapy in Practice* 2(2): 75–84.

Hall EJ and Cox JD (1994) Physical and biologic basis of radiation therapy. In: Cox JD (ed) *Moss's Radiation Oncology: Rationale, Technique, Results*, 7th edn. St. Louis: Mosby-Yearbook pp. 3–66.

Hayes SB, Freedman GM, Li T, Anderson PR and Ross E (2008) Does axillary boost increase lymphedema compared with supraclavicular radiation alone after breast conservation? *International Journal of Radiation Oncology, Biology and Physics* 72(5): 1449–1455.

Hilley C, Tutt A, Torres M and Palimieri C (2008) Adjuvant RT for breast cancer. *British Medical Journal* 337a: 2843.

HMSO (2000) *The Ionising Radiations (Medical Exposure) Regulations* No. 1059, London: HMSO.

Keisch M, Vicini F, Kuske RR *et al.* (2003) Initial clinical experience with the MammoSite breast brachytherapy applicator in women with early stage breast cancer treated with breast-conserving therapy. *International Journal of Radiation Oncology, Biology and Physics* 55: 289–293.

Langmack KA (1998) Factors influencing occupational radiation doses to brachytherapy nurses. *Radiography* 4: 141–146.

Maher EJ (1995) *Management of Adverse Effects following Breast Radiotherapy*. London: Maher Committee, Royal College of Radiologists.

Mangar S, Kumar S, Shentall G, Kirby M and Massey J (2002) Assessment of cardiac volume in tangential irradiation to the chest wall following mastectomy. Abstract for IPEM/RCR meeting, London: Breast Cancer: Advances in RT Planning and Treatment. *Clinical Oncology (Royal College of Radiologists)* 14: 174–177.

NHS Quality Improvement Scotland (2010) *Best Practice Statement: Skincare of Patients Receiving Radiotherapy*. Available: http://www.nhshealthquality.org.

Oliver G (1996) RT for Breast Cancer. In: Denton S (ed.) *Breast Cancer Nursing*. London: Chapman and Hall.

Orrechia R, Luini A, Veronesi P *et al.* (2006) Electron intraoperative treatment in patients with early stage breast cancer: data update. *Expert Review of Anticancer Therapy* 6(4): 605–611.

Overgaard M, Hansen PS, Overgaard J *et al.* (1997) Postoperative RT in high-risk premenopausal women with breast cancer who receive adjuvant chemotherapy. Danish Breast Cancer Cooperative Group 82b Trial. *New England Journal of Medicine* 337(14): 949–955.

Poirier P. (2007) Factors affecting performance of usual activities during radiation therapy. *Oncology Nursing Forum* 34(4): 827–834

Porock D and Kristjanson L (1999) Skin reactions during RT for breast cancer: the use and impact of topical agents and dressing. *European Journal of Cancer Care* 8(3): 143–153.

Price P, Hoskin PJ, Easton D, Austin D, Palmer SG and Yarnold JR (1986) Prospective randomised trial of single and multifraction RT schedules in the treatment of painful bony metastases *Radiation Oncology* 4: 247–255.

Ream E and Richardson A (1996) The role of information in patients' adaptation to chemotherapy and RT: a review of the literature. *European Journal of Cancer Care* 5: 131–13.

Regnard CFB and Tempest S (1998) *A Guide to Symptom Relief in Advanced Disease*. Cheshire: Hochland and Hochland.

Sainsbury JR, Anderson TJ and Morgan DA (2000) Breast cancer. In: Dixon JM (ed.) *ABC of Breast Diseases*. London: BMJ Publishing Group.

Souhami R and Tobias J (1995) *Cancer and its Management*, 2nd edn. Oxford: Blackwell Scientific Publications.

START Trialists Group (2008). The UK Standardisation of Breast RT (START) Trial B of RT Hypofractionation for the Treatment of Early Breast Cancer: a randomised trial. *The Lancet* 371: 1098–107.

Vaidya JS, Baum M, Tobias JS *et al.* (2001) Targeted Intraoperative RT (Targit): an innovative method of treatment for early breast cancer. *Annals of Oncology* 2: 1075–1080.

Verosesi U, Orrechia R, Luini A *et al.* (2001) A preliminary report on intraoperative RT (IORT) in limited-stage breast cancers that are conservatively treated. *European Journal of Cancer* 37: 2178–2183.

White BD, Stirling AJ, Paterson E *et al.* (2008) Diagnosis of patients at risk of or with metastatic spinal cord compression: a summary of NICE guidance. *British Medical Journal* 337: 1349–1352.

Yarnold JR (2002) Breast cancer: improvements in treatment planning and dosimetry. Abstract for IPEM/RCR Meeting, London: Breast Cancer: Advances in RT Planning and Treatment. *Clinical Oncology (Royal College of Radiologists)* 14: 174–177.

Yarnold JR, Price P and Steel GG (1995) Treatment of early breast cancer in the United Kingdom: RT Fractionation Practices. *Clinical Oncology (Royal College of Radiologists)* 5: 330–332.

10   Endocrine Treatment for Breast Cancer

Deborah Fenlon and Kay Townsend

INTRODUCTION

Women spend much of their lives aware of the rhythm and influences of their hormonal fluctuations. In today's society, it is customary to blame hormones for women's actions and behaviours, as if there were no other influences in their lives; if they are tired or irritable, their hormones are to blame, rather than stress, overwork, lack of sleep or any other possibilities. If men put on weight, it may be explained by decreased activity or increased calorific intake. If women put on weight, then it must be their hormones. Actual information about the way in which hormones work and their effects in the body is sadly lacking and inevitably, when breast cancer occurs, the same beliefs and attitudes will apply. Hormone replacement therapy (HRT) is often blamed for the occurrence of breast cancer, even if the woman has only been taking it for a few months. Many women automatically attribute weight gain to tamoxifen, irrespective of any other lifestyle changes that take place after breast cancer.

Conversely, health-care professionals frequently underestimate the impact that hormone therapies might have on an individual with breast cancer. For example, Fellowes *et al.* (2001) showed that 99% of women had side effects from treatment with tamoxifen or goserilin, but that only 89% were recorded in the medical notes.

It is important, therefore, that nurses and health-care professionals are adequately informed about hormonal treatments and their effects so that they can help women to understand the changes that they observe in their bodies after breast cancer treatment. Proper understanding can help women to make appropriate choices about the treatments they accept and will affect how they cope with any side effects from these treatments.

It will be clear to anyone working in this field that breast cancer is a complex disease. Nowhere is this more apparent than when considering hormonal manipulation as a treatment for breast cancer. This means that logical answers are not always the correct ones and that assumptions cannot be made about the way in which breast cancers will respond to the use of hormones. When answering patients' questions in relation to hormones, we must look to the findings of clinical trials. Where trial data are not available, then we can only say that we do not know the answer, rather than attempting to extrapolate from what is known.

Breast Cancer Nursing Care and Management, Second Edition, Edited by Victoria Harmer
© 2011 by Blackwell Publishing Ltd.

THE ROLE OF HORMONES IN THE EVOLUTION OF BREAST CANCER

The development of cancers such as breast cancer can be said to be an evolutionary one (Greaves, 2000), in that there are a number of barriers that cells need to overcome before they are able to grow and spread around the body. It is unlikely that a single genetic mutation will allow a cell to overcome all these barriers, and so there must be a succession of mutations enabling cell populations to evolve until they are ultimately able to establish as a cancer. This process is likely to take many years. Once a cancer has been detected and treated, there is no reason to assume that evolution does not continue. On the contrary, in the face of treatments that provide further barriers, it is more likely that further evolution will be stimulated. As a consequence, cancers that initially respond to hormone treatments may change and become resistant to that treatment. Moreover, it is possible that the cancer may evolve to the point where it can use the hormone as a stimulus for growth. Evidence for this apparently contrary situation comes from clinical practice, where it is occasionally seen that a breast tumour will shrink after a hormone treatment is withdrawn.

Key point

These principles (that cancer cells mutate to overcome barriers to growth, including a change in response to hormones) should be borne in mind when considering the use of hormone treatments. In practice, they mean that no assumptions can be made about the safety or efficacy of any hormone in the context of breast cancer. However, the reverse is also true – that assumptions cannot be made that hormones are not safe or that they will not be effective.

HORMONES AND THE RISK OF BREAST CANCER

It has been known for more than 100 years that oestrogen has an important role in breast cancer (Beatson, 1896), and oestrogen receptors were discovered in the 1960s (Jensen and Jacobson, 1962). Breast cancer is nearly always an adult tumour, and it becomes more common in older age; 80% of women diagnosed with breast cancer will be over 50 years old at the time of diagnosis (Cancer Research UK, 2006). This is logical as most of the risk factors for breast cancer are related to the amount of oestrogen that the body is exposed to during a lifetime (see Table 10.1). If breast cancer occurs at a young age, this points to early genetic damage, either due to an inherited mutation (Easton *et al.*, 1993) or to exposure to other agents that cause genetic damage, such as radiation (John and Kelsey, 1993). Breast cancer is not exclusively a disease of women, but it is rare in men.

Table 10.1 Oestrogen-related risk factors for breast cancer.

Risk factor	Source
Early menarche	Brinton *et al.*, 1988
Late age at first pregnancy or no pregnancies	Kelsey *et al.*, 1993
Late menopause and use of oral oestrogens (contraceptive pill or HRT)	Schairer *et al.*, 2000
Dietary factors and obesity	Mezzetti *et al.*, 1998

Dietary factors and obesity also increase the risk of breast cancer (Mezzetti *et al.*, 1998), but these can be argued to have a hormonal link. Cholesterol is a precursor of the sex hormones, and dietary fibre increases elimination of hormones from the body. Sex hormones are made in subcutaneous fat as well as in the gonads, and people with a high body-mass index have higher levels of circulating oestrogens (Prentice *et al.*, 1990). Thus a link can be demonstrated between high intake of saturated fats and increased hormones, especially oestrogen. All of these indicators point towards the role of oestrogens in the development of breast cancer.

This makes sense when considering the role of oestrogen within the body. The normal function of oestrogen is to cause breast and endometrial tissue to grow. During the first half of the menstrual cycle, follicle stimulating hormone (FSH) is released from the pituitary gland and stimulates the ovary to produce and develop a Graafian follicle. The ovary releases oestrogen at this time which, in turn, stimulates both the lining of the endometrium and ductal tissue within the breast to grow. Once the Graafian follicle has matured, it releases an egg into the fallopian tube ready for fertilisation, and the remaining follicle becomes the corpus luteum. The corpus luteum continues to be stimulated by the pituitary gland under the control of luteinising hormone (LH) and produces progesterone as the dominant hormone. Progesterone causes maturation of breast and endometrial tissue ready for the development and nurturing of a baby.

Key point

If cancers that arise within the breast are similar to the original tissue from which they have arisen, and normal breast tissue is stimulated to grow by oestrogen, then it can be postulated that oestrogen will also stimulate breast cancer to grow. Conversely, it might be suggested that depriving breast cancers of oestrogen will cause them to regress. These theories have been upheld in theoretical research and in clinical practice.

PRINCIPLES OF HORMONE THERAPY

The rationale for depriving breast tumours of oestrogen has been supported by the clinical observation, as long ago as 1899, when Beatson demonstrated that women with metastatic breast cancers could achieve remission of disease when their ovaries were removed (Forrest, 1982). In the 1970s, the mechanism for this was discovered when it was found that proteins on the surface of tumour cells could selectively bind with oestrogen and facilitate uptake of oestrogen into the nucleus of the cell. These were called oestrogen receptors (Barnes and Hanby, 2001). Tumours with oestrogen receptors are said to be ER+ve, and those without oestrogen receptors are ER−ve. About 75% of breast cancers are positive for the oestrogen receptor and/or progesterone receptor (PgR) (Johnston and Dowsett, 2003). Receptors have since been found for many other hormones and growth factors that act as physiological regulators. The action of oestrogen is to stimulate proliferation of ductal epthelial cells through the action of growth factors (Shao and Brown, 2003). Oestrogen receptors are a normal part of the cell and are found in cells throughout the body in nearly all the major organs, including the brain, skin, bones and periurethral tract.

Not all breast cancers contain oestrogen receptors, and those that are ER−ve are much less likely to respond to hormonal manipulation. Instead, these cancers have an over-expression of other cytokines which may account for the aggressive nature of these cancers (Chavery *et al.*, 2007). ER–ve cells are, therefore, independent from the effect of oestrogen.

Key point

Oestrogen has remained the most important hormone when considering treatment for breast cancer. All the hormonal treatments available are based on reducing the amount of oestrogen or opposing its action in some way There are three main ways in which this can be done: competing with oestrogen and therefore preventing its action, reducing levels of circulating oestrogen or opposing the actions of oestrogen.

Competing with oestrogen

There are a variety of molecules that are similar to oestrogen in their chemical structure, enabling them to bind to oestrogen receptors in the body. Once they have bound, they may trigger some of the normal oestrogen responses in the cell, but not all of them. This is known as a selective oestrogen receptor modifier (SERM) (Jordan *et al.*, 2001). This is potentially useful as SERMs may produce some of the beneficial effects of oestrogen without the harmful effects, most notably the production of growth factors.

The most widely used hormone which behaves in this way is tamoxifen (Tamofen, Soltamox and Nolvadex) (DeGregorio and Viebe, 1994). This is similar in many ways to oestrogen. It competes with oestrogen to bind to oestrogen receptors and is taken into the nucleus of the cell where it stimulates some of the changes in the same way as oestrogen. However, tamoxifen does not have all of the effects of oestrogen and, notably, does not encourage cancer cells to grow. It therefore works as an anti-oestrogen in relation to breast cancer. However, it continues to stimulate endometrial tissue in the same way as oestrogen and so menstrual irregularities may be seen. Uterine polyps and even uterine cancer may occur (van Leeuwen *et al.*, 1994).

An increase in deep vein thrombosis and pulmonary embolus has been noted with tamoxifen use (Fisher *et al.*, 2001b) and, although there is no significant increase in rates of stroke, the related drug raloxifene (Evista) has also been associated with a risk of fatal stroke and venous thromboembolism (Barrett-Connor *et al.*, 2006). Retinopathy may occur with high doses of tamoxifen use; however, at the normal dose of 20 mg daily, there appears to be no increase in this kind of damage above that which would be expected due to ageing (Lazzaroni *et al.*, 1998).

On the whole, the risks from tamoxifen are small when weighed against the benefits in terms of cancer treatment, and there are other benefits from tamoxifen that should be taken into consideration. It is possible that tamoxifen may have a long-term cardioprotective effect (Parton and Smith, 2008). Tamoxifen does appear to lower total cholesterol and low-density lipoprotein cholesterol (LDL) (Grey *et al.*, 1995) but, at present, an effect upon cardiovascular outcomes has yet to be seen in trials (Barrett-Connor *et al.*, 2006).

It is possible that tamoxifen acts to protect bones from post-menopausal osteoporosis (Love *et al.*, 1994), although bone loss has been observed in pre-menopausal women (Powles *et al.*, 1996). However, another SERM, raloxifene (Evista), has been licensed for the treatment and prevention of post-menopausal osteoporosis and has also been shown to reduce the risk of clinical vertebral fractures (Barrett-Connor *et al.*, 2006). It does not, however, prevent hot flushes and is not recommended for use either as HRT or for treating breast cancer. Current evidence suggests that raloxifene is as effective as tamoxifen in reducing the risk of invasive breast cancer and has a lower risk of adverse events, including uterine cancer, thromboembolic events and cataracts (Vogel 2009). Raloxifene has now been licensed for use to prevent breast cancer in the USA (Moen and Keating, 2008).

Experience from using tamoxifen has led scientists to search for the 'perfect SERM.' This would be a compound that is able to produce all the desired effects of oestrogen and none of the undesirable effects. Desirable effects include protection of bones, cardiovascular system, periurethral tissue, vagina and brain and the prevention of hot flushes. Undesirable effects are the stimulation of endometrial and breast tissue. Drugs that have been developed in the search for the perfect SERM include raloxifene (Evista), which has been used for bone health, and toremifene (Fareston), which has been licensed for treatment of advanced breast cancer.

Reducing oestrogen levels

Menopausal status is important when considering the most suitable therapy. Approximately 20% of all breast cancers occur in women under the age of 50 years (Cancer research UK, 2006). In a pre-menopausal woman, preventing the ovaries from working can eliminate 90% of circulating oestrogen. This can be done by surgically removing the ovaries, or by destroying them with radiation but, in the treatment of breast cancer, it is more normal to use drugs that 'switch off' the ovaries.

To understand how this 'switch off' is accomplished, it is necessary to understand the control of oestrogen production. Oestrogen is produced by the ovaries under the stimulation of the gonadotrophic hormones LH and FSH, released by the pituitary gland. In its turn, the pituitary gland is stimulated by luteinising hormone releasing hormone (LHRH), which comes from the hypothalamus. Synthetic analogues of LHRH have been developed which occupy and block all the receptors in the pituitary gland, thus rendering it insensitive to further stimulation from the hypothalamus. It then no longer releases any gonadotrophins (Cockshott, 2000). Once the ovary is not being stimulated, it ceases to produce any oestrogen. There are a variety of these LHRH analogues, such as goserilin (Zoladex), buserelin and leuprorelin. They will all induce a temporary menopause, together with its consequences, such as hot flushes (Matsumoto *et al.*, 2000).

Chemotherapy suppresses ovarian function and may also induce a temporary cessation of menstruation and hot flushes. Those women who are approaching the menopause may find that their periods do not return and that the menopause is permanent. Younger women usually find that menstruation does return, and so they cannot assume that they are not fertile during this time. The return of periods is significant when considering hormone treatments.

Aromatase inhibitors

Once the menopause is passed, the majority of naturally occurring oestrogen has gone. However, there are still small amounts of circulating oestrogens, which are produced mainly in subcutaneous tissue under the control of the adrenal gland. These are made by the conversion of the androgen androstenedione to oestrogen, by enzymes known as aromatase enzymes (Brodie and Njar, 2000). A variety of aromatase inhibitors have been developed that prevent this conversion from taking place, and so further reduce the amount of oestrogen in the body. The first of these was aminoglutethimide, but this was accompanied by high levels of toxicity, and so is now rarely used. The current third-generation medications now in use can be divided into non-steroidal inhibitors such as anastrozole (Arimidex) and letrozole (Femara) and steroidal inhibitors, such as formestane (Lentaron) and exemestane (Aromasin). Low levels of toxicity accompany these, and most women find them very acceptable.

As with other methods of oestrogen reduction, aromatase inhibitors cause oestrogen-withdrawal symptoms such as hot flushes and dry vagina. Long-term use may be associated with musculoskeletal changes, causing aching joints and bone changes. There is evidence that aromatase inhibitors cause accelerated loss of bone density and an increased risk of bone fracture. The relative risk is considered to be low, and current guidelines include monitoring those at risk with bone-density scans and giving treatment using anti-resorptive drugs (such as bisphosphonates), calcium and vitamin D supplements (Eastell and Hannon 2005; Perez 2006).

Opposing oestrogen

Due to the complex ways in which oestrogen and progesterone interact with each other, in some situations progesterone may act to inhibit the effect of oestrogen. Synthetic progesterones can be useful in the treatment of breast cancer. The main ones used are medroxyprogesterone acetate (Farlutal or Provera) (Pannuti *et al.*, 1993) and megestrol acetate (Megace) (Powles, 1993). The incidence of side effects is low, and some people experience a feeling of wellbeing when taking progesterones. This makes them particularly useful in palliative care. The main side effect noted is increased appetite and consequent weight gain. Long-term use may also result in Cushingoid changes, such as a redistribution of body fat, which results in a classic moon face and thoracic hump. Earlier changes noted may be increase in sebum production and thinning of hair. Glucose intolerance can be induced, so diabetes should be monitored for.

A summary of the most common hormone treatments used in breast cancer, and their major side effects, is given in Table 10.2.

Phytoestrogens

Some plants contain compounds that are similar in structure to animal oestrogens and may mimic some of the effects of oestrogen. Naturally occurring SERMs known as phytoestrogens, they are available in health food shops, with many claims made for their use as 'natural' remedies to 'balance' the body's hormones. If phytoestrogens do have any hormonal effects in the body, then it is just as likely that they will have the negative effects as well as the positive ones. As yet, there are few data to support either their safety or their efficacy. As they are classified as foods, they are not prepared to the rigorous standards required of drugs, and preparations may contain widely varying amounts of active ingredient. They may also be combined with other ingredients such as steroid hormones. It is certainly possible that they contain valuable compounds; however, caution should be used when considering their use until more research is available.

Some of these compounds are found in foodstuffs such as soy protein. It has been suggested that people who have high levels of soy in their diet have a low incidence of

Table 10.2 The most common hormone treatments used in breast cancer and their major side effects.

Class of action	Generic name	Trade name	Dose	Route	Side effects and notes
LHRH analogues	Goserilin	Zoladex	3.6 mg every 28 days	Subcutaneous	Menopause induced
Aromatase inhibitors	Aminoglutethimide	Orimeten	250 mg daily	Oral	Hot flushes, vaginal dryness Joint aches and pains Drowsiness, nausea, lethargy, diarrhoea, ataxia, depression Onset of fever and skin rash within 7-10 days, may settle if left Needs to be taken with hydrocortisone (withdraw gradually)
	Anastrozole	Arimidex	1 mg daily	Oral	Joint pain, hot flushes
	Letrozole	Femara	2.5 mg daily	Oral	Joint pain, hot flushes
	Formestane	Lentaron	250 mg every 2 weeks	Intra-muscular	Joint pain, hot flushes
	Exemestane	Aromasin	25 mg daily	Oral	Joint pain, hot flushes
Progesterones	Medroxyprogesterone acetate	Farlutal	500 mg^{-1} g daily	Oral	Nausea, fluid retention, weight gain. May experience withdrawal bleeding. Prolonged use in high doses may lead to Cushingoid effects. Can decrease glucose tolerance – monitor for diabetes.
		Provera	400–800 mg daily		
	Megestrol acetate	Megace	160 mg daily	Oral	
Selective oestrogen receptor modulators	Tamoxifen	Tamofen, Soltamox, Nolvadex	20 mg daily	Oral	Risk of increased endometrial changes, such as hyperplasia, polyps and cancer. Abnormal vaginal bleeding should be investigated. Hot flushes, vaginal discharge, alterations in menstrual flow. Rarely visual disturbances, thromboembolic events. Ovarian cysts.
	Toremifene	Fareston	60 mg daily	Oral	Hot flushes, vaginal discharge
	Raloxifene	Evista	60 mg daily	Oral	Used for osteoporosis. Increased risk of clotting. Hot flushes, sweating, leg cramps

breast cancer and menopausal hot flushes. It is certainly true that Japanese women, who traditionally have high intakes of soy, do have a low incidence of breast cancer, and this incidence rises on emigration to the USA where dietary changes are one of the main changes that occur (Kliewer and Smith, 1995). It is also the case that hot flushes are rarely recorded in the literature as a problem for Japanese women. There are some small studies that show a reduction in hot flushes in women who increase the proportion of their diet that contains soy (Albertazzi *et al.*, 1998) and others which show that soy does not help (Newton *et al.*, 2006). The role of soy is, as yet, unclear, and there may be other factors that have not yet been identified which may be more important to explain these phenomena.

Key point

The manipulation of hormones in the medical treatment of breast cancer is firmly based upon ongoing scientific research and is regulated by rigorous standards. Naturally occurring phytoestrogens may well have oestrogenic activity, both harmful and beneficial. They are often a mixture of molecules with complex actions, and there is insufficient evidence about their efficacy and safety.

HORMONE MANIPULATION IN CLINICAL PRACTICE

Prevention of cancer development

Before exploring the explicit manipulation of hormones in the prevention of cancer, it is worth revisiting the role that subcutaneous fat has in the production of hormones. There is a wealth of research in the relationship of nutrition, physical activity and weight management to cancer risk. A number of healthy lifestyle choices have been shown to reduce the risk of developing cancer, including:

- Being lean;
- Being physically active;
- Limiting the consumption of energy-dense foods and sugary drinks;
- Eating mostly plant-based foods;
- Limiting the amount of red meat and avoiding processed meat;
- Limiting the amount of alcohol consumed;
- Limiting salt intake;
- Breast feeding.
    (World Cancer Research Fund/American Institute for Cancer Research, 2007).

Some of these recommendations have an impact upon the amount of subcutaneous fat and, by implication, the production of oestrogen by androstenedione conversion. Others are more general to the risk of developing any cancers, and the opportunity to promote healthy behaviours at this point should not be missed.

The role of tamoxifen in preventing breast cancer has been explored by a number of studies (Veronesi *et al.*, 1998; Powles *et al.*,1998). It has now been established that the use of tamoxifen reduces the incidence in breast cancer by 38% (Cuzick *et al.*, 2003). However, a significant increase in the rates of endometrial cancer and thromboembolic events prevents the use of prophylactic tamoxifen as a standard measure (Cuzick *et al.*, 2007). Further studies are required to determine whether the benefits outweigh the risks for those at high risk of developing breast cancer and whether other means of hormone manipulation, such as aromatase inhibitors, would have better benefits versus risk.

Key point

While it seems possible that tamoxifen has a role to play in the prevention of breast cancer, it is clear that it is not without risk, and there are still many questions to be answered. There may, however, be a role for other SERMs, such as raloxifene, in preventing breast cancer. Further research is required and ongoing.

Adjuvant therapy

Once breast cancer has occurred and been treated by surgery, radiotherapy and chemotherapy, hormonal therapy is considered in order to reduce the possibility of recurrence. This is known as adjuvant therapy. Tamoxifen has been shown to reduce the chance of recurrence and mortality from breast cancer by 47% in those women whose tumours are shown to be oestrogen receptor–positive (Harvey *et al.*, 1999). An additional benefit is to reduce the incidence of new primaries in the other breast (Nayfield *et al.*, 1991). However, women who have ER−ve tumours do not benefit from tamoxifen (Fisher *et al.*, 2001a). The risk of thromboembolic events associated with tamoxifen rises when tamoxifen is given concurrently with chemotherapy. Pritchard *et al.* (1996) suggest that it is probably better to reserve tamoxifen use until after chemotherapy has been completed, as is current practice. However, the Early Breast Cancer Trialists' Collaborative Group (2005) report that there is no evidence for superiority with either concurrent or sequential use of tamoxifen and chemotherapy. (A concern is that effective treatment could be delayed with sequential therapy in sub-groups of patients who gain more from endocrine therapy than chemotherapy.)

Aromatase inhibitors have been shown to be at least as effective as tamoxifen in preventing breast cancer recurrence when used as primary adjuvant treatment of early ER+ve breast cancer (National Institute of Clinical Excellence [NICE], 2007). Aromatase inhibitors do not have the risks of endometrial cancer that are associated with tamoxifen (Baum, 2001). However, some women experience joint aches and pains, and an increased risk of osteoporosis (Eastell and Hannon 2005; Perez 2006). If tamoxifen has been used as a first-line adjuvant hormonal therapy, there is benefit to switching to an aromatase inhibitor; exemestane following 2–3 years of adjuvant tamoxifen therapy, or letrozole following standard tamoxifen therapy (National Institute of Clinical Excellence NICE, 2007).

Ovarian ablation, either by surgery or through use of LHRH analogues, may also be recommended as an adjuvant treatment for pre-menopausal women (Baum, 2001). The benefit of this has been disputed, as it could be argued that chemotherapy that suppresses ovarian function has a hormonal effect as well as a direct cytotoxic effect.

Key point

Decisions regarding the appropriate adjuvant hormonal therapy should be made with regard to an individual's clinical history and concerns about side effects.

Metastatic disease

Once metastatic disease has been diagnosed in women with breast cancer, it is not possible to completely eliminate the disease. The balance of treatment therefore shifts from increasing length of life to maintaining the quality of life. Hormonal therapies can be invaluable in this setting as they have relatively low side effects and may achieve useful responses in ER+ve disease. If the disease is not life-threatening, for example it is confined to bone or soft tissue, hormonal therapy should be regarded as the treatment of choice.

Women who are pre-menopausal should undergo oophorectomy, either surgically or with LHRH analogues. For post-menopausal women, tamoxifen has been used for many years as the first-line treatment, although some studies have now demonstrated anastrozole to be equally as effective as tamoxifen (Bonneterre *et al.*, 2000). Almost all patients with advanced breast cancer who initially respond to tamoxifen therapy will eventually develop resistance to the therapy. The resistance is not due to a change in the oestrogen receptor status, and tumour response is still seen with second-line hormone therapy in the majority of cases (Shao and Brown, 2003).

Hormones can be given sequentially and should be continued until disease progression. Once tamoxifen and the aromatase inhibitors have been used, progesterones may also be useful, with the use of androgens, high-dose oestrogen and aminoglutethimide now becoming rare. The response rate for ER+ve tumours is around 70%, and the duration of response is about 20 months.

Key point

Hormone therapies do increase survival and time to disease progression. No one treatment is considered of more benefit than another at this time, and studies which take into account quality of life, as well as time gained, need to be carried out and reviewed.

Hormone replacement therapy

HRT remains a contentious issue within breast cancer. It is almost certain that long-term use slightly increases the occurrence of primary breast cancer (see Table 10.3) (Schairer *et al.*, 2000), although it has been argued that most of these tumours are low grade, carrying a good prognosis (Holli *et al.*, 1998). HRT may also increase the risk of ovarian cancer, but may reduce the risk of colorectal cancer (Marsden, 2000). The little available evidence from randomised controlled trials suggests that HRT increases the risk of recurrence in women who have had breast cancer by a factor of 3.4 (Col *et al.*, 2005). Conversely, there

Table 10.3   Increased risk of breast cancer with HRT use (Collaborative Group on Hormonal Factors in Breast Cancer, 1997).

Use of HRT	Number of women who develop breast cancer (per 1000)
No use	45
5 years	47
10 years	51
12 years	57

is a potential for skeletal and coronary health benefits with the use of long-term HRT, but the evidence for this is still controversial (Barlow, 2008).

Key point

Women should be given available information about the risks and benefits of HRT, so that they can assess for themselves whether they wish to take it. For some women, menopausal difficulties are severe after breast cancer, and they may wish to take on an unknown risk for the future in order to alleviate present suffering.

Male breast cancer

There are no controlled studies to determine the most appropriate adjuvant treatment for male breast cancer. However, 85% of male breast cancers are ER+ve and 70% are progesterone receptor–positive (Jaiyesimi *et al.*, 1992). As response to hormone therapy correlates to the presence of receptors, it is presumed that there is a survival benefit to giving adjuvant tamoxifen to men. It is associated with a high rate of symptoms, such as hot flushes and impotence (Anelli *et al.*, 1994).

In metastatic disease, orchidectomy or the use of LHRH analogues may be useful. Tamoxifen, progesterones and aromatase inhibitors may also be used in the same way as for female breast cancer.

IMPLICATIONS FOR NURSING PRACTICE

Hormone therapies are often given alongside other treatments, and so separating out the effects of the hormone therapy from the other treatments can be difficult and sometimes impossible. Women who enter an early menopause owing to adjuvant therapy will often assume it is due to the tamoxifen, as that is hormonal treatment, rather than to chemotherapy. The reverse is usually the case. It is rare to enter the menopause as a consequence of being treated with tamoxifen unless the woman is about to enter menopause anyway. Chemotherapy suppresses ovarian function and can reduce oestrogen levels to less than normal post-menopausal levels. Dry vagina and loss of libido are more common on chemotherapy than on hormone therapy (Biglia *et al.*, 2003). The combination of tamoxifen and chemotherapy appears to make hot flushes not only more likely, but also more severe (Biglia *et al.*, 2003). Older women who are well past the menopause may find that hot flushes return. Women as old as 82 years of age have been observed to have hot flushes on tamoxifen.

Women who are feeling tired and depressed may blame hormonal imbalances, forgetting that they have been through a major life-threatening illness with aggressive concomitant treatments, all of which frequently result in feeling tired, anxious and depressed. Weight gain is automatically blamed onto tamoxifen, although it is almost certainly not the culprit (Kumar *et al.*, 1997). One should not dismiss hormones as a possible cause of depression and weight gain, but these problems should not be taken in isolation from other events that are occurring.

Many common side effects of hormone therapies are similar to the effects that are experienced during menopause. As menopause is a natural process, many women prefer not to think of these difficulties as symptoms, as this is a term associated with disease and disorder. Menopause is, rather, a time of change often accompanied by a variety of bodily experiences, such as hot flushes, which may be difficult and unpleasant for some women. When experienced as a direct consequence of treatment, women may regard these experiences as side effects. While these bodily changes may be materially very similar to those in a normal menopause, there is evidence to suggest that, for some, they may be more frequent and more severe (Fenlon *et al.*, 2009). Menopausal issues will be addressed first in this chapter, and then other side effects of hormone therapy that are not necessarily associated with menopause will be considered.

MENOPAUSE IN ASSOCIATION WITH BREAST CANCER

It has been now been established that menopausal problems are an issue for a majority of women treated for breast cancer (Fenlon *et al.*, 2009; McPhail, 2000; Canney and Hatton, 1994) and that around 65% will experience hot flushes (Carpenter and Andrykowski, 1999; Harris *et al.*, 2002). These difficulties may be due to the suppression of the ovaries by medical intervention such as goserilin or chemotherapy. Thirty percent of all pre-menopausal women will be amenorrhoeic 1 year after chemotherapy, and many more will suffer disruptions to the menstrual cycle (Lower *et al.*, 1999). The nearer to natural menopause, around the age of 50 years, the more likely it is that menopause will occur and be permanent (Goodwin *et al.*, 1999b). A further group of women will be undergoing their natural menopause and will be denied the use of HRT. Those who have been taking HRT and are advised to stop when breast cancer occurs will frequently experience hot flushes. It is a commonly held misconception that tamoxifen causes menopause. Unless the woman is near to natural menopause anyway, then this is not the case (see Table 10.4). However, it is the case that tamoxifen can cause hot flushes in some women (Powles *et al.*, 1994).

Carpenter and Andrykowski (1999) have described the physical effects of menopause experienced by women with breast cancer (Table 10.4).

Table 10.4 Symptoms attributed to menopause by women with breast cancer (Carpenter and Andrykowski, 1999).

Symptom	Percentage reporting symptoms
Joint pain	77%
Feeling tired	75%
Difficulty sleeping	68%
Hot flushes	66%
Headaches	55%
Irritable and nervous	54%
Depressed	51%
Numbness and tingling	40%
Vaginal dryness	36%
Dizzy spells	25%
Pounding heart	25%
Painful intercourse	21%
Skin crawls (formication)	18%

The list of symptoms described in Table 10.4 is similar to those given for normal menopause, although Ganz *et al.* (1998) found that breast cancer survivors experienced an increased incidence of joint pains, headaches and hot flushes when compared with a group of post-menopausal women of the same age who did not have breast cancer. A study by Duffy *et al.* (1999) showed a very high level of depression, insomnia and hot flushes in women who experienced a premature menopause due to breast cancer treatment.

It may be difficult for women with breast cancer to interpret some of the symptoms that they experience. Some menopausal signs could be confused with effects from treatment or symptoms caused by the cancer itself. For example, sensations of prickling experienced in the upper chest (formication) may be interpreted as cancer recurrence, and the increase in joint aches and pains raises anxiety about bone metastases.

The onset of menopause may also be a reminder for women that they are getting older. They may have hoped not to have to face the menopause for a few more years yet, and this represents another change in life. Women experiencing premature menopause interviewed by Singer and Hunter (1999) describe having to redefine themselves – suddenly they are a different person, an older, less attractive person and less of a woman. For some, it caused a dramatic loss of self-esteem. Additionally, those women who have never had children, whether by choice or not, may also need to grieve the loss of the possibility of children. It is clear that both breast cancer and menopause cause alterations to body image and may require adjustments in role function. All human beings need to face their own ageing and mortality. However, to have this imposed on them, and to need to address both issues at the same time, may cause particular difficulties with adjustment.

Women undergoing the menopause need to be assessed in a holistic fashion so that they can be helped to understand the changes that are occurring in their bodies, and specific interventions may be suggested to help women to adjust to these changes.

Key point

Menopause and menopausal symptoms are very frequently associated with breast cancer, either by coincidence or by associated treatment. Although the menopause is a naturally occurring phenomenon in all women, it may be worse for women who have had breast cancer, as they have fewer treatment options available to them.

Hot flushes

Hot flushes are a commonly reported sign of menopause, but vary widely in their manifestation. For many, they are likely to be little more than an irritation; however, there is a significant minority that find them troubling (Hunter and Liao, 1995). After breast cancer, women are more likely to experience hot flushes (McPhail 2000; Fenlon *et al.*, 2009, with one study showing that 80% of women taking tamoxifen had hot flushes (Hunter *et al.*, 2004). Most of the literature discussing relief of hot flushes focuses on pharmacological interventions, but women with breast cancer are less likely to take medication for flushes, and are more likely to take herbal remedies (Carpenter and Andrykowski, 1999; Harris *et al.*, 2002), preferring self-help management (Hunter *et al.*, 2004).

Although many women find flushing to be a problem, many feel that they are not taken seriously by health-care professionals. In 250 breast cancer survivors, Biglia *et al.* (2003) found that 50% consulted a physician about long-term heath issues and chemotherapy-induced menopause, but that 21% found their doctors deemed their complaints 'irrelevant'.

Box 10.1

'It's as though somebody has built a furnace inside of you and it's your whole body. It starts almost at your feet and works up and you just feel as though you are literally on fire inside and it's trying to escape and you just want to escape but you can't escape, there's nowhere to go and nothing to do.' (Fenlon and Rogers, 2007)

Hot flushes can be frequent and severe and have been reported with up to 240 occurring in a 24-hour period (Levine-Silverman, 1989). One study of 150 breast cancer patients found that the median number of flushes per day was five, ranging from one to 30 flushes per day (Fenlon *et al.*, 2009). Descriptions vary from being a mild feeling of warmth in the upper body and face, with mild perspiration, through to severe flushes that feel like 'a furnace' (Fenlon and Rogers 2007) or 'burning up' (Finck *et al.*, 1998) (see Box 10.1).

While day-time flushes may be problematic, many women describe night sweats as more troubling, with 72% of women with flushes having disrupted sleep (Fenlon *et al.*, 2009). Sleep disruption is frequent, with more than one hour's sleep lost in more than a third of disturbed nights (Fenlon *et al.*, 2009) (see Box 10.2).

The impact of hot flushes can be far-reaching, affecting the ability to work and having an impact on personal relationships with, for many, an effect on self-image and self-esteem (see Box 10.3).

Women manage hot flushes with a variety of coping mechanisms. These can be largely divided into physical cooling strategies and cognitive strategies. Cooling strategies that are employed include the use of sprays and fans and choice of appropriate clothing. One study asked women what they did to manage flushes and found that the most frequently described method was to drink plenty of cold water (Fenlon, 2005). Choices of clothing and bed-clothing were about using absorbent materials, such as cotton and silk; wearing layers of thin clothing that are easier to adjust, and wearing loose-fitting clothing, which is less restrictive than tailored clothes. However, some women may feel disadvantaged by the necessity to wear less feminine clothing and may not wish to alter their clothing, but would rather maintain their normal social image.

Many women describe how they learn not to fight hot flushes, which can then spiral out of control. They learn to relax and just let the flush wash over them. Concentration may be lost for a few seconds but, when this is accepted, it is found that it soon passes. Some women describe how they reinterpret the heat as a positive experience, for example reminding themselves of enjoyable summer holidays (see Box 10.4).

Box 10.2

'The hot flushes during the day I could cope with. I just feel I would like to have more . . . I suppose in the last eight years, six or more hours sleep I've probably had a dozen times. Um . . . you know waking up is, is quite frequent. It might just be um, might just be enough to know that I've woken up and then I would go back to sleep within a minute. Other times you know what it is like if you've got things on your mind, if you're woken up during the night it's very difficult to get back to sleep.' (Fenlon and Rogers, 2007)

> **Box 10.3**
>
> 'I could no sooner have a man sleeping in my bed than fly to the moon.' (Fenlon and Rogers, 2007)

Fears of being unable to cope in social situations are common and are often accompanied by embarrassment and inability to concentrate on tasks at hand. Some women are able to challenge these fears by asking for honest feedback from those they trust about socially embarrassing occurrences such as body odour. Coping strategies, such as going back over work done during a flush, or taking a few minutes out for deep breathing, can also help minimise distress.

Interviews with breast cancer survivors who experience hot flushes suggest that taking control is important. Women take control by adjusting their environment, their clothing and their lives, which may be a high cost; even to the point of giving up social life or work. Fenlon and Rogers (2007) suggest that ultimately control is best gained through a state of mind, rather than by actions (see Box 10.5).

As well as managing the stress of individual hot flushes, it may be appropriate to lower stress levels in daily life in general. It is known that women who are more stressed experience more hot flushes in a 24-hour period (Freedman and Woodward, 1992). Relaxation therapy has been shown to be effective in reducing both the incidence and severity of flushes in women who have had breast cancer, and this is accompanied by a reduction in the distress due to flushing (Fenlon et al., 2008a). It is possible that learning self-management techniques, such as relaxation, result in an increased sense of control, which may also contribute to decreasing the distress caused by flushing. Finally, one of the most distressing problems caused by hot flushes is sleep disturbance and resulting chronic tiredness. Daily relaxation may help to improve sleep and increase feelings of being rested and, again, increase tolerance of difficult symptoms.

Drugs that are available to treat hot flushes are variable and all have side effects. HRT is widely regarded as the most effective treatment for hot flushes (Bachmann 2005), but is generally contraindicated after breast cancer due to the theoretical risk of increasing cancer recurrence (Adelson et al., 2005). Some women may choose to take this risk if their perspective suggests that life in the long term is irrelevant if life in the short-term is not worth living (Fenlon and Rogers, 2007).

Clonidine 0.1 mg per day is effective in reducing hot flushes in tamoxifen-induced hot flushes by nearly 40% (Goldberg et al., 1994), although some women have headaches or dry mouth and some experience difficulty sleeping. Some studies have shown that selective serotonin-reuptake inhibitors (SSRIs) may be effective in reducing hot flushes. Pilot studies have been conducted using venlafaxine (Loprinzi et al., 1998) and paroxetine (20 mg daily)

> **Box 10.4**
>
> 'I think that one has to accept that hot flushes are going to be a part of your life and you can either go with it, and let them just, you know, be there, (not that you like them) or you can get more het up about them and they can be a great inconvenience.' (Fenlon and Rogers, 2007)

> **Box 10.5**
>
> '... obviously things like just accepting that those hot flushes are there, and just trying to um, just trying to stay calm when they happen, not try to fight them. Because I think they get worse if you try and fight them.' (Fenlon and Rogers, 2007)

(Stearns *et al*., 2000). These pilot studies showed that 55–67% of women show at least a 50% reduction in the incidence of hot flushes and a 58–73% reduction in the severity of hot flushes. Unwanted effects of these drugs include dry mouth, nausea, somnolence, nightmares, disorientation and a stimulation of anxiety. While these early studies appear promising, personal experience has shown a high level of side effects that women find totally unacceptable. Progesterone therapy, such as Megace, has been found to be effective in reducing hot flushes in women with breast cancer (Loprinzi *et al*., 1994). However, there are few data on the long-term safety of the use of progesterone after primary breast cancer.

Many women have used complementary therapies, such as herbal remedies, homeopathy and acupuncture to help relieve hot flushes. Research on these approaches is notoriously difficult, and there is very little evidence available to support their use. There is a growing body of anecdotal evidence that supports benefits from these approaches, and they may increase a sense of control and wellbeing in women that use them. Herbal remedies may be regarded by women as *'natural'* and therefore safe or *'not so strong'* (Fenlon and Rogers, 2007), and many women choose to use these. There is a theoretical rationale for the use of some herbal remedies; however, there are very few data available on their precise mechanism of action, efficacy and safety. Herbal remedies that contain phytoestrogens are often recommended for menopausal difficulties.

Phytoestrogens are found in herbal remedies and throughout the human diet and include many substances, which are classified as lignans, isoflavones and coumestrans. Intestinal flora convert inactive plant precursors into compounds that are active in the human. The biological actions of these compounds are extremely complex and very variable. They are found in a variety of plant food sources, such as red clover, dong quai, liquorice and soy protein. Most studies have not shown any reduction in hot flushes with phytoestrogens, either using supplements (Eden, 1998; Baber *et al*., 1999; Knight *et al*., 1999) or by incorporating soy flour into the diet (Murkies *et al*., 1995). One study showed a reduction in the frequency of hot flushes by about 45% by the addition of soy powder (60 g daily) to the diet (Albertazzi *et al*., 1998). There is some indication that phytoestrogens may have an influence on the maturation of the lining of the vagina (Wilcox *et al*., 1990), but these are inconsistent and do not correlate with serum levels of phytoestrogen in those who are taking soy supplements (Albertazzi *et al*., 1999).

As suggested above, the long-term safety of phytoestrogens is unknown. If they have an oestrogenic effect in the body to prevent hot flushes, then it is theoretically possible that they also have an oestrogenic effect in stimulating breast cancer. Until more evidence is available, it cannot be assumed that the use of herbal preparations for the relief of hot flushes is safe.

Evening primrose oil is often recommended for hot flushes, but there is little evidence to support this. Vitamin E supplements have been shown to decrease the number of flushes experienced, although this is a small effect (Barton *et al*., 1998). Smoking increases the number of hot flushes that women have (Obermeyer *et al*., 1999), so smoking cessation should be encouraged.

Key point

Although the literature suggests that menopausal difficulties are minor when compared to cancer (Fenlon and Rogers, 2007; Knobf 2001), hot flushes may be troubling, and women want their concerns to be taken seriously. It is therefore important for nurses to take the time to discuss these issues.

Vaginal dryness

While it is clear that vaginal dryness may lead to dyspareunia (painful sexual intercourse) and thus interfere with sexual relationships, this again cannot be taken in isolation from the other changes that are occurring in a woman's life at this time. Work done by Cawood and Bancroft (1996) showed that the most important predictors of sexuality in menopausal women were not physiological but social. These were other aspects of the sexual relationship, sexual attitudes and measures of wellbeing. The best predictor of both wellbeing and depression was tiredness (Cawood and Bancroft, 1996). Therefore, while advising on vaginal dryness, this should not be taken in isolation from a general assessment and discussion regarding general health and wellbeing.

About 36% of women experience vaginal dryness. This may be a mild irritation or can be severe, causing pain and inhibiting intercourse. The use of simple moisturisers and gels may be beneficial (see Table 10.5). A polycarbophil moisturising gel such as Replens can improve vaginal moisture and elasticity and is found to be of benefit in up to 80% of women (Gelfand and Wendman, 1994). Several studies found this to be an effective alternative to local oestrogen therapy (Nachtigall, 1994; Bygdeman and Swahn, 1996).

For some women, it may be appropriate to consider the use of local oestrogen. This is poorly absorbed and, indeed, when the vagina is particularly dry will not be absorbed at all. Oestrogen preparations should be chosen with care as some are larger doses which

Table 10.5 Preparations available to use for vaginal dryness.

Generic (proprietary name)	Formulation	Regimen	Notes
Astroglide, Gyne-moistrin and Moist Again	Gel moisturiser	As required	No oestrogen
Vaginal moisturising gel (Replens)	Polycarbophil gel	Use applicator-insert gel three nights per week	No oestrogen. May be retained in the vagina for longer
Oestradiol tablet (Vagifem)	25 μg oestradiol	Insert one tablet daily for 2 weeks, then reduce to one tablet twice weekly; discontinue after 3 months to assess need for further treatment	Low levels of oestrogen detectable in the blood stream
Oestradiol ring (Estring)	Silicone elastomer ring with core that contains 2 mg oestradiol (released as 7.5 μg/24-hour period)	To be inserted into upper third of vagina and worn continuously; replace every 90 days	Maximum duration of continuous treatment is 2 years; lack of data regarding systemic absorption

may be absorbed and raise serum oestrogen levels, for example oestrogen creams such as Ovestine (oestriol 0.1%). It has now been shown that all vaginal oestrogen preparations are associated with raised oestrogen levels in the blood stream (Kendall *et al.*, 2006). Some preparations, such as the oestradiol tablet Vagifem, may result in low levels of circulating oestrogen, but this may still be contraindicated, especially where the aim of treatment is to minimise oestrogen levels, as with the aromatase inhibitors. Other women may feel that the gain is worth the potential risks, especially if only taken over a short period of time.

Osteoporosis

Some women who experience early menopause due to cancer treatment may be concerned about the possibility of developing osteoporosis in later life, especially if this is a known problem in their families. Those at high risk of developing osteoporosis include: over 65 years of age; early menopause; known osteopenia; low dietary calcium intake; smoking; excessive alcohol intake; weight less than 57 kg. In these cases, a baseline bone mineral density measurement should be considered, and scans repeated every 18 to 24 months (Royal College of Nursing, 2005).

Tamoxifen helps to prevent bone loss in post-menopausal women, and aromatase inhibitors and LHRH inhibitors increase bone loss. If women are considering using HRT after breast cancer, then one of the benefits is the reduction in bone loss and therefore a reduction in the risk of fracture. However, this protection is only given while hormones are still being taken, and the incidence of fractures after the age of 75 years, when most fractures occur, is unchanged (te Velde and van Leusden, 1994). Weight-bearing exercise will prevent bone loss, although it will not increase bone density (Sharkey *et al.*, 2000). Such exercise can also help to improve fitness and muscle strength, which will contribute to the prevention of falls and a lower risk of fracture (Forwood and Larsen, 2000). In conjunction with advice to increase dietary calcium and oral calcium and vitamin D supplements, exercise plays a significant part in a lifestyle prescription for reducing fractures in later life. Willett *et al.* (2000) suggest that hormones should not be used routinely, even in the non-cancer population, for fractures and coronary heart disease, because avoidance of smoking, performance of regular exercise and a good diet are effective preventive measures. There are also other non-hormonal drugs that are effective against osteoporosis and so, while HRT could be considered for the relief of menopausal distress, it should not be used as a prophylactic against osteoporosis in breast cancer patients.

Joint pains

Carpenter and Andrykowski (1999) described joint pains as the most common menopausal problem after breast cancer, affecting 77% of women. This has since been confirmed by Fenlon *et al.* (2008b), who demonstrated that joint pains are more frequent in women who have had breast cancer than those who have not. The exact aetiology of this is unknown, although decreased oestrogen levels are likely to be a contributory factor (Franco *et al.*, 2005). Joint pains appear to be a particular problem in women taking aromatase inhibitors, where oestrogen levels are very low, with as many as 82% of women reporting joint pain (Crew *et al.*, 2006) and 15% discontinuing treatment for this reason (Felson and Cummings, 2005). As yet, there is little known about how this pain might be managed.

Key point

It has been seen that menopause is a complex phenomenon and that, within the context of breast cancer, it is even more so. There is much that is still not clearly understood about the way in which women view this transition and the meanings for them when experienced with breast cancer. Very little is reported in the literature about the ways in which women would prefer to manage the difficulties that they may experience. Current advice must be to explore the phenomenon with each individual to help them understand what is happening to them and to identify options and the way in which they will want to manage their difficulties.

While menopause may be a difficult time for some women, most hormone therapies are generally low in side effects. A number of effects can occur with or without the menopause, and these are covered in the next section.

OTHER HORMONAL EFFECTS

Weight gain

An increase in appetite and subsequent gain in weight are clearly associated with the use of progesterone. However, other weight gain is not clearly related to hormone use. It is the norm for women to increase their weight with age and, after the menopause, the distribution of body fat will change so that it is more concentrated around the abdomen (Astrup, 1999). Davies *et al.* (2001) showed that weight gain is an age-related effect and is not influenced either by cessation of ovarian function or by the use of HRT. A number of studies have shown that it is common to gain weight during the year following a diagnosis of breast cancer, whether adjuvant treatment is given or not (Goodwin *et al.*, 1999a; Kumar *et al.*, 1997; Hoskin *et al.*, 1992), although the use of chemotherapy is closely correlated with weight gain (McInnes and Knobf, 2001). Goodwin *et al.* (1999a) showed that weight gain is greatest for those who have chemotherapy (1.6 kg) and least for those who have no adjuvant therapy (0.6 kg). Women on tamoxifen gained an average of 1.3 kg. Pre-menopausal women gain more weight than post-menopausal women. The most important controlling factor in weight gain is physical exercise (Simkin-Silverman and Wing, 2000). DeGeorge *et al.* (1990) showed that exercise and dietary measures could be effective in controlling weight gain even after breast cancer treatment.

Body image changes

Although the relative contributions of hormone therapy, chemotherapy and menopause are unclear, it is the case that weight gain does occur in women undergoing adjuvant therapy for breast cancer. Western societies put undue pressure on women to conform to the ideal of young, slim and beautiful (Greer, 1991). To increase weight is to emphasise change and loss in women who are already undergoing significant change and losses due to facing a life-threatening illness. It may be possible for women to reduce weight by a programme of exercise and dieting, but this may also be very difficult in the face of a regimen of aggressive treatments that have debilitating effects.

Some women also suffer other body image changes, such as thinning hair, with tamoxifen and an increase in oily skin with progesterones. If androgens are used in women, then virilisation will occur. This takes the form of an increase in body and facial hair, male-pattern hair loss, an increase in oily skin and a lowering of the voice. It may also be accompanied by an increase in libido.

The process of undergoing menopause may also contribute to significant body image change in some women. Most cancer treatments are for a defined period, something to be endured and which ultimately come to an end, but menopause is an irreversible change to the body. The woman may feel that she is no longer the person that she used to be. She must now think of herself as an old woman instead of a young woman. Menopause is a constant reminder of all the losses due to the cancer experience (Davis *et al.*, 2000).

Men who are being treated with female hormones may experience gynaecomastia, which can be distressing, especially within the context of a 'female' disease. It is possible to prevent this from occurring by using radiation.

Sexuality

Changes in sexuality can occur with hormone treatments, but are more likely to be part of the overall changes that occur at this time. Cancer treatment can have an impact on the quality of sexual relationships due to the discomfort of breast surgery, the fatigue of chemotherapy and the disruption to sleep caused by hot flushes. Alterations in circulating sex hormones are only one of the contributing factors to changing sexual relations (Greendale *et al.*, 2001). The use of androgens can increase libido in women, and the use of oestrogens in men will decrease libido.

Treatments that induce early menopause can cause sexual difficulties due to a dry and painful vagina (see above). Goserilin increases sexual dysfunction during treatment among patients without chemotherapy, but the disturbances of sexual functioning are reversible. The use of adjuvant chemotherapy is associated with continued sexual problems, even after 3 years (Berglund *et al.*, 2001).

Flare

Tumour flare is a rare phenomenon that may happen in patients with metastatic disease. The use of oestrogen, LHRH analogues or, rarely, tamoxifen may cause an initial worsening of the disease due to a temporary surge of circulating oestrogen. In women with bone disease, this may cause an increase in pain and a release of calcium into the blood stream. This can result in hypercalcaemia, which is potentially life-threatening. Women should be taught to be aware of the effects of hypercalcaemia and to report them immediately.

Thromboembolism

Oestrogens increase the risk of embolism and cause a rise in deep vein thrombosis and pulmonary embolism. A small rise in thromboembolic events has also been observed with tamoxifen (Fisher *et al.*, 1998).

CONCLUSION

Hormone therapies are effective in reducing breast cancer recurrence and can help both to lengthen and to improve the quality of life for women with metastatic disease. As they are not curative, due weight should be given to side effects, but many women will find them to be a valuable alternative to other breast cancer treatments. The role of nurses in caring for women having hormone therapies for breast cancer has several components. The nurses need to ensure that they are adequately informed so that they can help the women to understand the changes that are taking place in their bodies. They need to be prepared to listen to women's accounts of their problems and to make full assessments of their difficulties. They then need to be aware of a range of strategies to help each individual woman work out for herself the best path to take to deal with these problems. Because it is rarely curative, hormone therapy is one treatment modality where it is clear that the woman being treated needs to make her own decision about quality of life, side effects and the benefits to be gained from treatment.

REFERENCES

Adelson KB, Loprinzi CL and Hershman DL (2005) Treatment of hot flushes in breast and prostate cancer. *Expert Opinion on Pharmacotherapy* 6(7): 1095–1106.

Albertazzi P, Pansini F, Bonaccorsi G, Zanotti L, Forini E and De Aloysio D (1998) The effect of dietary soy supplementation on hot flushes. *Obstetrics and Gynecology* 91(1): 6–11.

Albertazzi P, Pansini F, Bottazzi M, Bonaccorsi G, De Aloysio D and Morton MS (1999) Dietary soy supplementation and phytoestrogen levels. *Obstetrics and Gynecology* 94(2): 229–231.

Anelli TF, Anelli A, Tran KN, Lebwohl DE and Borgen PI (1994) Tamoxifen administration is associated with a high rate of treatment-limiting symptoms in male breast cancer patients. *Cancer* 74(1): 74–77.

Astrup A (1999) Physical activity and weight gain and fat distribution changes with menopause: current evidence and research issues. *Medicine and Science in Sports and Exercise* 31(Suppl. 11): S564–567.

Baber RJ, Templeman C, Morton T, Kelly GE and West L (1999) Randomized placebo-controlled trial of an isoflavone supplement and menopausal symptoms in women. *Climacteric* 2(2): 85–92.

Bachmann GA (2005) Menopausal vasomotor symptoms: a review of causes, effects and evidence-based treatment options. Journal of Reproductive Medicine 50(3): 155–165.

Barlow DH (2008) The medical management of menopause: to treat or not to treat? *Annals of the New York Academy of Science* 1127: 134–139.

Barnes DM and Hanby AM (2001) Oestrogen and progesterone receptors in breast cancer: past, present and future. *Histopathology* 38(3): 271–274.

Barrett-Connor E, Mosca L, Collins P *et al.* (2006) Effects of raloxifene on cardiovascular events and breast cancer in postmenopausal women. *New England Journal of Medicine* 355(2): 125–137.

Barton DL, Loprinzi CL, Quella SK *et al.* (1998) Prospective evaluation of vitamin E for hot flashes in breast cancer survivors. *Journal of Clinical Oncology* 16(2): 495–500.

Baum M (2001) A vision for the future? *British Journal of Cancer* 85(Suppl. 2): 15–18.

Beatson GT (1896) On the treatment of inoperable cases of carcinoma of the mamma: suggestions for a new method of treatment with illustrative cases. *The Lancet* 2: 104–107; 162–165.

Berglund G, Nystedt M, Bolund C, Sjoden PO and Rutquist LE (2001) Effect of endocrine treatment on sexuality in premenopausal breast cancer patients: a prospective randomized study. *Journal of Clinical Oncology* 19(11): 2788–2796.

Biglia N, Cozzarella M, Cacciari F *et al.* (2003) Menopause after breast cancer: a survey on breast cancer survivors. *Maturitas* 45(1): 29–38.

Bonneterre J, Thurlimann B, Robertson JF *et al.* (2000) Anastrozole versus tamoxifen as first-line therapy for advanced breast cancer in 668 postmenopausal women: results of the Tamoxifen or Arimidex Randomized Group Efficacy and Tolerability Study. *Journal of Clinical Oncology* 18(22): 3748–3757.

Brinton LA, Schairer C, Hoover RN and Fraumeni JF, Jr (1988) Menstrual factors and risk of breast cancer. *Cancer Investigation* 6(3): 245–254.

Brodie AM and Njar VC (2000) Aromatase inhibitors and their application in breast cancer treatment. *Steroids* 65(4): 171–179.

Bygdeman M and Swahn ML (1996) Replens versus dienoestrol cream in the symptomatic treatment of vaginal atrophy in postmenopausal women. *Maturitas* 23(3): 259–263.

Cancer Research UK (2006) *UK Breast Cancer Incidence Statistics* Available at http://info. cancerresearchuk.org/cancerstats/types/breast/incidence.

Canney PA and Hatton MQ (1994) The prevalence of menopausal symptoms in patients treated for breast cancer. *Journal of Clinical Oncology* 6(5): 297–299.

Carpenter JS and Andrykowski MA (1999) Menopausal symptoms in breast cancer survivors. *Oncology Nursing Forum* 26(8): 1311–1317.

Cawood EH and Bancroft J (1996) Steroid hormones, the menopause, sexuality and well-being of women. *Psychological Medicine* 26(5): 925–936.

Chavey C, Bibeau F, Gourgou-Bourgade S *et al.* (2007) Oestrogen receptor negative breast cancers exhibit high cytokine content. *Breast Cancer Research* 9(1): R15.

Cockshott ID (2000) Clinical pharmacokinetics of goserelin. *Clinical Pharmacokinets* 39(1): 27–48.

Col N, Kim J and Chlebowski R (2005) Menopausal hormone therapy after breast cancer: a meta-analysis and critical appraisal of the evidence. *Breast Cancer Research* 7(4): R535–540.

Collaborative Group on Hormonal Factors in Breast Cancer (1997) Breast cancer and hormone replacement therapy: collaborative reanalysis of data from 51 epidemiological studies of 52,705 women with breast cancer and 108,411 women without breast cancer. *The Lancet* 350(9084): 1047–1059.

Crew K *et al.* (2006) Prevalence of joint symptoms in postmenopausal women on aromatase inhibitors for early stage breast cancer. In: Proceedings of the 29th San Antonio Breast Cancer Symposium, San Antonio.

Cuzick J, Forbes JF, Sestak I *et al.* (2007) Long-term results of tamoxifen prophylaxis for breast cancer – 96 month follow-up of the randomised IBIS-I trial. *Journal of the National Cancer Institute* 99(4): 272–282.

Cuzick J, Powles T, Veronesi U *et al.* (2003) Overview of the main outcomes in breast cancer prevention trials. *The Lancet* 361(9354): 296–300.

Davies KM, Heaney RP, Recker RR, Barger-Lux MJ and Lappe JM (2001) Hormones, weight change and menopause. *International Journal of Obesity and Related Metabolic Disorders* 25(6): 874–879.

Davis CS, Zinkand ZE and Fitch MI (2000) Cancer treatment-induced menopause: meaning for breast and gynecological cancer survivors. *Canadian Oncology Nursing Journal* 10(1): 14–21.

DeGeorge D, Gray JJ, Fetting JH and Rolls BJ (1990) Weight gain in patients with breast cancer receiving adjuvant treatment as a function of restraint, disinhibition, and hunger. *Oncology Nursing Forum* 17(Suppl. 3): 23–28; discussion 28–30.

DeGregorio M and Viebe V (1994) *Tamoxifen and Breast Cancer* New Haven and London: Yale University Press.

Duffy LS, Greenberg DB, Younger J and Ferraro MG (1999) Iatrogenic acute estrogen deficiency and psychiatric syndromes in breast cancer patients. *Psychosomatics* 40(4): 304–308.

Early Breast Cancer Trialists' Collaborative Group (2005) Effects of chemotherapy and hormonal therapy for early breast cancer on recurrence and 15-year survival: An overview of the randomised trials. *The Lancet* 365: 1687–1717.

Eastell R and Hannon R (2005) Long term effects of aromatase inhibitors in bone. *The Journal of Steroid Biochemistry and Molecular Biology* 95: 151–154.

Easton D, Ford D and Peto J (1993) Inherited susceptibility to breast cancer. *Cancer Surveys* 18: 95–113.

Eden J (1998) Phytoestrogens and the menopause. *Baillière's Clinical Endocrinology and Metabolism* 12(4): 581–587.

Fellowes D, Fallowfield LJ, Saunders CM and Houghton J (2001) Tolerability of hormone therapies for breast cancer: how informative are documented symptom profiles in medical notes for 'well-tolerated' treatments? *Breast Cancer Research and Treatment* 66(1): 73–81.

Felson DT and Cummings SR (2005) Aromatase inhibitors and the syndrome of arthralgias with estrogen deprivation. *Arthritis and Rheumatism* 52(9): 2594–2598.

Fenlon D (2005) *Menopause after Breast Cancer: A Randomised, Controlled Trial of Relaxation Training to Reduce Hot Flushes*. Southampton: School of Nursing and Midwifery.

Fenlon D, Addington-Hall J and Simmonds PD (2008a) Case controlled, cross-sectional survey of joint and muscle aches, pains and stiffness in women with primary breast cancer. Proceedings San Antonio Breast Cancer Symposium. San Antonio.

Fenlon D, Corner JL and Haviland J (2009) Menopausal hot flushes after breast cancer. *European Journal of Cancer Care* 18(2): 140–148.

Fenlon DR and Rogers AE (2007) The experience of hot flushes after breast cancer. *Cancer Nursing* 30: E19–26.

Fenlon DR, Corner JL and Haviland JS (2008b) A randomized controlled trial of relaxation training to reduce hot flashes in women with primary breast cancer. *Journal of Pain and Symptom Management* 35: 397–405.

Finck G, Barton DL, Loprinzi CL, Quella SK and Sloan JA (1998) Definitions of hot flashes in breast cancer survivors. *Journal of Pain and Symptom Management* 16(5): 327–333.

Fisher B, Anderson S, Tan-Chiu E *et al.* (2001a) Tamoxifen and chemotherapy for axillary node-negative, estrogen receptor-negative breast cancer: findings from National Surgical Adjuvant Breast and Bowel Project B-23. *Journal of Clinical Oncology* 19(4): 931–942.

Fisher B, Costantino J, Wickerham D *et al.* (1998) Tamoxifen for prevention of breast cancer: report of the National Surgical Adjuvant Breast and Bowel Project P-1 Study. *Journal of the National Cancer Institute* 90(18): 1371–1388.

Fisher B, Dignam J, Bryant J and Wolmark N (2001b) Five versus more than five years of tamoxifen for lymph node-negative breast cancer: updated findings from the National Surgical Adjuvant Breast and Bowel Project B-14 Randomized Trial. *Journal of the National Cancer Institute* 93(9): 684–690.

Forrest AP (1982) Beatson: hormones and the management of breast cancer. *Journal of the Royal College of Surgeons Edinburgh* 27(5): 253–263.

Forwood MR and Larsen JA (2000) Exercise recommendations for osteoporosis. A position statement of the Australian and New Zealand Bone and Mineral Society. *Australian Family Physician* 29(8): 761–764.

Franco S *et al.* (2005) Drawbacks of ovarian ablation with goserelin in women with breast cancer. (Published in Portugese). *Acta Médica Portugesa* 18(2): 123–127.

Freedman RR and Woodward S (1992) Behavioral treatment of menopausal hot flushes: evaluation by ambulatory monitoring. *American Journal of Obstetrics and Gynecology* 167(2): 436–439.

Ganz PA, Rowland JH, Meyerowitz BE and Desmond KA (1998) Impact of different adjuvant therapy strategies on quality of life in breast cancer survivors. *Recent Results in Cancer Research* 152: 396–411.

Gelfand MM and Wendman E (1994) Treating vaginal dryness in breast cancer patients: results of applying a polycarbophil moisturizing gel. *Journal of Women's Health* 3(6): 427–434.

Goldberg R, Loprinzi C and O'Fallon J (1994) Transdermal clonidine for ameliorating tamoxifen-induced hot flashes. *Journal of Clinical Oncology* 12: 155–158.

Goodwin PJ, Ennis M, Pritchard KI *et al.* (1999a) Adjuvant treatment and onset of menopause predict weight gain after breast cancer diagnosis. *Journal of Clinical Oncology* 17(1): 120–129.

Goodwin PJ, Ennis M, Pritchard KI, Trudeau M and Hood N (1999b) Risk of menopause during the first year after breast cancer diagnosis. *Journal of Clinical Oncology* 17(8): 2365–2370.

Greaves M (2000) *Cancer: The Evolutionary Legacy* Oxford: Oxford University Press.

Greendale GA, Petersen L, Zibecchi L and Ganz PA (2001) Factors related to sexual function in post-menopausal women with a history of breast cancer. *Menopause* 8(2): 111–119.

Greer G (1991) *The Change: Women, Ageing and the Menopause*, London: Penguin.

Grey AB, Stapleton JP, Evans MC and Reid IR (1995) The effect of anti-estrogen tamoxifen on cardiovascular risk factors in normal postmenopausal women. *Journal of Clinical Endocrinology and Metabolism* 80: 3191–3195.

Harris PF *et al.* (2002) Prevalence and treatment of menopausal symptoms among breast cancer survivors. *Journal of Pain and Symptom Management* 23(6): 501–509.

Harvey JM, Clark GM, Osborne CK and Allred DC (1999) Estrogen receptor status by immunohistochemistry is superior to the ligand-binding assay for predicting response to adjuvant endocrine therapy in breast cancer. *Journal of Clinical Oncology* 17(5): 1474–1481.

Holli K, Isola J and Cuzick J (1998) Low biologic aggressiveness in breast cancer in women using hormone replacement therapy. *Journal of Clinical Oncology* 16(9): 3115–3120.

Hoskin PJ, Ashley S and Yarnold JR (1992) Weight gain after primary surgery for breast cancer – effect of tamoxifen. *Breast Cancer Research and Treatment* 22(2): 129–132.

Hunter M and Liao K (1995) Problem-solving groups for mid-aged women in general practice: a pilot study. *Journal of Reproductive and Infant Psychology* 13: 147–151.

Hunter MS *et al.* (2004) *Menopausal symptoms in women with breast cancer: prevalence and treatment preferences*. Psycho-Oncology 13(11): 769–778.

Jaiyesimi IA, Buzdar AU, Sahin AA and Ross MA (1992) Carcinoma of the male breast. *Annals of Internal Medicine* 117(9): 771–777.

Jensen E.V and Jacobson HI (1962) Basic guides to the mechanism of estrogen action. *Recent Progress in Hormone Research* 18: 387–414.

John EM and Kelsey JL (1993) Radiation and other environmental exposures and breast cancer. *Epidemiologic Reviews* 15(1): 157–162.

Johnston SR and Dowsett, M (2003) Aromatase inhibitors for breast cancer: lessons from the laboratory. *Nature Reviews Cancer* 3(11): 821–831.

Jordan VC, Gapstur S and Morrow M (2001) Selective estrogen receptor modulation and reduction in risk of breast cancer, osteoporosis, and coronary heart disease. *Journal of the National Cancer Institute* 93(19): 1449–1457.

Kendall A, Dowsett M, Folkerd E and Smith I (2006) Caution: Vaginal estradiol appears to be contraindicated in postmenopausal women on adjuvant aromatase inhibitors. *Annals of Oncology* 17(4): 584–587.

Kelsey JL, Gammon MD and John EM (1993) Reproductive factors and breast cancer. *Epidemiologic Reviews* 15(1): 36–47.

Kliewer EV and Smith KR (1995) Breast cancer mortality among immigrants in Australia and Canada. *Journal of the National Cancer Institute* 87(15): 1154–1161.

Knight DC, Howes JB and Eden JA (1999) The effect of Promensil, an isoflavone extract, on menopausal symptoms. *Climacteric* 2(2): 79–84.

Knobf MT (2001) The menopausal symptom experience in young mid-life women with breast cancer. *Cancer Nursing* 24(3): 201–210; quiz 210–211.

Kumar NB, Allen K, Cantor A *et al.* (1997) Weight gain associated with adjuvant tamoxifen therapy in stage I and II breast cancer: fact or artifact? *Breast Cancer Research and Treatment* 44(2): 135–143.

Lazzaroni F, Scorolli L, Pizzoleo CF *et al.* (1998) Tamoxifen retinopathy: does it really exist? *Graefe's Archive for Clinical and Experimental Ophthalmology* 236(9): 669–673.

Levine-Silverman S (1989) The menopausal hot flash: a procrustean bed of research. *Journal of Advanced Nursing* 14(11): 939–949.

Loprinzi CL, Michalak JC, Quella SK *et al.* (1994) Megestrol acetate for the prevention of hot flashes. *New England Journal of Medicine* 331(6): 347–352.

Loprinzi CL, Pisansky TM, Fonseca R *et al.* (1998) Pilot evaluation of venlafaxine hydrochloride for the therapy of hot flashes in cancer survivors. *Journal of Clinical Oncology* 16(7): 2377–2381.

Love RR, Barden HS, Mazess RB, Epstein S and Chappell RJ (1994) Effect of tamoxifen on lumbar spine bone mineral density in postmenopausal women after 5 years. *Archives of Internal Medicine* 154(22): 2585–2588.

Lower EE, Blau R, Gazder P and Tummala R (1999) The risk of premature menopause induced by chemotherapy for early breast cancer. *Journal of Women's Health and Gender-Based Medicine* 8(7): 949–954.

Marsden J (2000) Hormone replacement therapy and breast cancer. *Maturitas* 34(Suppl. 2): S11–S24.

Matsumoto M, Miyauchi M, Yamamoto N, Shishikura T and Imanaka N (2000) Investigation of menstruation recovery after LH-RH agonist therapy for premenopausal patients with breast cancer. *Breast Cancer* 7(3): 237–240.

McInnes JA and Knobf MT (2001) Weight gain and quality of life in women treated with adjuvant chemotherapy for early-stage breast cancer. *Oncology Nursing Forum* 28(4): 675–684.

McPhail G and Smith LN (2000) Acute menopause symptoms during adjuvant systemic treatment for breast cancer: a case-control study. *Cancer Nursing* 23(6): 430–443.

Mezzetti M, La-Vecchia C, Decarli A, Boyle P, Talamini R and Franceschi S (1998) Population attributable risk for breast cancer: diet, nutrition and physical exercise. *Journal of the National Cancer Institute* 90(5): 389–394.

Moen MD and Keating GM (2008) Raloxifene: a review of its use in the prevention of invasive breast cancer. *Drugs* 68(14): 2059–2083.

Murkies AL, Lombard C, Strauss BJ, Wilcox G, Burger HG and Morton MS (1995) Dietary flour supplementation decreases post-menopausal hot flushes: effect of soy and wheat. *Maturitas* 21(3): 189–195.

Nachtigall LE (1994) Comparative study: Replens versus local estrogen in menopausal women. *Fertility and Sterility* 61(1): 178–180.

National Institute for Health and Clinical Excellence (2007) *NICE Technology Appraisal Guidance 112: Hormonal Therapies for the Adjuvant Treatment of Early Oestrogen-Receptor-Positive Breast Cancer.* London: NICE.

Nayfield SG, Karp JE, Ford LG, Dorr FA and Kramer BS (1991) Potential role of tamoxifen in prevention of breast cancer. *Journal of the National Cancer Institute* 83(20): 1450–1459.

Newton KM *et al.* (2006) Treatment of vasomotor symptoms of menopause with black cohosh, multibotanicals, soy, hormone therapy, or placebo: a randomized trial. *Annals of Internal Medicine* 145(12): 869–879.

Obermeyer CM, Ghorayeb F and Reynolds R (1999) Symptom reporting around the menopause in Beirut, Lebanon. *Maturitas* 33(3): 249–258.

Pannuti F, Martoni A, Zamagni C and Melotti B (1993) Progestins I: Medroxyprogesterone acetate. In: T. Powles and I. Smith (eds), *Medical Management of Breast Cancer* Cambridge: Dunitz.

Parton M and Smith IE (2008) Controversies in the management of patients with breast cancer: adjuvant endocrine therapy in premenopausal women. *Journal of Clinical Oncology* 26(5): 745–762.

Perez E (2006) The balance between risks and benefits: long-term use of aromatase inhibitors. *European Journal of Cancer Supplements* 4(9): 16–25.

Powles T (1993) Progestins II: Megestrol acetate. In: T. Powles and I. Smith (eds), *Medical Management of Breast Cancer*. Cambridge: Dunitz.

Powles T, Eeles R, Ashley S *et al.* (1998) Interim analysis of the incidence of breast cancer in the Royal Marsden Hospital tamoxifen randomised chemoprevention trial. *The Lancet* 352(9122): 98–101.

Powles TJ, Hickish T, Kanis JA, Tidy A and Ashley S (1996) Effect of tamoxifen on bone mineral density measured by dual-energy X-ray absorptiometry in healthy premenopausal and postmenopausal women. *Journal of Clinical Oncology* 14(1): 78–84.

Powles TJ, Jones AL, Ashley SE *et al.* (1994) The Royal Marsden Hospital pilot tamoxifen chemoprevention trial. *Breast Cancer Research and Treatment* 31(1): 73–82.

Prentice R, Thompson D, Clifford C, Gorbach S, Goldin B and Byar D (1990) Dietary fat reduction and plasma estradiol concentration in healthy postmenopausal women. The Women's Health Trial Study Group. *Journal of the National Cancer Institute* 82(2): 129–134.

Pritchard KI, Paterson AH, Paul NA, Zee B, Fine S and Pater J (1996) Increased thromboembolic complications with concurrent tamoxifen and chemotherapy in a randomized trial of adjuvant therapy for women with breast cancer. National Cancer Institute of Canada Clinical Trials Group Breast Cancer Site Group. *Journal of Clinical Oncology* 14(10): 2731–2737.

Royal College of Nursing (2005) *Breast Cancer and Bone Health*. London: Royal College of Nursing.

Schairer C, Lubin J, Troisi R, Sturgeon S, Brinton L and Hoover R (2000) Menopausal estrogen and estrogen-progestin replacement therapy and breast cancer risk. *Journal of the American Medical Association* 283(4): 485–491.

Shao W and Brown M (2003) Advances in estrogen receptor biology: prospects for improvements in targeted breast cancer therapy. *Breast Cancer Research* 6: 39–52.

Sharkey NA, Williams NI and Guerin JB (2000) The role of exercise in the prevention and treatment of osteoporosis and osteoarthritis. *Nursing Clinics of North America* 35(1): 209–221.

Simkin-Silverman LR and Wing RR (2000) Weight gain during menopause. Is it inevitable or can it be prevented? *Postgraduate Medicine* 108(3): 47–50: 53–56.

Singer D and Hunter M (1999) The experience of premature menopause: a thematic discourse analysis. *Journal of Reproductive and Infant Psychology* 17(1): 63–81.

Stearns V, Isaacs C, Rowland J *et al.* (2000) A pilot trial assessing the efficacy of paroxetine hydrochloride (Paxil) in controlling hot flashes in breast cancer survivors. *Annals of Oncology* 11(1): 17–22.

te Velde E and van Leusden H (1994) Hormonal treatment for the climacteric: alleviation of symptoms and prevention of postmenopausal disease. *The Lancet* 343: 654–658.

van Leeuwen FE, Benraadt J, Coebergh JW *et al.* (1994) Risk of endometrial cancer after tamoxifen treatment of breast cancer. *The Lancet* 343(8895): 448–452.

Veronesi U, Maisonneuve P, Costa A *et al.* (1998) Prevention of breast cancer with tamoxifen: preliminary findings from the Italian randomised trial among hysterectomised women. Italian Tamoxifen Prevention Study. *The Lancet* 352(9122): 93–97.

Vogel VG (2009) The NSABP Study of Tamoxifen and Raloxifene (STAR) trial. *Expert Reviews of Anticancer Therapy* 9(1): 51–60.

Wilcox G, Wahlqvist ML, Burger HG and Medley G (1990) Oestrogenic effects of plant foods in post-menopausal women. *British Medical Journal* 301(6757): 905–906.

Willett WC, Colditz G and Stampfer M (2000) Postmenopausal estrogens – opposed, unopposed, or none of the above. *Journal of the American Medical Association* 283(4): 534–535.

World Cancer Research Fund/American Institute for Cancer Research (2007) *Food, Nutrition, Physical Activity, and the Prevention of Cancer: A Global Perspective*. Washington, DC: AICR.

11   Lymphoedema and Breast Cancer

Mary Woods

INTRODUCTION

Cancer-related lymphoedema can occur after treatment for a variety of cancers, but most commonly occurs after treatment for breast cancer. The swelling can appear at any time after lymph node intervention and may involve all, or part, of the limb next to the treated breast. The breast itself and adjacent chest wall can also be involved. The experience of lymphoedema is unique to the person affected and has the potential to influence different aspects of life, including physical ability and body image. However, the degree to which the patient is affected is not necessarily dependent upon the size of the swollen arm, but on individual perceptions of the swelling and the coping mechanisms employed to assist in the treatment and necessary adaptation to a chronic condition. Successful management of lymphoedema involves a combination of approaches, but it is essential that the person affected is actively involved in employing self-care strategies aimed at gaining maximum improvement and long-term control of the swelling.

In this chapter, the reader will be introduced to the physiology underlying the development of lymphoedema in order to understand how it occurs following treatment for breast cancer, and to be able to identify patients at risk of its development. The physical, psychological and psychosocial problems that can occur will then be discussed and an overview provided of the range of treatment strategies employed to manage lymphoedema.

Many health-care professionals come into contact with breast cancer patients during their journey with cancer, and all have a role to offer in the education, treatment and support of the patient who has developed lymphoedema.

THE DEVELOPMENT OF LYMPHOEDEMA

Oedema can appear in the body for several reasons, and it is important that the patient is fully assessed in order to establish the cause of the oedema that is present and to identify the most appropriate strategy of management. Oedema can be of an acute nature, occurring as a result of trauma, and can also develop in response to chronic physiological changes in the body.

Lymphoedema is described by the British Lymphology Society (2007) as swelling that develops as a failure of lymph drainage.

Breast Cancer Nursing Care and Management, Second Edition, Edited by Victoria Harmer
© 2011 by Blackwell Publishing Ltd.

The lymphatic system consists of a network of vessels which are present throughout the body and are found in vascularised tissue. The superficial lymphatic system drains the tissues of the skin, and the deeper lymphatic system is found in skeletal muscle (CREST, 2008)

Larger lymphatic vessels contain smooth muscle and are able to contract. These larger lymphatic vessels act as collecting vessels, whilst smaller lymphatics are responsive to pressure changes and propel lymph by muscular movement, arterial pulsation and joint movement (Stanton, 2000). The role of the lymphatic system is to move fluid from within the interstitial spaces into the lymphatics in a unidirectional flow, until it reaches the efferent lymphatics, before finally draining into the bloodstream via the thoracic duct (Mortimer *et al.*, 1996).

The lymphatic system serves two main functions (Mortimer, 1990):

1 The regulation of homeostasis:
   • Large molecules, such as proteins, are returned to the circulation;
   • Unwanted cellular by-products are removed from the tissues;
   • Excess fluid is drained from the interstitium.
2 An immunological function:
   • Functioning lymph nodes are maintained;
   • Foreign material is removed and processed;
   • An appropriate auto-immune response is generated where necessary.

Lymph drainage can fail when damage or obstruction of the lymphatic system alters the available drainage routes and results in a reduced lymphatic system transport capacity (Woods, 2000). This may occur following treatment for breast cancer when the lymph node area of the axilla undergoes surgery or radiotherapy treatment. As a result, the lymph flow becomes restricted and swelling can appear in the tissues of the arm, the breast itself or the adjacent part of the trunk.

INCIDENCE AND PREVALENCE OF LYMPHOEDEMA

All patients with breast cancer who have undergone axillary intervention, are at risk of developing lymphoedema, which may appear many years after the initial breast cancer treatment and in the absence of recurrent disease.

Studies reporting the incidence of breast cancer–related lymphoedema vary considerably, and Keeley (2000) suggests that it is difficult to draw firm conclusions from them because of the different variables used in data collection. A recent review of research evidence on secondary lymphoedema suggests that, from 6 months post-surgery, one in five patients treated for breast cancer will experience secondary lymphoedema and that the number of patients with lymphoedema increases with time from surgery (National Breast and Ovarian Cancer Centre, 2008). Armer and Stewart (2005) looked at the risk of lymphoedema following breast cancer, using objective criteria to determine the presence of lymphoedema and, at 12 months post-surgery, found the incidence ranged from 42% to 70%. Francis *et al.* (2006), using the criteria for determining the presence of lymphoedema as a circumferential difference between the arms greater than 5%, found that 47% of women had lymphoedema 12 months post-surgery.

The well-recognised pattern of delay in the appearance of lymphoedema is not acknowledged in many studies of incidence where patients frequently complete a short follow-up period not exceeding 12 months (Keeley, 2000), and relatively few studies follow patients at risk of developing lymphoedema for a sufficiently long period to detect its development later on. Williams *et al.* (2005), in a review of epidemiological figures for lymphoedema, conclude that the overall incidence of lymphoedema is 30%, but a clearer picture of the incidence of lymphoedema developing after treatment for breast cancer requires additional prospective studies using standard diagnostic criteria and large cohorts of patients.

RISK FACTORS ASSOCIATED WITH THE DEVELOPMENT OF LYMPHOEDEMA

Although it is not possible to predict which patients will develop lymphoedema following breast cancer treatment, factors frequently thought to be involved in the development, progression and severity of the condition include:

- The type of breast cancer treatment that the patient receives;
- Post-operative events;
- The use and care of the 'at risk' arm.

Evidence-based support for these assertions, however, is weak and confined to suspected associations experienced primarily in clinical practice. In a systematic review of risk factors associated with lymphoedema, Cole (2006) stated that it is essential to separate the cause of lymphoedema from the risk of its development.

Type of breast cancer treatment

There is no clear indication that the type of surgical incision used can influence the risk of lymphoedema developing, but any intervention of the axillary lymph nodes during surgery or radiotherapy results in trauma to the lymphatic system and can alone be responsible for the subsequent development of lymphoedema (Stanton *et al.*, 1996). In a study by Clarke *et al.* (2005), more extensive breast cancer treatment was shown to increase the incidence of lymphoedema. More conservative treatment, however, may reduce the risk of lymphoedema, but does not protect patients from secondary lymphoedema, and procedures such as sentinel lymph node biopsies frequently progress to more extensive treatment in the axilla.

Post-operative events

The development of lymphoedema has been related to several post-operative events including wound complications, seroma formation and cording (Keeley, 2000). It is thought that the occurrence of one or more of these events may place the patient at greater risk of the development of lymphoedema later on. Infection is reported as a significant risk factor (Mozes, 1982), but Cole (2006) suggested that a clearer distinction is required between wound infection, occurring at the time of surgery and infection, reported as a trigger factor in the later development of lymphoedema.

Additional trigger factors

Additional trigger factors that are considered to be related to the development of lymphoedema following treatment for breast cancer include increasing age (Clarysse, 1993), and venepuncture in the affected arm (Smith, 1998; Harlow, 2001).

The relationship between a higher body mass index (BMI) and an increased risk of lymphoedema is unclear, but an association has long been suspected (Segerstrom *et al.*, 1992). The National Breast and Ovarian Cancer Centre (2008) conclude that a high BMI is not associated with a reduced risk of lymphoedema, but maintenance of a healthy BMI with its associated general health benefits should be promoted. However, further research is required in these areas.

IDENTIFYING LYMPHOEDEMA

Lymphoedema is characterised by the appearance of swelling which develops over a period of time. During the early stages, clothing or jewellery may become tighter and, there may be an ache or sense of fullness in the affected area. Visible swelling may be transient and mild but, as the condition progresses, the swelling becomes more evident and does not resolve. The skin becomes dry and thickened and the tissues harden. Left untreated, the swollen limb becomes mis-shapen as skinfolds develop, and the hardened, thickened skin gives rise to warty growths and hyperpigmentation.

Specific criteria for diagnosing lymphoedema do not exist, and the diagnosis is most frequently made on the basis of the patient's medical history and a full physical examination (CREST, 2008). Lymphoscintigraphy may be used to confirm the diagnosis, and Keeley (2006) suggests that this can be particularly useful when there is bilateral lower-limb oedema, or lower-limb oedema of uncertain origin. Circumferential measurement of the affected and unaffected upper limbs, using a tape measure, can indicate whether there is a difference between the sizes of the two limbs, but it can be difficult to draw conclusions from the measurement if both arms are swollen. In addition, there is a natural difference between the upper limbs of many women due to hand dominance.

The International Society of Lymphology (ISL) (2003) outlines a three-stage developmental process for lymphoedema, based on physical signs and symptoms associated with the oedema (Table 11.1). Whilst this is useful to identify the physical extent of the problem, it must be acknowledged that consideration is not made of the psychological and psychosocial impact of the swelling for the person concerned.

Table 11.1 International Society of Lymphology (2003) staging of lymphoedema.

Stage 1	Tissues are soft with no fibrosis Oedema pitts on pressure and reduces with limb elevation Limb volume difference <20%
Stage 2	Substantial fibrosis Tissues feel firm Oedema does not pitt on pressure or reduce on elevation Risk of infection is increased Limb volume difference >20%
Stage 3	Severe skin changes; hyperkeratosis and papillomatosis Skin loses elasticity Skin folds develop Risk of infection increases Limb volume difference >40%

Reproduced with permission from Woods, M (2007) *Lymphoedema Care.* Copyright © Wiley-Blackwell.

THE PHYSICAL EFFECTS OF LYMPHOEDEMA

Lymphoedema may involve all, or part of a limb (Fig. 11.1), the breast and the adjacent truncal quadrant. At an early stage, the swelling may be palpable and soft, responding well to treatment designed to reduce the volume of the limb. But as time passes, the tissues can become hardened and fibrosed, making the swelling more difficult to reverse. Physical changes which occur in the limb due to lymphoedema can influence a person's quality of life. This often presents personal challenges and can become a constant reminder of the breast cancer treatment.

Effects on the skin

The connective tissue in the dermis of the skin contains collagen and elastin fibres to give the skin its shape and to enable it to move over the subcutaneous tissues (Linnitt, 2000). As stasis of lymph occurs in the limb, fibrin and collagen are deposited in the subcutaneous tissues, causing the skin to become hardened and fibrosed. As the swelling progresses further, a loss of limb shape develops, accompanied by skin folds and deep crevices. In advanced lymphoedema, a warty, scaly appearance to the skin can develop (hyperkeratosis), and dilated skin lymphatics can give the appearance of blisters on the skin (lymphangiomata) (Linnitt, 2007).

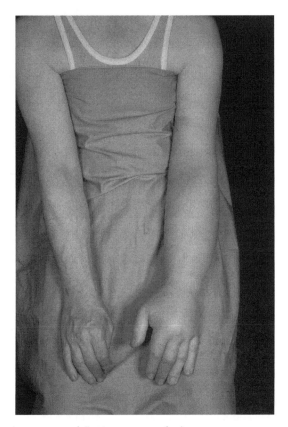

Fig. 11.1   Lymphoedematous arm following treatment for breast cancer.

Effects on limb function

A swollen arm may feel uncomfortable and heavy and, if the hand and fingers are swollen, fine finger movements may also become impaired. Studies have shown that the weight of a swollen limb can influence shoulder movement (Tobin *et al.*, 1993; Casley-Smith, 1994), and larger limbs result in greater physical problems.

THE PSYCHOLOGICAL EFFECTS OF LYMPHOEDEMA

Studies which have considered the psychological impact of breast cancer–related lymphoedema have identified a significant number of ways in which women can be affected by their swelling (McWayne and Heiney, 2005) Lymphoedema can have a negative impact upon daily life and can result in a mixture of emotions. These vary between individuals and are shaped by factors such as culture, upbringing and support from friends and family. Knowledge and understanding of the condition and how it can be managed also influences the response to it.

Tobin *et al.* (1993) suggested that women with lymphoedema following breast cancer suffer significantly greater depression and poorer adjustment to their illness than patients with breast cancer who have not developed lymphoedema This psychological handicap appears to be related to changes in body image and limb function, coupled with the associated effects that these problems can have upon social activities, occupation and personal relationships (Woods *et al.*, 1993; Maunsell *et al.*, 1993). Poorer illness adjustment leads to anger, depression and anxiety related to the loss of control and changes in body image. The suffering is intensified when there are difficulties accessing treatment and a lack of information and support by health-care professionals (Greenslade and House, 2006).

In a study of women with breast cancer–related arm swelling, Johanssen *et al.* (2003) identified two coping strategies that women developed in order to deal with their swelling in everyday life.

- Emotion-focused coping was most commonly used and involved a regulation of the emotions associated with the swelling. Patients described how they tried to adjust their personal values to accept the swelling or 'played down' its influence upon their life by trying to carry on as before (Johanssen *et al.*, 2003).
- Problem-focused coping involved making deliberate changes to the environment where significant problems were being experienced in order to make life easier (Johanssen *et al.*, 2003).

The visible change in the size and shape of a limb when lymphoedema develops can influence how patients perceive their body image. Whilst the effects of the original surgery remain hidden by clothing, the swollen arm can attract questions from others and serve as a visible reminder of the cancer and its treatment. Culture, upbringing and the media influence individual perceptions of body image, and reactions to an altered body image depend primarily upon the person's usual coping mechanisms.

Price (1990) outlines three components to body image:

1 Body reality: how the body is.
2 Body ideal: how we would like our body to look and function.
3 Body presentation: how we present ourselves to the world in order to balance body reality with body ideal.

Lymphoedema can be difficult to disguise and lead to a negative self-image. Body presentation may require great changes to a preferred style of dress (Woods *et al.*, 1993) and can sometimes lead to a complete loss of interest in dress and appearance (Tobin *et al.*, 1993).

THE PSYCHOSOCIAL EFFECTS OF LYMPHOEDEMA

For some patients, the effects of lymphoedema are far reaching, touching many areas of their lives. McWayne and Heiney (2005) highlight the threat of impaired quality of life due to role changes, disability and a lack of social support whilst Williams *et al.* (2004) in their study of patients with lymphoedema noted social stigma and social isolation to be a recurring theme among the research participants In many cases individual adaptation occurs as difficulties arise and the support of family and friends is required to make adaptation possible.

Occupation

Women, who have developed lymphoedema following breast cancer treatment and work outside the home, have been shown to have significantly larger swollen arms than women who do not work (Woods *et al.*, 1993). Combining the demands of a chosen occupation with other roles may mean that less time is available to care for the swollen arm. The type of occupation followed may also have an impact on the degree of swelling present with more sedentary occupations preferable to those requiring exertive, strenuous activities with the swollen arm which may increase the likelihood of problematic swelling.

Relationships and social activities

The uniqueness of each individual may mean that many different problems are encountered by the woman with breast cancer–related arm swelling. Personal and social relationships may suffer if there are difficulties with self image and Williams *et al.* (2004) describe how patients found it difficult to talk to others about their condition. The demands of coping with lymphoedema and a loss of self-esteem can place tremendous pressure upon relationships of a personal, sexual and social nature and difficulties in function may influence the work and home environment. The quality and quantity of understanding and support from others has been shown by Passik *et al.* (1995) to influence the degree of psychological distress experienced and Mason (2000) suggests that support received from others can influence how receptive the patient is to a suggested programme of care.

THE MANAGEMENT OF LYMPHOEDEMA

Foeldi, a German physician, developed an effective strategy of management for lymphoedema in Europe during the 1970s. Based on the experience of Emil and Estrid Vodder, who had developed a technique of lymphatic massage to increase the transport of lymphatic fluid, Foeldi's method comprised four main elements of treatment, used in combination, which he termed Complex Decongestive Physiotherapy (Foeldi *et al.*, 1985). Today, this method of treatment can also be termed complex physical therapy (Mason, 1993) complex decongestive therapy (Daane, 1998) and complex lymphoedema therapy (Johansson *et al.*, 1999), but the four elements of skin care, exercise and movement, lymph drainage and external containment continue and are regarded by the British Lymphology Society as a desirable approach to the management of lymphoedema in this country (British Lymphology Society, 2007; Lymphoedema Framework, 2006).

The treatment of lymphoedema is not curative, due to the disruption that has occurred within the lymph channels. The aim is to maximise lymph drainage so that a reduction in the swelling can be achieved based on the potential of the individual patient. Appropriate care of the swollen limb ensures that the likelihood of problematic complications occurring is minimised.

Assessment

Lymphoedema is a long-term chronic condition in which the patient should become an active participant in its management. A full and accurate assessment of the patient should therefore include the identification of personal priorities and goals so that the patient and therapist can work together in partnership to achieve maximum improvement and long-term control of the swelling. Mason (2000) in an article which explores rehabilitation in lymphoedema management, suggests that patient-centred decisions regarding treatment should recognise individual experiences, problems and coping mechanisms. Goal-setting then becomes relevant and the patient can develop a sense of ownership in the decision making process, which encourages compliance with treatment (Mason, 2000).

Rather than a single event, assessment of the patient with lymphoedema is an ongoing event which incorporates subjective and objective aspects. Based on the work by Alfaro-Lefevre (1999) a five-stage model for the assessment process was outlined by Webb (2004) and can be applied to the assessment of the patient with lymphoedema:

- **Stage 1: Assessment.** To highlight the cancer treatment that the patient has received and identify risk factors for the development of lymphoedema.
- **Stage 2: Problem identification.** To identify actual and potential problems based on a physical examination of the swollen area and consideration of the impact and influence of the swelling on the patient's daily life.
- **Stage 3: Planning.** To utilise patient strengths in making decisions regarding the choice of treatment for the lymphoedema based on clear patient focused goals.
- **Stage 4: Implementation.** Implementing appropriate aspects of treatment and modifying them when required.
- **Stage 5: Evaluation.** Progress is assessed at regular intervals to encourage motivation and compliance and also to ensure the treatment strategies remain appropriate.

With the patient's views and wishes fully respected, Woods stresses that the burden of treatment should not exceed the benefit to be gained and that realistic expectations of the outcome of treatment are fully discussed (Woods, 2000).

The two phases of treatment

The four elements of treatment; skin care, exercise and movement, lymph drainage and external containment are organised into two phases of care described by Jenns (2000) and Lymphoedema Framework (2006)

Phase 1: The intensive phase

The intensive phase is a short planned period of therapist-led treatment, in which specific goals are mutually agreed between the patient and the therapist. Treatment is usually carried out daily to include multi-layer compression bandaging and additional elements of treatment depending upon the patient's needs.

Indications for this phase of treatment include:

- Large limbs;
- Mis-shapen limbs;
- Severe lymphoedema with skin changes;
- Damaged or fragile skin;
- Lymphorrhoea;
- Support and comfort in the palliative care setting.

Treatment may include some, or all of the following elements of treatment:

- Skin hygiene and care;
- Limb movement and exercise;
- Manual lymph drainage;
- External containment using multi-layer compression bandaging.

Phase 2: The maintenance phase

The concept of self-care is promoted to enable the patient to become independent in the long-term control and management of their swelling. The therapist provides advice and support for the patient, evaluating progress at regular intervals to ensure that any problems are identified early and that compression garments remain appropriate and are replaced when necessary.

Indications for this phase of treatment include:

- Mild/moderately swollen limbs;
- Normal limb shape;
- Patient ability to follow a self-care regime;

Treatment may include some, or all of the following elements of treatment:

- A skin-care regime;
- Limb movement and exercise regime;
- Simple lymph drainage;
- External containment using compression garments.

Many patients will embark upon a maintenance phase of treatment for their swelling without the need for an intensive course of treatment.

Elements of treatment

Skin care

A number of skin conditions and potential skin problems are associated with lymphoedema Reduced local immunity following the removal or irradiation of lymph nodes means there is an increased risk of infection in the limb (Lymphoedema Framework, 2006) and a loss of natural elasticity develops with lymph stasis.

The aim of skin care is:

- To promote skin integrity;
- To minimise the risks of infection.

A daily skin hygiene regime is recommended (Rich, 2007) which includes meticulous hygiene, inspection and observation of the skin, coupled with the application of emollients to provide a protective lipid layer and prevent water loss and subsequent dehydration of the skin. Patients should also be advised to take precautions to ensure that the integrity of their skin is not compromised during activities likely to place them at risk.

The advice to patients with arm lymphoedema is as follows:

- Wash the skin gently and dry thoroughly.
- Moisturise daily with a bland, non-perfumed cream or lotion.
- Take care to avoid trauma to the skin when cutting nails and removing unwanted body hair.
- Use gloves to protect the hands when gardening, washing up or reaching in to a hot oven.
- Use an antiseptic cream if trauma to the skin does occur.
- Avoid extremes of temperature such a very hot baths and saunas.
- Protect the skin from insect bites and sunburn during the summer months and when on holiday.
- Avoid any kind of venepuncture in the affected arm through injections or the giving/taking of blood.
- Ask for blood pressure recordings to be taken on the other arm.

A number of skin problems can develop, as listed below.

Fungal infections

Common fungal infections include athlete's foot and thrush, which can occur in deep skin folds or between swollen fingers. The skin appears moist, white, scaly and macerated and may be extremely itchy. If left untreated, fungal infections can increase the risk of the development of cellulitis. Treatment is with anti-fungal agents available via the pharmacy.

Cellulitis

A feature of lymphoedema are attacks of apparent infection in the swollen arm, preceded by symptoms associated with influenza. The patient feels unwell with a fever, which progresses to pain and redness in the affected limb coupled with an increase in swelling. Although attacks can occur suddenly and without warning, they are frequently associated with a recent accidental skin injury in the affected arm and can sometimes be severe enough to require hospitalisation. Treatment is with antibiotics administered orally or intravenously for a 2-week period. The patient should be encouraged to rest during the acute phase of the attack. Recurrent attacks may require control with long-term antibiotics (Mortimer, 2000).

A consensus document is available to guide practitioners in the management of cellulitis in lymphoedema. This document clearly outlines the appropriate treatment protocol to be followed when cellulitis occurs (British Lymphology Society/Lymphoedema Support Network).

Dry skin

Stretched skin due to swelling can become inelastic and feel tight and uncomfortable. If left to progress, the skin can become flaky and scaly with an increasing risk of bacterial entry if cracks in the skin develop. The use of bland, unperfumed emollient lotions or creams soothes and rehydrates dry, irritated skin. A skin-care regime of hygiene and moisturising adopted daily can promote healthy skin.

Lymphorrhoea

A leakage of lymph through the surface of the skin can develop spontaneously if the skin it tight and fragile. It can also occur following an injury to the skin where skin integrity becomes compromised. Lymphorrhoea poses an infection risk, and the persistent leakage of lymph fluid can result in skin excoriation and breakdown. The management of this condition is reported to vary between professionals. Ling *et al.* (1997) and Benbow (2002) identified seven different dressings which could be used for lymphorrhoea. Non-adherent dressings and light compression applied to the limb for 24–48 hours can achieve considerable success in terminating the leakage of lymph fluid and allowing the condition of the skin to improve (Gilbert and Mortimer, 2001; Renshaw, 2007).

Exercise and movement

Joint mobility and lymph drainage can be promoted through movement and appropriate exercise of the swollen arm as the action of the muscle pump stimulates superficial lymphatics to drain. The effect is enhanced whilst compression garments are worn.

The research available to assist the therapist in identifying a safe, effective exercise regime for patients with lymphoedema supports a gradual, controlled exercise programme, tailored to the patient's life-style and interests (McKenzie and Kalda, 2003; Lane *et al.*, 2005) and the avoidance of over vigorous, isometric (static) activities e.g. carrying heavy shopping bags which can increase blood flow, overwhelm the lymphatics and make the swelling worse.

Isotonic exercises, such as those carried out against a fixed resistance, shorten or lengthen the muscle, allowing the initial lymphatics to open as the connective tissue moves and interstitial fluid is permitted to enter (Lane, 2005).

Davies and Desborough (2008) believe that patients with breast cancer–related lymphoedema can have a combination of problems including shoulder problems, stiffness and weakness, which require a full assessment and holistic approach with an individual programme of exercise to suit their needs.

Lymph drainage

In lymphoedema management, lymph drainage refers to a particular type of skin massage called manual lymph drainage, which has also been adapted into a simplified form called simple lymph drainage.

Manual lymph drainage

Manual lymph drainage (MLD) is a unique method of massage in which specialised movements of the thumbs, fingers and hand are used to exert gentle and smooth pressure on the skin. Originally used by beauticians and masseurs within a framework of classical massage, MLD is now used for a range of medical conditions where lymph drainage routes have *not* been impaired by medical intervention. In order to treat lymphoedema, MLD therapists must undergo additional specific training in order to understand abnormal or altered lymph flow.

The aim of MLD is:

- To improve the function of the normal lymphatics;
- To encourage superficial lymph channels to find alternative drainage routes;
- To stimulate lymph flow and drainage away from congested areas.

As an aspect of treatment for lymphoedema, there have been reports of significant improvements in swelling following a 3-week course of daily treatment (Pearson, 1995; Jackson, 1995). However, MLD is felt to be most effective when used in combination with multi-layer compression bandaging (Jenns, 2000).

There remains limited scientific research to support the use of MLD in lymphoedema management, but it is frequently used to treat long-standing swelling that has become complex and complicated or where there is congestion evident at the root of the limb, which is impeding the drainage of lymph. It is vital that the therapist performing MLD has undergone appropriate specialist training.

Simple lymph drainage

Simple lymph drainage (SLD) has evolved from MLD to be easily accessible to patients and their relatives. Based on the principles of MLD, with simplified hand movements, it is only used on areas where normal lymph drainage exists (British Lymphology Society, 2001).

The aim of SLD is:

- To stimulate normal draining lymphatics;
- To 'milk' fluid away from congested areas;
- To improve superficial lymph drainage.

Most patients with lymphoedema can benefit from using SLD within a self-care programme of management for their swelling. However, the success with which it can be applied is dependent upon the ability of the therapist to teach the technique and the motivation and confidence of the patient (Bellhouse, 2000). SLD can be taught to a relative or friend so that they can use it on the patient if there are difficulties with movement restricting the patient from using the technique independently.

Compression therapy

In the management of lymphoedema, compression therapy refers to the enclosing of a limb within bandages or garments in order to reduce or control swelling. It is a widely used aspect of treatment for lymphoedema, which is acknowledged as particularly beneficial for the majority of patients (Todd, 2000; Lymphoedema Framework, 2006).

Compression bandages

Low-stretch, inelastic bandages are used within the intensive phase of lymphoedema treatment to act as a counterforce to voluntary muscular activity. They can provide an effective means of management for lymphoedema where the limb size, shape and condition are compromised or complicated by severe swelling.

The use of bandages within this phase of treatment is a specialist technique requiring skills and knowledge in the application of the bandages, and should not be attempted by health-care professionals without the supervision of an experienced therapist. The therapist has a responsibility to ensure that he/she has a sound knowledge of bandaging theory and a good technique in bandage application as the inappropriate use of bandages, or their poor application, can result in skin and tissue damage.

The suitability of a patient for a course of bandaging should be carefully considered during a full assessment to ensure that it is appropriate to their needs. Education and advice will be required regarding appropriate clothing to accommodate the bulk of the bandages, personal hygiene whilst the bandages are in place and the impact that the bandages may have upon activities of daily living.

For bandaging to be effective in reducing swelling, a number of physical principles must be considered.

The pressure provided by the bandages on the swollen arm must be evenly distributed. Where the normal limb shape has become distorted by swelling, it can be corrected by the use of foam and padding underneath the bandages to provide an even profile upon which the bandages can be applied.

The pressure must be graduated along the length of the swollen arm to ensure that the most pressure is achieved distally and the least proximally, to aid lymph drainage. This can be achieved by selecting the correct bandage width for the size of the swollen arm and ensuring that the bandage overlap is greatest towards the distal part of the arm and less towards the root of the arm. Graduated pressure can also be achieved by using more than one layer of bandages and controlling the amount of tension applied to the bandages.

The pressure exerted on the limb must be adequate to counter the limb circumference. When the circumference of the swollen arm is significant, greater pressure will be required in order to influence the swelling. This can be achieved by the use of more than one layer of bandages and the correct choice of bandage width for the circumference of the arm.

Low-stretch bandages provide a low resting pressure enabling them to be comfortable whilst the patient is at rest. During muscular activity however, a high working pressure is provided by the bandages, as the muscle works against the support provided by the bandages. For this reason, the patient should be aware of the importance of exercise whilst the arm is bandaged to ensure maximum effectiveness from their use. The bandages should not be painful or uncomfortable, but if discomfort occurs at any time they should be removed.

Compression garments

Graduated compression garments are used in the maintenance phase of lymphoedema management alongside skin care, exercise and simple lymph drainage. By compressing the tissues, they limit the formation of lymph and, by maximising the effect of the muscle pump, the flow of lymph towards the root of the limb is increased.

Compression garments are manufactured as either round knit or flat bed knit. Round knit garments are produced in one piece and are readily available as 'off-the shelf' garments at reasonable cost. Synthetic materials are used to produce these garments in order to make them aesthetically pleasing and easy to wear. A wide range of sizes and styles are available to accommodate the needs of most patients.

Flat bed knit garments are made as one piece garments joined with a seam. These are usually specifically 'made-to-measure' for a patient, and therefore accurate measurements of the swollen arm are necessary to ensure that the finished garment fits. These garments can be useful when round knit garments cannot meet specific patient requirements.

The therapist choosing a compression sleeve for a patient with arm lymphoedema, should possess sound knowledge concerning the different types, styles and sizes of the garments available. A full assessment and discussion with the patient should highlight any concerns regarding the safe application and removal of the garments each day and all swollen areas must be included within the garment chosen.

Garments should *not* be fitted if:

- The limb size is > 20% excess volume (Badger *et al.*, 2000).
- The limb shape is irregular, particularly if there are deepened skin folds.
- The skin condition is poor with fragile or damaged areas of skin.
- The patient is suffering an acute infective episode (cellulitis).
- There is arterial or venous insufficiency.

Once chosen, the therapist should evaluate the fitted garment to satisfy him/herself that it will meet the role for which it is intended.

- The garment should fit snugly and be comfortable to wear.
- The garment should not cut into the limb, causing a tourniquet effect, or have loose pockets where excess fluid can accumulate.
- The fingers should remain pink and warm with normal sensations.
- The garment should include all parts of the limb where swelling is present.
- The garment should be the correct length and not be allowed to crease or be turned over at the top.

The application of compression garments can be assisted with the use of an ordinary household rubber glove, which facilitates the even distribution of material along the length of the limb. There are also several commercially made aids available if greater assistance is required. The use of creams and oils on the skin should be avoided prior to the application of the garments as these can damage the fabric.

Compression garments are most effective when worn every day, particularly when the arm is most active.

CONCLUSION

As a chronic condition, which can develop following treatment for breast cancer, the impact of lymphoedema upon the patient's life should not be underestimated. Lymphoedema is not 'a small price to pay' for the cancer treatment received, as some patients are still unfortunately lead to believe. The literature discussed in this chapter illustrates how the development of swelling can influence many different areas of the individual's life. Indeed adaptation to some aspects of daily life is even required by those who are 'at risk' of developing lymphoedema if they are to minimise the risks of problematic swelling occurring in the future.

Individual needs and coping mechanisms are very different, and therefore the key to true holistic and patient-centred care for the patient with lymphoedema is not just an assessment of their physical symptoms, in order to apply the different physical treatment strategies outlined, but the inclusion of an assessment of psychological and psychosocial needs also. The therapist must seek to understand the patient's individual story in order to adopt an approach to management of the swelling that is acceptable for the patient and promotes independence and confidence in their ability to manage the swelling during everyday life.

REFERENCES

Alfaro-Lefevre R (1999) Critical thinking. In: *Nursing: A Practical Approach*, 2nd edn. Philadelphia: W.B. Saunders.

Armer J and Stewart B (2005) A comparison of four diagnostic criteria for lymphoedema in a post-breast cancer population. *Lymphatic Research and Biology* 3(4): 208–217.

Badger C, Peacock J and Mortimer P (2000) A randomised controlled parallel-group clinical trial comparing multi-layer bandaging followed by hosiery versus hosiery alone in the treatment of patients with lymphoedema of the limb. *Cancer* 88(12): 2832–2837.

Bellhouse S (2000) Simple lymphatic drainage. In: R Twycross, K Jenns and J Todd (eds) *Lymphoedema*. Oxford: Radcliffe Medical Press Ltd.

Benbow M (2002) Swollen, leaking legs. *Nurse 2 Nurse* 2(8): 34–38.

British Lymphology Society (2007) *Strategy for Lymphoedema Care*. Cheltenham: British Lymphology Society Administration Centre.

British Lymphology Society (2001) *Guidelines for the Use of Manual Lymph Drainage (MLD) and Simple Lymph Drainage (SLD) in Lymphoedema*. Caterham: British Lymphology Society Administration Centre.

British Lymphology Society/Lymphoedema Support Network (2005) *Consensus Document on the Management of Cellulitis in Lymphoedema*. Available: http://www.lymphoedema.org/lsn.

Casley-Smith JR and Casley-Smith J (1994) *Modern Treatment for Lymphoedema*. Adelaide: The Lymphoedema Association of Australia.

Clarke B, Sitzia J and Harlow W (2005) Incidence and risk of arm oedema following treatment for breast cancer; a three year follow-up study. *Quarterly Journal of Medicine* 98: 343–348.

Clarysse A (1993) Lymphoedema following breast cancer treatment. *Acta Clinica Belgica Supplementum* 15: 47–50.

Cole T (2006) Risks and benefits of needle use in patients after axillary node surgery. *British Journal of Nursing* 15(18): 969–979.

CREST (2008) *Guidelines for the diagnosis, assessment and management of lymphoedema*. Available: http://www.cancerni.net/publications/crestguidelinesonthediagnosisassessmentandmanagementoflymphoedema.

Daane S (1998) Post mastectomy lymphoedema management: evolution of the of the complex decongestive therapy technique. *Annals of Plastic Surgery* 40: 323–327.

Davies R and Desborough S (2008) Lymphoedema. In: J Rankin, K Robb, N. Murtagh, J Cooper and S Lewis (eds) *Rehabilitation in Cancer Care*. Oxford: Wiley-Blackwell.

Foeldi E, Foeldi M and Weissleder H (1985) Conservative management of lymphoedema of the limbs *Angiology – Journal of Vascular Diseases* 36(3): 171–180.

Francis W, Abghari P, Du W, Rymal C, Suna M and Kosir M (2006) Improving surgical outcomes: standardising the reporting of incidence and severity of acute lymphoedema after sentinel lymph node biopsy and axillary lymph node dissection. *American Journal of Surgery* 192(5): 636–639.

Gilbert J and Mortimer P (2001) Current views on the management of breast cancer related lymphoedema. *CME Breast* 1(1): pp. 14–17.

Greenslade M and House C (2006) Living with lymphoedema: a qualitative study of women's perspectives on prevention and management following breast cancer related treatment *Canadian Oncology Nursing Journal* 16(3): 165–179.

Harlow W (2001) Venepuncture – a causative factor in the development of arm oedema following breast cancer treatment. *British Lymphology Society Annual Conference; Innovations in Practice* 1–2 October.

International Society of Lymphology (2003) The diagnosis and treatment of peripheral lymphoedema. Consensus document of the International Society of Lymphology. *Lymphology* 36(2): 84–91.

Jenns K (2000) Management strategies. In: R Twycross, K Jenns and J Todd (eds) *Lymphoedema*. Oxford: Radcliffe Medical Press Ltd, pp. 97–117.

Johansson K, Albertsson M, Ingvar C and Ekdahl C (1999) Effects of compression bandaging with or without manual lymph drainage treatment in patients with post-operative arm lymphoedema. *Lymphology* 32: 103–110.

Johansson K, Holmstrom H, Nilsson I, Ingvar C, Albertsson M and Ekdahl C (2003) Breast cancer patient's experiences of lymphoedema. *Scandinavian Journal of Caring Science* 17: 35–42.

Keeley V (2000) Classification of lymphoedema. In: R Twycross, K Jenns and J Todd (eds) *Lymphoedema*. Oxford: Radcliffe Medical Press Ltd.

Keeley V (2006) The use of lymphoscintigraphy in the management of chronic oedema. *Journal of Lymphology* 1(1): 42–57.

Lane K, Jespersen D and McKenzie D (2005) The effect of a whole body exercise programme and dragon boat training on arm volume and arm circumference in women treated for breast cancer. *European Journal of Cancer Care* 14: 353–358.

Ling J, Duncan A, Laverty D and Hardy J (1997) Lymphorhoea in palliative care. *European Journal of Cancer Care* 4(2): 50–52.

Linnitt N (2000) Skin management in lymphoedema. In: R Twycross, K Jenns and J Todd (eds) *Lymphoedema*. Oxford: Radcliffe Medical Press Ltd, pp. 118–129.

Linnitt N (2007) Complex skin changes in chronic oedemas. *British Journal of Community Nursing: The Lymphoedema Supplement* (April) S10–S15.

Lymphoedema Framework (2006) *Best Practice for the Management of Lymphoedema, International Consensus.* London: Medical Education Partnership (MEP) Ltd.

Mason W (2000) Exploring rehabilitation within lymphoedema management. *International Journal of Palliative Nursing* 6(6): 265–273.

Maunsell E, Brisson J and Deschenes L (1993) Arm problems and psychological distress after surgery for breast cancer. *Canadian Journal of Surgery* 36: 315–320.

McKenzie D and Kalda A (2003) Effect of upper extremity exercise on secondary lymphoedema in breast cancer patients: a pilot study *Journal of Clinical Oncology* 21(3): 463–466.

McWayne J and Heiney S (2005) Psychological and social sequelae of secondary lymphoedema–a review. *Cancer* 104(3): 457–466.

Mortimer PS (1990) Investigation and management of lymphoedema. *Vascular Medicine Review* 1: 1–20.

Mortimer PS (2000) Acute inflammatory episodes. In: R Twycross, K Jenns and J Todd (eds) *Lymphoedema*. Oxford: Radcliffe Medical Press Ltd, pp. 130–139.

Mortimer PS, Bates D, Brassington H, Stanton A, Strachan D and Levick J (1996) The prevalence of arm oedema following treatment for breast cancer. *Quarterly Journal of Medicine* 89: 377–380.

Mozes M (1982) The role of infection in postmastectomy lymphoedema. *Surgery Annual* 14: 73–83.

National Breast and Ovarian Cancer Centre (2008) *Review of Research Evidence on Secondary Lymphoedema: Incidence, Prevention, Risk Factors and Treatment.* Surrey Hills, New South Wales: NBOCC. Available: http://www.nbocc.org.au/view-document-details/slerw-review-of-research-evidence-on-secondary-lymphoedema.

Passik S, Newman M, Brennan M and Tunkel R (1995) Predictors of psychological distress, sexual dysfunction and physical functioning among women with upper extremity lymphoedema related to breast cancer. *Psycho-Oncology* 4: 255–263.

Price B (1990) A model for body-image care. *Journal of Advanced Nursing* (15): 585–593.

Renshaw M (2007) Lymphorrhoea: leaky legs are not just the nurse's problem. *British Journal of Community Nursing: The Lymphoedema Supplement* (April) S18–S21.

Rich A (2007) How to care for uncomplicated skin and keep it free from complications. *British Journal of Community Nursing: The Lymphoedema Supplement* (April) S6–S9.

Segerstrom K, Bjerle P, Graffman S and Nystrom A (1992) Factors that influence the incidence of brachial oedema following treatment of breast cancer. *Scandanavian Journal of Plastic and Reconsructive Surgery and Hand Surgery* 26: 223–227.

Smith J (1998) The practice of venepuncture in lymphoedema. *European Journal of Cancer Care* 7: 97–98.

Stanton A (2000) How does tissue swelling occur? In: R Twycross, K Jenns and J Todd (eds) *Lymphoedema*. Oxford: Radcliffe Medical Press Ltd.

Stanton A, Levick J and Mortimer P (1996) Current puzzles presented by postmastectomy oedema (breast cancer related lymphoedema) *Vascular Medicine* 1: 213–225.

Tobin M, Lacey H, Meyer L and Mortimer P (1993) The psychological morbidity of breast cancer-related arm swelling. *Cancer* 72(11): 3248–3252.

Todd J (2000) Containment in the management of lymphoedema. In: R Twycross, K Jenns and J Todd (eds) *Lymphoedema*. Oxford: Radcliffe Medical Press Ltd.

Webb C (2004) Communication and assessment. In: L Dougherty and S Lister (eds) *The Royal Marsden Manual of Clinical Nursing Procedures*, 6th edn. Oxford: Blackwell Publishing, pp. 27–37.

Williams A, Franks P and Moffatt C (2005) Lymphoedema: estimating the size of the problem *Palliative Medicine* 19: 300–313.

Williams A, Moffatt C and Franks P (2004) A phenomenological study of the lived experiences of people with lymphoedema. *International Journal of Palliative Nursing* 10(6): 279–286.

Woods M (2000) Lymphoedema. In: J Cooper (ed.) *Stepping into Palliative Care; A Handbook for Health Care Professionals*. Oxford: Radcliffe Medical Press Ltd.

Woods M, Tobin M and Mortimer PS (1993) The psychosocial morbidity of breast cancer patients with lymphoedema. *Cancer Nursing* 18(6): 467–471.

12   Fungating Wounds

Victoria Harmer (previous contribution by Rachael King)

INTRODUCTION

Fungating wounds are distressing and often complex as there is a need to manage them from both the patient and carer perspective. Fungating wounds present many challenges to nursing staff, because they rarely heal, and they produce a multitude of problems, which often recur and are difficult to manage (Laverty *et al.*, 2000). They are often an indication that the patient has reached the end stage, or has an advanced primary cancer, and that alone is a serious concern for the patient. There is little research in this area, and much of the work is based on anecdotal evidence and case studies. It is imperative to encourage a multidisciplinary approach to care for this group of patients, in order to ensure that the progression in their wound care is of the optimum. Effective wound care in the community, or indeed in hospital outpatient clinics, may result in reducing hospital admissions and allow patients more independence.

Radiotherapy, chemotherapy and hormone therapy may have some effect on reducing the size and symptoms of these wounds, but the benefits of these treatments need to be balanced against their potential side effects (Naylor, 2001). The main priorities within the assessment and management of this type of wound on this type of patient is to ensure that not only the wound itself is dressed in the most appropriate fashion, but that the patient's body image and self-esteem are managed effectively as well.

DEFINITION OF A FUNGATING WOUND

Fungating wounds occur due to the related changes in the cells and tissues from a cancerous growth. Owing to the involvement of the deeper tissues, there are large amounts of exudate.

A fungating wound develops from the extension of a malignant tumour into the structures of the skin, producing a raised or ulcerating necrotic lesion (Moody and Grocott, 1993; Bennett and Moody, 1995; Mortimer, 1998). Fungating wounds are described as 'fungus-like' or 'cauliflower-like' growths because of their appearance (Grocott, 1999). There is some controversy in the available literature in this field as to whether the correct terminology for these types of wounds should be a fungating lesion, malignant lesion or skin ulceration, and all have been identified as being dependent on the stage at which the fungating wound

Breast Cancer Nursing Care and Management, Second Edition, Edited by Victoria Harmer
© 2011 by Blackwell Publishing Ltd.

is (Haagenson, 1971; Petrek *et al.*, 1983; Sims and Fitzgerald, 1985; Bale and Harding, 1987; Carville, 1994). It is important to mention that the appearance and presentation of the wound will differ significantly from patient to patient (Grocott, 1999).

AETIOLOGY OF FUNGATING WOUNDS

Fungating malignant wounds are a result of the infiltration of the skin and its supporting blood and lymph vessels by a local tumour, or of metastatic spread from a primary tumour (Grocott, 2000). They will occur along blood and lymph capillaries and between tissue planes (Moseley, 1998). A reduction in oxygen diffusion will lead to tissue hypoxia and, ultimately, will lead to tissue breakdown. The consequences of this will be a build up of anaerobic and aerobic bacteria at the tumour site, which is the cause of the characteristic malodour, and large amounts of exudate production are often associated with fungating malignant wounds. There will be an increased level of proteases that will also lead to further breakdown. Regnard and Tempest (1992) claim that the cause of the easy bleeding associated with this type of wound is the fragility of the capillaries contained within the mass. There is a high risk to life when the tumour infiltrates into major blood vessels, causing a great risk of massive haemorrhage.

APPEARANCE OF A FUNGATING WOUND

It is recognised that a fungating wound can appear in the form of a nodule with the appearance of fungus, or it may appear as an ulcerating crater resulting from ignored cancer. It is generally characterised by the 'lip' that surrounds the margin of the wound and by its nature and complexity (Naylor, 2001). Fungating wounds are often associated with carcinoma of the breast, but can also be the result of sarcomas, squamous cell carcinomas or melanomas (Hallett, 1995) (see Plate 4).

INCIDENCE OF FUNGATING WOUNDS

The true incidence of fungating malignant wounds is unknown (Grocott, 1995). A retrospective survey carried out by Thomas (1992) provides the most reliable of recent data available. This shows that, over a 1-year period, community nurse practitioners could visit in the region of 2 500 patients with fungating wounds; the most prevalent location for this type of wound was on the breast.

THE SKIN

The skin is the largest organ of the body. It measures 1.5–2 m^2 and is home to about 3 000 000 micro-organisms per cm^2, which feed on its secretions and scales. The skin holds the body contents together and is designed to limit the loss of essential body fluids whilst providing a defensive shield against hazardous effects of physical, chemical and biological influences from the environment. It is made up of two layers, epidermis and dermis, which are anchored to the subcutaneous layer.

NORMAL WOUND HEALING

The healing process commences following a break in the skin. The degree of tissue damage, the cause of the wound, the general condition of the patient and ongoing management of care are all variables which influence the length of time the wound will take to heal (Benbow, 2008).

Platelets stem bleeding, resulting in haemostasis. Platelets also control cellular injury, contain blood loss and prepare a clean bed for wound repair (Waldrop and Doughty, 2000). The platelets release cytokines, which attract other cells, ready for the inflammatory phase of healing. The platelets then release serotonin and vasoconstrictors. Vasoconstriction occurs to limit blood loss and a clot will form, acting as a temporary bacterial barrier and a framework for migrating cells. The clot is lysed by plasmin once it has achieved its purpose (Kindlen and Morison, 1997).

Wound healing is a complex physiological process that is dependent on a number of inter-related factors. The process of wound healing can be divided into four overlapping phases ((Kindlen and Morison, 1997)):

- Acute inflammatory phase;
- Destructive phase;
- Proliferative phase;
- Maturation phase.

Acute inflammatory phase of healing (0–3 days)

The acute inflammatory phase of healing is the initial phase that commences the process of wound healing. When the skin becomes subject to trauma, bleeding will occur. The damaged ends of the blood vessels will constrict in order to minimise blood loss, blood clots will occur, allowing a temporary closure of the wound and a scab will form. The bleeding will also help to cleanse the wound of any debris and bacteria that may have entered the wound as a result of the injury.

Healing occurs as a result of complex relationships between inhibitory and stimulatory chemical mediators, and this inflammatory phase is to prepare the injured tissue for the next phases of healing. Damaged cells release mediators such as histamine, and white cells and dilated blood vessels cause the characteristics of redness, swelling, pain, loss of function and oedema (Kindlen and Morison, 1997).

This inflammatory phase of healing lasts about 3–4 days, after which time the blood vessels return to their normal size, the signs of inflammation reduce and fibroblasts infiltrate to assist in reconnecting the tissue (Bale and Jones, 2000).

As this phase of healing demands much energy, it is important that the patient is eating and resting well. If the patient has diabetes or anaemia, this inflammatory phase will be prolonged, and thus there will be a delay in healing (Benbow, 2008).

Destructive phase of healing (2–6 days)

During the destructive phase of healing, the wound is cleared of debris and unwanted material. Macrophages engulf and digest bacteria, removing excess fibrin, producing growth factors and stimulating the production of fibroblasts. Fibroblasts give strength and structure to the wound as they stimulate cell migration, angiogenesis, embryonic development and wound healing. They are involved in soft tissue growth and regeneration (Collins *et al.* 2002).

The repair and production of new collagen-rich tissue (scar tissue) occurs during this phase of healing through cellular activity (Benbow, 2008).

Proliferative phase of healing (3–24 days)

During the proliferative phase of healing, the wound is filled with new connective tissue. New forming capillaries infiltrate the wound, providing nourishment and encouraging the development of connective tissue through angiogenesis. This is the stage of healing when the base of the wound may become irregular and sloughy or may contain necrotic tissue (Harding, 1996).

Granulation tissue is the fragile, bright red tissue in the wound. A range of growth factors (more than 20 in number) stimulate activities within different cells in order for wound nourishment to occur.

The proliferative phase of healing is illustrated with a decrease in the wound size as granulation, contraction and epithelialisation occur. The wound is strengthened, the dead space is filled out, and it is shrunk by contraction (Harding, 1996).

Maturation phase of healing (3 weeks to months/years)

In healthy individuals, the maturation phase of healing begins after about 20 days of injury and may last for months or even years in complex wounds (Clark, 1988). Scar tissue will be formed, reducing in size and colour with time. Scar formation is a normal consequence of the process of wound healing in adults.

As the wound covers with re-epithelialisation (new skin), there is tissue contraction and reorganisation of the healing tissue within the wound. The wound must provide the conditions that promote easy movement of epithelial cells, i.e. be warm and moist (Winter, 1962). Microfibroblasts contract to decrease the size of the wound, which changes colour from red to white as the amount of blood vessels reduce and return to normal. Fibroblasts stimulate the production of collagen, which increases the strength of the wound, although the scar tissue is never as strong as the original tissue (Kindlen and Morison, 1997).

Healing is said to be complete when the skin surface has reformed and the skin has regained most of its tensile strength (Davis *et al.*, 1992).

Many wounds heal without complications. However, there are many factors that can delay the healing process. Local factors such as wound infection, mechanical stress, use of toxic cleansing agents and the presence of foreign bodies can prolong healing. External factors, such as smoking, poor nutrition, age, drug therapy and disease will also slow the wound-healing process. Socio-economic and psychological factors can have a detrimental effect on the rate of repair (Kiecolt-Glaser *et al.*, 1995).

In patients who have a fungating wound, healing will be affected by the concomitant therapies, such as radiotherapy and chemotherapy.

Anaemia may be a common problem in patients who have cancer, and this can directly reduce the oxygen supply to the wound bed, ultimately reducing the rate of healing if not corrected.

Healing which involves cellular activity is optimal at normal body temperature; if there is a variation in temperature, healing will be compromised (Dealey, 2000). It has been suggested that stress and anxiety can affect wound healing (Kiecolt-Glaser *et al.*, 1995), and patients who live with fungating wounds may feel the effects of stress and anxiety, along with the psychological impact.

ASSESSMENT OF PATIENTS WITH A FUNGATING WOUND

As with all aspects of wound care, it is vital to consider the holistic needs of a patient in order to optimise wound healing. A fungating wound may need additional palliative management, as the wound is often the secondary focus of care. In order to ensure that a holistic approach to the care of the wound is taken, it is essential that a thorough assessment be made. Assessment should encompass the following areas (Hallett, 1995):

- History relating to the present wound – this will identify factors that may have influenced the disease process.
- Cause and stage of disease – may indicate the origin of the cancer and, if appropriate, its expected progression.
- Present treatment, if any – importantly radiotherapy, chemotherapy, hormone therapy, laser treatment or surgery. It is imperative to have a history of any adverse reactions to any of the treatments.
- Physical limitations – location and range of the wound may affect the dressing choice and the treatment options available.
- Nutritional assessment – current nutritional intake is vital information at this stage, as deficiencies in vitamins and minerals will be detrimental to wound care. It will also be important to establish if there is poor appetite, anorexia, nausea and/or weight loss.
- Emotional considerations – depression, social stigma, guilt or shame are often associated with malodorous wounds. Relationships with loved ones and partners can also be affected due to the lack of confidence and sexual expression. Fear of the unknown, pain and death may also be common.
- Self-perception of wound and body image – altered body image should be considered, especially when considering dressings that are cosmetically acceptable.
- Knowledge of diagnosis – establish the amount of knowledge and information that the patient and family have on the disease process.
- Family/carer influences – establish if family and friends are able to cope with the likely increase in vented anger towards them and that they are aware of the networks available to help them.
- Support networks and systems in place – establish whether there is a need for the multidisciplinary team to be involved whenever the patient needs it.
- Local wound condition and associated symptoms – a full assessment of the wound should include the size, location, shape, colour of the wound bed, pain, exudates levels, odour, infection and bleeding.

It is vital at this stage that members of the multidisciplinary team are involved and informed of any decisions with the treatment. This will ensure that the optimum care can and will be given to the patient.

The use of photography (with patient consent) can be a useful method by which to monitor the condition the wound. It should be done with caution as it can be an encouragement to the patient if the wound is improving, but may be disheartening if the wound deteriorates.

Schultz *et al.* (2003) developed the TIME framework, which is a practical guide to direct the management of patients with wounds:

- T – for tissue (non-viable or deficient);
- I – for infection/inflammation;
- M – for moisture imbalance;
- E – for edge, which is not advancing or undermining.

Complications that commonly accompany malignant ulcers

There are a number of complications and consequences that a person with a fungating wound may experience. Some are listed below (Naylor, 2002; Schulz *et al.*, 2002).

Psychological distress

People with malignant ulcers often become depressed, anxious, embarrassed and ashamed. They may have difficulties with body image and sexuality. The appearance and smell of the wound is a constant reminder of their disease, and they may need to alter their style of dress to camouflage bulky dressings.

Social withdrawal

Social withdrawal may result from embarrassment about possible unpleasant smell and appearance.

Exudate

Exudate may soil or stain clothing and bedding, and may require frequent, bulky dressing changes.

Bleeding

Bleeding may also cause staining of clothes and bedding. Bleeding can be profuse and difficult to control.

Pain

Pain is common, and is often due to infiltration or compression of nerves and surrounding tissues.

Pruritus

Pruritus is less common than pain. Pruritus can be caused by excoriation of the skin surrounding the ulcer. It can also be caused by skin infiltration by the associated tumour, particularly with inflammatory breast carcinoma.

Malodour

Malodour is common. The blood supply to some parts of malignant tumours is often impaired, and this results in areas of hypoxic or necrotic tissue. These areas become infected with anaerobic bacteria, which release malodorous volatile fatty acids as a metabolic by-product.

MANAGEMENT OF FUNGATING WOUNDS

Aims of managing a fungating wound

The aims of wound management for fungating wounds where healing is unlikely should focus on comfort, improving quality of life, controlling the symptoms and promoting confidence and a sense of wellbeing (Moody and Grocott, 1993). These aims should be met through appropriate use of dressings and interventions.

In many instances, it is not always possible to provide a cure for the underlying disease. Therefore, the aim of the nursing management of the fungating wound may be palliative, and in an effort to improve the patient's quality of life (Hallett, 1995).

Wound cleansing

The use of warmed normal saline to cleanse a wound has long been an established and well-recognised method. It can also be useful in the removal of existing dressings that may have stuck and, if not removed carefully, may cause pain and trauma. Warming the saline before cleansing will be gentler to the patient, and it will also ensure that the temperature of the wound is not lowered, thus continuing with an environment for optimal for wound healing.

In light of the fact that many of this group of patients will be nursed at home, health-care professionals should be encouraging patients to shower the wound thoroughly in warmed water. This will enhance the psychological wellbeing of the patient as well as ensuring the wound is cleaned to the optimum.

Management of necrotic tissue

Among the goals for the wound care of patients with fungating wounds is the management of the necrotic tissue caused by the lack of oxygen supply to the tumour area. Surgical debridement may prove beneficial if the patient's condition allows (Fairburn, 1993). If surgical debridement is not suitable, conservative management may be necessary through the use of dressings and other treatments.

The use of hydrogels and hydrocolloids are useful as they have a high water content and will allow the rehydration of the necrotic tissue. Hydrogels are available in either sheet or gel format. The hydrogel sheets are used for shallow wounds such as fungating wounds, and the gels are more suitable for cavities and dense areas of eschar. A secondary dressing should always be used to keep the dressing in place. There can be problems associated with the use of hydrogels. Peri-wound maceration and excoriation can be experienced as a result of leakage of the gel if an appropriate secondary dressing is not used. The use of a barrier film can combat this. Owing to the high water content of the hydrogel, the wound can be subject to a very wet environment that is conducive to breed infection; in light of this, it is imperative that the wound bed is cleansed and inspected frequently.

Hydrocolloids create an environment that encourages the removal of sloughy or necrotic wounds. There is also evidence that hydrocolloids reduce pain in wounds (Rousseau, 1991), an important aspect to consider when choosing the correct dressings. The additional advantage of hydrocolloids is their absorptive capabilities, ensuring the wound is maintained in a moist environment. These dressings are waterproof, which enables the patient to bath or shower without removing them.

The use of honey, icing sugar and sugar paste have been shown to be effective in encouraging autolytic debridement of necrotic tissue in fungating wounds. They also have the benefit of reducing any malodour (Sims and Fitzgerald, 1985; Thomas, 1992).

Larval therapy is a method of treatment that will debride necrotic tissue. The larvae break down and liquefy dead tissue rapidly by depositing powerful proteolytic enzymes. Although larval therapy is back in vogue and is effective at the debridement of necrotic tissue, some patients and nursing staff do not like the thought of it. Its place should be considered carefully for use on necrotic tissue in fungating wounds.

It should be remembered that, with the use of any debriding agents on necrotic tissue, there is an expected larger area that will remain once the necrotic tissue is removed. This is normal and should not cause concern. It is important that this is considered and that the patient is fully informed to expect this larger area following removal of the necrotic tissue, and that it is a sign of improvement to the wound, not deterioration.

Management of a bleeding or haemorrhaging fungating wound

Haemorrhage may occur as a result of a ruptured or eroded major blood vessel local to the tumour, due to their weakened state. The use of alginates, particularly Kaltostat and sorbsan, are extremely effective in controlling localised bleeding, as well as allowing the wound area to continue to be moist (Thomas, 1992).

When carrying out a dressing change, it is important to do so gently and with care to reduce trauma and damage. The use of warmed normal saline will aid the removal of any stuck dressings, as well as providing a soothing environment around the wound for the patient.

When the wound is bleeding profusely, more extreme measures may need to be taken but with caution and careful monitoring. The use of topical adrenaline solution (1 in 1000 for injection) may be used, and this may cause localised ischaemic necrosis due to onset of vasoconstriction. Oral or topical tranexamic acid solution (for injection) may be used; as could the cauterisation of bleeding vessels, however, due to the increase and availability of modern dressing products, this method is not used as frequently. Ligation of the bleeding vessels by the surgeon may also be used to stop bleeding (Naylor, 2001).

Radiotherapy, given as a single dose, may also be used. This will reduce the tumour size, with a consequent reduction in the symptoms including bleeding (Young, 1997).

Management of infection in a fungating wound

Infection will often occur as a result of the build up of aerobic and anaerobic bacteria in the necrotic tissue. Wound infection is a problem, as it will prevent a wound from healing. Infection may also lead to further breakdown and extension of the wound; it can also increase patient discomfort, pain, disability, smell and other serious complications that may lead to septicaemia and death.

A swab of the wound should be taken if it shows signs of clinical infection, in order for systemic antibiotics to be administered, with the correct sensitivity to that specific organism. The signs of clinical infection could be the presence of pus, increased exudate levels, an increase in pain, a change in appearance, or an increase in any malodour (Cutting and Harding, 1994).

There is some controversy around the use of topical antibacterial agents to help treat wound infection. A recent report concluded 'Topical antibiotics are inappropriate for wounds and ulcers, although they are widely promoted for this purpose' (Drug and Therapeutics Bulletin, 1991). The exception to this is for the use of topical metronidazole gel on malodorous wounds, which has been shown to be effective in reducing and preventing odour (Lancet, 1990).

Management of malodour in a fungating wound

Odour at the wound site could possibly be one of the most distressing associated symptoms for a patient with a fungating wound. Patients have described the effect that a malodorous wound has on their lives as being embarrassing, socially isolating and often distressing, as a result of the continuous leaking of exudate that stains clothes and sheets (Neal, 1991; Boardman et al., 1993). There is stigma associated with malodorous wounds that may inhibit sexuality and intimacy (Clark, 1992). A number of products are available that will reduce the odour. Treatment should depend on the cause of the odour (Haughton and Young, 1995). Some recommend the use of external odour absorbers, such as cat litter or activated charcoal. A bowl of this under the bed has been shown to be beneficial (McDonald and Lesage, 2006; Seaman, 2006).

Malodour can also be distressing to the nurse, and this distress and fear is felt by the patient (Hastings, 1993).

Odour will often be present in a fungating wound as a result of infection due to the rise in aerobic and anaerobic bacteria. This results in the formation of necrotic tissue in the wound, owing to poor tissue oxygenation at the site of the tumour.

The most effective way of managing malodorous wounds is to prevent or eradicate the infection responsible for the odour. The administration of systemic antibiotics and antimicrobial agents may be effective in some cases (Thomas, 1998).

Exudate management

Wound exudate in a fungating wound is difficult to predict or control. The exudate that is produced by the wound is as a result of the wound infection/colonisation (Gottrup, 1997; Harding, 1997) and the wound type. Lymphatic drainage problems can occur following surgery for cancer which can increase exudate (Gottrup, 1997). If colonisation is reduced, exudate will decrease. It is important to maintain a moist environment whilst diminishing the need for dressing changes and, at the same time, ensuring there is no maceration around the wound.

A number of dressings are available that will cope with moderate to very high levels of exudate. When choosing the dressing, it is imperative that all aspects of the holistic assessment are considered.

Management of the peri-wound skin

Care is required when managing wound margins. This vulnerable skin should be protected from maceration from skin stripping during dressing removal or from the corrosive properties from chronic wound exudate.

High levels of wound exudate increase the risk of skin breakdown. This, along with ill-fitting dressings or dressings that do not adequately manage the amount of fluid expelled from a wound, allowing it to be retained on nearby health skin, put this fragile skin at an increased risk of breakdown (Hollinworth, 2009). In turn, the breakdown of this skin would increase wound size and exacerbate wound pain (Mudge *et al* 2008).

While non-adhesive dressings are generally used for the person with the fungating breast lesion, the majority of these still require adhesive tapes to secure them in some way to the body. Care should be taken that this is not simply relocating the potential for tissue trauma a little further away from the wound (Hollinworth 2009).

DRESSINGS

Where possible, the wound should be kept in a moist environment in order to maximise the healing potential of the wound (Winter, 1962) and to allow the migration of the epithelial cells across the wound's surface at a faster rate. The ideal dressing should have the following properties (also see Table 12.1).

- Provides the optimum environment for wound healing;
- Allows gaseous exchange;
- Is acceptable to the patient;
- Maintains a moist environment;
- Is impermeable to micro-organisms/bacteria;
- Is free from particulate contaminants;
- Is safe to use;
- Is highly absorptive;
- Can carry medications;
- Allows monitoring of the wound;
- Provides protection;
- Is capable of standardisation and evaluation;
- Does not harm;
- Is non-adherent;
- Is thermally insulating;
- Is non-toxic and non-allergenic;
- Is comfortable;
- Is conforming;
- Can protect the wound from further trauma;
- Is cost effective;
- Is available;
- Has properties that remain constant;
- Is non-inflammable;
- Is sterilisable.

Table 12.1   Dressing the fungating wound.

Symptom	Management
Necrotic tissue	Surgical debridement
	Hydrogels and hydrocolloid dressings contain high water content that allow rehydration of necrotic tissue
	Larval therapy – consider implications carefully
Bleeding wound	Alginate dressings control localised bleeding and allow wound to be moist
	Warmed normal saline assists removal of dressings that have stuck
	Use topical adrenaline solution (1 in 1000 for injection) to cause localised ischemic necrosis due to vasoconstriction
	Oral/topical tranexamic solution (for injection) may cauterise bleeding vessels (used infrequently due to availability of modern dressings)
	Give a dose of radiotherapy to reduce symptom
Infection	Take a swab
	Administer systemic antibiotics sensitive to correct sensitivity to organism
Malodour	Administer systemic antibiotics and antimicrobial agents
	Metronidazole gel reduces and prevents odour
	Combine metronidazole with intrasite gel
	Use charcoal dressings to stop odour
	Honey and sugar paste, although less conventional, can be used
	Could use aromatherapy oils on dressings to disguise odours
Exudate	Use hydrofibres, foams or alginates plus a secondary absorbent dressing
	Drainage bags could also be used if the exudate demands it
Itchy surrounding skin	Hydrogel sheets could be applied to cool the skin
	Oral antihistamines may be useful
Fragile surrounding skin	A tight-fitting garment, almost like a 'sleeveless T-shirt', can be used to secure dressings, protecting skin and dispensing with the need for adhesive tapes and dressings

Adapted from King (2003) and Harmer (2008).

The choice of dressing should limit the frequency of dressing changes, whilst enabling maximum exudate management to prevent peri-wound maceration as well as ensuring that the risk of infection is kept to a minimum.

Odour-absorbing dressings

The use of the antibiotic metronidazole has been shown to be effective in the treatment of anaerobic infections (Thomas, 1989; Thomas, 1988). The use of topical metronidazole gel has been shown to reduce the level of bacteria present in the wound, and is now the preferred treatment over oral or intravenous metronidazole in the treatment of fungating wounds (Sims and Fitzgerald, 1985; Thomas, 1992; Saunders and Reguard, 1989; Morgan, 1992).

The combined use of metronidazole gel and intrasite gel has been shown to be an effective treatment regimen (Thomas, 1992; Boardman *et al.*, 1993). The intrasite gel will encourage autolytic debridement, and the metronidazole gel will combat malodour. The use of a non-adherent absorbent dressing should be used as a secondary dressing.

The application of honey is a less conventional method that has been used to manage malodorous wounds. It has been shown in a number of laboratory studies to completely inhibit the wound-infecting bacteria, therefore reducing the malodour associated with the infection produced (Molan, 1999; White and Molan, 2005). Additionally, the antimicrobial property of honey can help to eradicate odour (Molan, 2005), and the antioxidant capacities reduces inflammation in the wound bed (Sharp, 2009).

The use of sugar paste to control odour has been recommended in the literature (Chirife *et al.*, 1982) because of its antimicrobial properties. Sugar will encourage the removal of exudate and tissue fluid, which will subject the bacteria to an increase in osmotic pressure; this will result in cell injury and death and ultimately inhibit bacterial growth. The negative aspect of using sugar is that it is most effective after 3 to 4 hours of application; this means that the dressing treatment should be applied twice daily, something that may be impossible if the patient is being managed in the community. It is not recommended for use on patients who have diabetes. It is, however, self-sterilising, inexpensive and will mould to any wound type.

More recently, larval therapy has been shown to be an effective way of eliminating wound infection and odour from extensive necrotic wounds (Thomas *et al.*, 1996; Evans, 1997; Thomas, 1998).

The use of a charcoal dressing may also be considered to reduce the odour from a fungating wound. This method of combating wound odour was discovered by Butcher *et al* in 1976. Since then, a number of odour-absorbing dressings have become available, with Actisorb the first manufactured charcoal dressing. A number of dressings containing activated charcoal have been developed and, depending on the individual dressing's ability to absorb, odour will depend on whether it can be used as a primary or secondary dressing. The dressings will dampen the odour and absorb exudate, but will not treat the cause of the odour. As previously mentioned, some charcoal dressings can only be used as a secondary dressing. This may add bulk to the wound site and cause more reason for the patient to be concerned about their appearance, something practitioners should be avoiding. Many charcoal dressings cannot be cut to size, again restricting the sites at which they can be used and also increasing unnecessary bulk to the dressing. Charcoal dressings are ineffective once they are wet, however, and may require frequent changing.

Since the original charcoal dressing, there have been a number of developments that include the use of silver and alginates impregnated within the charcoal dressing. Actisorb Plus and Acticoat are examples of charcoal dressings impregnated with silver, which not only combat malodour but will also fight the levels of bacteria on the wound. This has been seen to be of greater benefit, as the odour will be addressed, whilst fighting its cause at the same time.

Carboflex uses a combination of alginate and charcoal. This limits the need for a primary dressing, and issues of exudate management and odour absorption have been addressed.

It is imperative to encourage bedding and clothes to be changed once exudate has come into contact with them. The use of aromatherapy should be considered with caution as this will only reduce the smells, not treat the cause, and may leave the patient associating that particular smell with the wound (Haughton and Young, 1995).

TYPES OF DRESSINGS SUITABLE FOR FUNGATING WOUNDS

Hydrofibres

Aquacel Hydrofibre stands out as being of exceptional performance in providing an optimum healing environment as well as a pain-free removal. It will absorb rapidly and retain exudate; it is highly effective at exudate control without having the risk of maceration. Aquacel has been shown to control the release of bacteria, which may reduce the risk of cross-infection in the clinical setting (Bowler, 2000). This is an important aspect to consider, especially as the patient may be immunocompromised as a result of the adjunctive therapy they may be receiving.

Alginates

Alginates were first used in the 1940s (Thomas and Loveless, 1992). They are made from seaweed and can be composed of galuronic acid and mannuronic acid. The amount of each type of acid in the alginate will give rise to the 'gelling' abilities that the dressing has; this in turn will reflect the ease of removal of the dressing, an important aspect in reducing pain and trauma to the wound bed. Some alginates have haemostatic properties, and this is of additional advantage to the fungating wounds, as uncontrolled bleeding is often a common problem. Alginates are best used in highly exuding wounds as they are very absorbent. If the wound is too dry, the alginate will adhere to the wound bed and cause trauma to the wound on removal. This could restart bleeding in a fungating wound. A secondary dressing will need to be applied over the alginate to secure it in place. The level of exudate produced from the wound should determine dressing change.

Foams

Foams are formed using a polymer technology. They can absorb large amounts of exudate and are non-adherent to the wound bed. They can be used as a primary or secondary dressing. Many foam dressings are on the market, and the amount of exudate that can be absorbed will depend on which one is used and, ultimately, this will determine the length of time needed in between each dressing change.

Allevyn hydrocellular and Allevyn cavity have both been shown to absorb larger amounts of exudate than other low-adherent absorbent padding (Boardman *et al.*, 1993), allowing fewer dressing changes for the patient that will ultimately increase their quality of life.

Two-layer permeable system

The use of a perforated non-adherent contact layer, Mepitel, protects the wound bed, whilst allowing for inspection of the wound bed, and enabling exudate to pass through the dressing. It therefore allows the use of cheaper absorbent dressing pads that will absorb the high level of exudate whilst controlling the expenditure of the total treatment costs. This dressing is gentle on removal and only needs to be changed every 7 days, reducing the trauma to the local wound area and ultimately reducing pain at dressing changes for the patient. The negative aspect of Mepitel is that is not recommended for use on bleeding wounds, which are often a symptom of the fungating wound. However, if used appropriately, it has a large number of positive features missed in other dressings.

Drainage bags

Drainage bags can also be used with a barrier cream to prevent maceration of the surrounding skin (Hallett, 1995). Butterfly drains inserted into the dressings to allow further drainage of exudate have had a limited effect (Grocott, 1991). This would not be considered to be the optimal management, as issues associated with body image and self-respect may not have been met.

Cosmetic appearance

It is imperative that the cosmetic appearance of the dressing used is considered, to allow the patient to continue to dress in the same way they did prior to the development of the fungating wound.

Care of the surrounding skin

Local trauma to the surrounding skin can occur from repeated dressing application. It is important to try to dress the wound and to keep the dressings applied to the surrounding skin to a minimum. The detrimental effects of moisture on the surrounding skin of a vulnerable patient can cause maceration, excoriation and dermatitis (Benbow, 2008). Early application of a skin barrier film can minimise these risks. It is important to treat the underlying clinical condition when addressing moisture imbalance in a wound (Newton and Cameron, 2003).

MANAGEMENT OF PAIN

Pain in fungating wounds is often as a result of the erosion and breakdown of the nerve endings, which often cannot be repaired (Naylor, 2001). Pain may also be due to further invasion or growth of the tumour. The degree of pain will depend on the site of the wound, the degree of the disease and the involvement of nerves, soft tissue damage and past experience of pain. It is imperative that this is established throughout the assessment process.

If pain is continuously felt at dressing change, a review of dressing treatment may be necessary to ensure that the appropriate dressing is being used and one that is not sticking and causing pain as a result of removal of a stuck dressing. Exudate levels may have reduced over time, and therefore pain may be an indication that a change of dressing is required.

Lignocaine gel may be applied directly to the wound surface (Rang, 1995) to help reduce the wound pain. This will act by blocking the message of pain reaching the brain. If this is not adequate, the use of topical opioids, such as diamorphine or morphine, mixed with a soluble medical lubricant or hydrogel and applied topically to the wound may reduce pain at the wound site (Naylor, 2001). This should be used with caution as it may make the wound sensitive to topical opioids (Stein, 1995). It is also unclear as to whether the opioids provide a true analgesia effect or whether they provide a more anti-inflammatory effect that ultimately reduces the pain (Stein, 1995).

It is important to ensure that adequate oral analgesia/opioids have been taken far enough in advance of the dressing change to ensure the analgesia has had time to work.

The use of entinox is short acting and may be effective in reducing pain as a result of dressing change (Naylor, 2001). The use of a barrier film around the wound site will prevent maceration resulting from poor exudate management associated with the pain. Non-steroidal anti-inflammatory drugs could be used with caution to reduce the amount of pain that may be a result of localised inflammation.

MANAGEMENT OF ITCHING AND PRURITUS

Itching may be a further complication as a result of the tumour nodules beginning to emerge under the surrounding skin. The stretching of the skin irritates nerve endings and may cause a biochemical reaction leading to local inflammation (Naylor, 2001). The use of oral anti-histamines may be of some help. There is documentation that suggests the use of hydrogel sheets helps with this as they have a cooling (especially if they have been refrigerated prior to use) and soothing effect on the irritable skin. They can be covered with a film dressing to prevent them from dehydrating, or they can be used with a secondary absorbent dressing if the wound is exuding (Naylor, 2001). Naylor (2001) also suggests the use of menthol in aqueous cream. The menthol has a cooling effect and can be applied to the itching areas two to three times a day. It should not be applied to any broken areas of skin.

Transcutaneous nerve stimulation (TENS) has been used effectively to relieve pruritis (Grocott, 1999).

ADJUNCTIVE TREATMENT

Radiotherapy

Radiotherapy may reduce the size of the tumour and should therefore reduce the levels of exudate associated with the wound, making the wound more manageable.

Hormone therapy

Hormonal therapy for breast cancer will be given if the index oestrogen-receptor protein is positive, and surgery will not be, or has already been, performed.

Chemotherapy

Chemotherapy may be given immediately after surgery to eliminate micrometastasis. Chemotherapy may also be given pre-operatively to reduce the bulk of a fungating wound in the hope that an inoperable lesion becomes operable.

Nutritional supplements

Nutritional levels may be depleted or compromised as result of the disease process; there-fore, fluid and nutritional supplements of protein, vitamins and minerals should be encour-aged.

Complementary treatments

Anecdotal evidence exists to support the use of essential oils, and individuals are free to use them for their own benefit (Baker, 1998). It is imperative that a safe and suitable education programme is developed to ensure the safe use of the oils. It is also suggested that a stronger evidence base for the use of essential oils in wound care is established before extending their use in practice (Baker, 1998).

PSYCHO-SOCIAL ASPECTS OF MANAGING FUNGATING WOUNDS

Compliance

Involving the patient and family with the decision process regarding the choice of dressing is important to ensure compliance. This should include time needed to carry out dressing changes, frequency of dressing changes and location of dressing changes, (whether at home, hospital or doctor's surgery.) Importantly, the cosmetic image of the dressing is essential in order to maintain compliance.

Body image

Illness and radical surgery can directly affect the development and stability of an individual's body image. The breast will carry a special meaning for a woman due to their reproductive and nurturing functions. Wounds resulting from surgery, infection or malignancy to this area have added problems associated with the actual or perceived loss of femininity.

When the wound becomes smelly or unsightly in an area that is not normally exposed, such as the breast, more problems are likely to arise. Touching and exposure of this part of the body would normally only be permitted to those close to the patient. Suddenly, this part of the body is expected to be exposed at regular intervals to a large number of medical and nursing staff.

Dressing choice will be fundamental to ensure that the patient is still able to carry on normal activities of daily living, and that she is not restricted in what to wear because of the bulkiness of the dressing.

It should never be assumed that it is acceptable to carry out a dressing change. It is essential that the patient is asked if it is a convenient time. If there are any other members of the team who would like to view the wound, it is important that the permission is sought from the patient and that her wishes respected.

When the dressing requires changing, it may be an idea to coordinate an appropriate time with other members of the team, as they may wish to monitor the progress of the wound. This will limit the number of dressing changes needed and will ensure that the patient's best interests are met. Ultimately, if the whole team is present at this time, it is easier to discuss the next step for the treatment all together.

CONCLUSION

Fungating wound management is a multidisciplinary responsibility. It is imperative that symptom control is managed effectively to ensure that all treatment regimes are given the opportunity to be as successful as possible. The health-care professional is the most suitable link between the patient and the advancing scientific technologies and knowledge, and providing specialist care in this area can mean the difference between wounds deteriorating, healing or maybe re-developing (Stephen-Haynes, 2008). Wound care is complex, and the health-care professional providing this care must be armed with up-to-date information and knowledge on wound healing, pain, pharmacology, dressing products, microbiology and psychosocial ethics, as well as possessing good communication skills (Stephen-Haynes, 2008). Applying this specialist knowledge can promote wound healing, result in less painful dressing changes for the patient and reduce scarring. It is the responsibility of the individual practitioner to ensure that these elements are in place before they manage patients with fungating wounds (Benbow, 2008).

A number of modern dressings are available which have been shown to enhance the healing process of a fungating wound. It is essential that the practitioner is aware of all the advantages and disadvantages of each dressing in order to ensure an optimum wound-healing environment.

Effective management of a fungating wound may increase the psychosocial wellbeing of the patient, and enable them to more freely take part in the activities of daily living. The importance of empowering a patient through effective wound management and use of the dressings available should not be underestimated.

REFERENCES

Baker J (1998) Essential oils: a complementary therapy in wound management. *Journal of Wound Care* 7(7): 355–357.

Bale S and Harding KG (1987) Fungating breast wounds. *Journal of District Nursing* 9(12): 4–5.

Bale S and Jones V (2000) *Wound care nursing: a patient centred approach.* London: Bailliere Tindall.

Benbow M. (2008) Exploring the concept of moist wound healing and its application in practice. *British Journal of Nursing* (Tissue Viability Supplement) 17(15): S4–S16.

Bennett G and Moody M (1995) *Wound Care for Health Professionals.* London: Chapman and Hall.

Boardman M, Mellor K, and Neville B (1993) Treating a patient with a heavily exuding malodorous fungating wound. Journal of Wound Care 2(2): 74–77.

Bowler P (2000) Infection control properties of wound dressings. In: *Aquacel: New Dimensions in the Treatment of Post-Surgical Wounds. Proceedings from the 10th Conference of the EWMA.* Holsworthy: Medical Communications.

Butcher G, Butcher JA and Maggs FAP (1976) The treatment of malodorous wounds. *Nursing Mirror* 142: 76.

Carville K (1994) Assessment and management of cancerous wounds. Primary Intention *February* 20–26.

Chirife J, Scarmato G and Herszage L (1982) Scientific basis for the use of granulated sugar in treatment of infected wounds. *The Lancet* 6; 1(8271): 560–561.

Clark RAF (1988) Overview and general considerations of wound repair. In: RAF Clark and PM Henson (eds) *The Molecular and Cellular Biology of Wound Repair.* New York: Plenum.

Clark L (1992) Caring for fungating tumours. *Nursing Times* 88(12): 66–70.

Collins F, Hampton S and White R (2002) *A–Z Dictionary of Wound Care.* London: Quay Books.

Cutting KF and Harding K (1994) Criteria for identifying wound infection. *Journal of Wound Care* 3(4): 194–201.

Davis M, Dunkley P, Harden RM *et al.* (1992) *The Wound Programme.* Dundee: Centre for Medical Education.

Dealey C (2000) *The Care of Wounds. A Guide for Nurses.* Oxford: Blackwell Science.

Drug and Therapeutics Bulletin (1991) Local applications to wounds: 1 Cleansers, antibacterials, debriders. *Drug and Therapeutics Bulletin* 29(24): 93–95.

Evans H (1997) A treatment of last resort. *Nursing Times* 9(23): 62–67.

Fairburn K (1993) Towards better care for women: understanding fungating breast lesions. *Professional Nurse* 9(3): 204–212.

Gottrup F (1997) Is exudate a clinical problem? A surgeon's perspective. In: C Cherry and K Harding (eds) *Management of Wound Exudate: Proceedings of Joint Meeting of EWMA and ETRS*. London: Churchill Communications.

Grocott P (1991) Application of the principles of modern wound management for complex wounds in palliative care. In: KG Harding, DL Leaper and TD Turner (eds) *Proceedings of the First European Conference on Advances in Wound Management* 96–97.

Grocott P (1995) The palliative management of fungating malignant wounds. *Journal of Wound Care* 4(5): 240–242.

Grocott P (1999) The management of fungating wounds. *Journal of Wound Care* 8(5): 232–234.

Grocott P (2000) The palliative management of fungating malignant wounds. *Journal of Wound Care* 9(1): 4–9.

Haagenson CD (1971) *Diseases of the breast*, 2nd edn. Eastbourne: W B Saunders.

Hallett A (1995) Fungating wounds. *Nursing Times* 91(39): 81–83.

Harding K (1997) Is exudate a clinical problem? A Specialist physician's perspective. In: C Cherry and K Harding (eds) *Management of Wound Exudate: Proceedings of Joint Meeting of EWMA and ETRS*. London: Churchill Communications.

Harding, KG (1996) Managing wound infection. *Journal of Wound Care* 5(8): 391–392.

Harmer V (2008) Breast cancer. Part 3: Advanced cancer and psychological implications. *British Journal of Nursing* 17(17): 1088–1097.

Hastings D (1993) Basing care on research. *Nursing Times* 89(13): 70–74.

Haughton W and Young T (1995) Common problems in wound care: malodorous wounds. *British Journal of Nursing* 4(16): 959–963.

Hollinworth H (2009) Challenges in protecting peri-wound skin. *Nursing Standard* 24(7): 53–62.

Kiecolt-Glaser JK, Marucha PT, Malarkey WB, Mercado AM and Glaser R (1995) Slowing of wound healing by psychological stress. *The Lancet* 346: 1194–1196.

Kindlen S and Morison M (1997) The physiology of wound healing. In: M Morrison, C Moffatt, J Bridel-Nixon, and S Bale (eds) *Nursing Management of Chronic Wounds*. Mosby: London: 1–26.

King R (2003) Fungating wounds. In: V Harmer (ed.) *Breast Cancer: Nursing Care and Management*. London: Whurr Publishers Ltd.

Lancet (1990) Management of smelly tumours (editorial). *The Lancet* 335: 141–142.

Laverty D, Cooper J and Soady S (2000) Wound management. In: J Mallett and L Dougherty (eds) *The Royal Marsden Hospital Manual of Clinical Nursing Procedures*, 5th edn. Oxford: Blackwell Science.

McDonald A and Lesage P (2006) Palliative management of pressure ulcers and malignant wounds in patients with advanced illness. *Journal of Palliative Medicine* 9(2): 285–295.

Molan PC (1999) The role of honey in the management of wounds. *Journal of Wound Care* 8(8): 415–418.

Molan PC (2005) Re-introducing honey in the management of wounds and ulcers – theory and practice. *Ostomy Wound Management* 48(11): 28–40.

Moody M and Grocott P (1993) Let us extend our knowledge base: assessment and management of fungating malignant wounds *Professional Nurse* 8(9): 586, 588–590.

Morgan DA (1992) *Formulary of Wound Management Products: A Guide for Healthcare Staff*, 5th edn. Aldershot: BritCair.

Mortimer P (1998) Skin problems in palliative care: medical aspects. In: D Doyle, G Hanks and N Macdonald (eds) *Oxford Textbook of Palliative Medicine*. Oxford: Oxford Medical Publications.

Moseley JG (1998) *Palliation in Malignant Disease*. Edinburgh: Churchill Livingstone.

Mudge EJ, Meaume S, Woo K, Sibbald RG and Price EP (2008) Patients' experience of wound-related pain: an international perspective. *European Wound Management Association Journal* 8(2): 19–28.

Naylor W (2001) Management of fungating wounds. In: W Naylor, D Laverty and J Mallett (eds) *The Royal Marsden Hospital of Wound Management in Cancer Care* Oxford: Blackwell Science.

Naylor W (2002) Part 1: Symptom control in the management of fungating wounds. *World Wide Wounds*. Available: http://www.worldwidewounds.com/2002/march/Naylor/Symptom-Control-Fungating-Wounds.html.

Neal K (1991) Treating fungating lesions. *British Journal of Nursing* 4(16): 958–963.

Newton H and Cameron J (2003) *Skin Care in Wound Management*. London: Medical Communications Ltd.

Petrek JA, Glen PD and Cramer AR (1983) Ulcerated breast cancer: patients and outcome. *The American Surgeon* 49(4): 187–191.

Rang H (1995) *Pharmacology*, 3rd edn. Edinburgh: Churchill Livingstone.

Regnard CF and Tempest S (1992) *A Guide to Symptom Relief in Advanced Cancer*, 3rd edn. London: Haigh and Hochland.

Rousseau P (1991) Comparison of the various physiochemical properties of various hydrocolloid dressings. *Wounds* 3(1): 43–48.

Saunders J and Reguard C (1989) Management of malignant ulcers and flow diagram. *Palliative Medicine* 2: 153–155.

Seaman S (2006) Management of malignant fungating wounds in advanced cancer. *Seminars in Oncology Nursing* 22(3): 185–193.

Schultz GS, Sibbald RG, Falanga V *et al.* (2003) Wound bed preparation: systematic approach to wound management. *Wound Repair and Regeneration* 11 (Suppl 1): S1–28.

Schulz V, Triska OH and Tonkin K (2002) Malignant wounds: caregiver-determined clinical problems. *Journal of Pain and Symptom Management* 24(6): 572–577.

Sharp A (2009) Beneficial effects of honey dressings in wound management. *Nursing Standard* 24(7): 66–74.

Sims R and Fitzgerald V (1985) *Community Nursing Management of Patients with Ulcerating/Fungating Malignant Breast Disease*. London: RCN Oncology Nursing Society.

Stein C (1995) The control of pain in peripheral tissue by opioids. *The New England Journal of Medicine* 332(25): 1685–90.

Stephen-Haynes J (2008) What's affecting future care delivery in tissue viability? *British Journal of Nursing* (Tissue Viability Supplement) 17: 15 S3.

Thomas M (1988) Coping with distressing symptoms. In: J Wilson (ed.) *Nursing Issues and Research in Terminal Care*. Chichester: John Wiley and Sons.

Thomas S (1989) Treating malodorous wounds. *Nursing Times (Community Outlook)* 85(10): 27–30.

Thomas S (1992) *Current Practices in the Management of Fungating Lesions and Radiation Damaged Skin*. Bridgend: Mid Glamorgan Surgical Materials Testing Laboratories.

Thomas S (1998) Odour-absorbing dressings. *Journal of Wound Care* 7(5): 246–250.

Thomas S and Loveless P (1992) Observations on the fluid handling properties of alginate dressings. *Pharmaceutical Journal* 248: 672–675.

Thomas S, Jones M, Shutler S and Jones S (1996) Using larvae in modern wound management. *Journal of Wound Care* 5(2): 60–69.

Waldrop J and Doughty D (2000) Wound healing-physiology. In: R Bryant (ed.) *Acute and Chronic Wounds. Nursing Management*, 2nd edn. London: Mosby, pp. 17–39.

White R and Molan P (2005) A summary of published clinical research on honey in wound management. In: R White, R Cooper and P Molan (eds) *Honey: A Modern Wound Management Product*. Aberdeen: Wounds UK, pp. 130–142.

Winter G (1962) Formation of the scab and rate of epitheliazation of superficial wounds in the skin of a young domestic pig. *Nature* 193: 293–294.

Young T (1997) Wound care: the challenge of managing fungating wounds. *Community Nurse* 3(9): 41–44.

13 Advanced Disease

Elizabeth Sumner

INTRODUCTION

Even after treatment, many patients diagnosed with breast cancer live with the fear that, at some point in their lives, the cancer will return. For some, this fear is unfounded. However, figures show that, for just over half of these patients, their fears will come true and, despite having surgery and/or radiotherapy, they will go on to develop metastatic disease (Smith and de Boer, 2000).

For nurses to provide high-quality, evidence-based care, they need to have access to information on advanced breast cancer. This chapter will cover topics that are related to every aspect of the disease. It will discuss local and loco-regional recurrence as well as metastatic disease. It will discuss principles that can be applied when caring for patients with advanced breast cancer. Most importantly, it will focus on the symptoms associated with advanced breast disease, looking at what effect these symptoms will have on a patient, both physically and emotionally. The help and support that we, as nurses, can give to the patient and their family/carers will be discussed.

THE PATTERN OF CLINICAL SPREAD

In 2005, 10 900 women in England and Wales died as a result of breast cancer (Office for National Statistics, 2008). It is thought that about 10% of women diagnosed with breast cancer also initially present with metastatic disease (National Institute for Health and Clinical Excellence, 2006; Overmoyer, 1995). Of those remaining, a large proportion will go on to develop metastases, months or even years after being diagnosed.

Advanced disease in breast cancer can take two forms, that of local or loco-regional recurrence and systemic recurrence (i.e. metastases). The two forms are very different and have different implications for the patient, as patients usually die from metastases, but not from local recurrence (Souhami and Tobias, 1995).

Breast Cancer Nursing Care and Management, Second Edition, Edited by Victoria Harmer
© 2011 by Blackwell Publishing Ltd.

LOCAL RECURRENCE

In itself, isolated local breast cancer recurrence does not seem to be a threat to survival. However, it is a well-documented fact that local recurrence is a predictor of distant metastases which, although often asymptomatic, should be actively looked for in any presenting patient (Dixon and Sainsbury, 1998).

Often, despite optimum treatment, residual tumour cells may remain at the original site or in lymph nodes situated within the local area. These residual cells can lead to a recurrence of the cancer in the remaining breast tissue, in the chest wall, or in the regional lymph nodes. Local recurrence is usually picked up clinically and is confirmed by carrying out a fine-needle aspiration or biopsy.

Once local recurrence has been confirmed, there are several different treatment options depending on what treatment has been given in the past, where the secondaries are situated and whether there are singular or multiple nodules.

Surgery, chemotherapy, radiotherapy and hormone therapy can all be used individually or in combination to control and treat local recurrence.

SYSTEMIC METASTATIC DISEASE

Metastasis means the spread of cancer, and occurs when cancer cells detach from a primary tumour and travel via the lymphatic system or blood stream to other parts of the body (Fig. 13.1). In breast cancer, an obvious route of spread is through the lymph nodes and channels that supply the breast tissue. However, it is also possible for the cancer to engulf blood vessels within the breast, thus allowing the cancer cells to enter the blood stream and spread throughout the body.

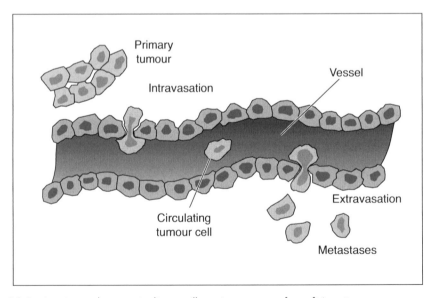

Fig. 13.1   Invasion and metastatic disease. Illustration courtesy of sanofi-Aventis.

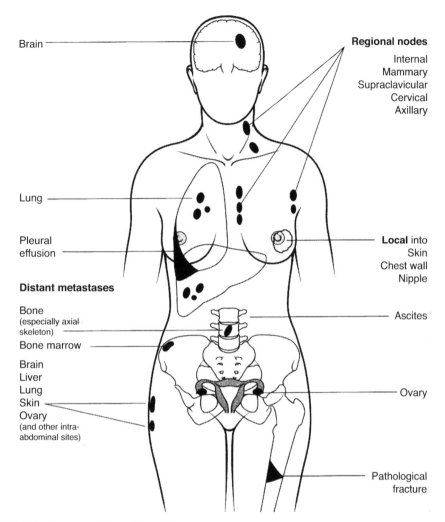

Fig. 13.2 Diagram of clinical spread.

Metastatic disease can occur weeks, months or years after an initial diagnosis of breast cancer. Unlike local recurrence, which is commonly asymptomatic, it is often not until the patient presents with a distressing symptom such as bone pain, confusion and breathlessness, that metastatic breast cancer is diagnosed (McGinn and Moore, 2001).

The most common sites of metastatic spread for patients with primary breast cancer are to the lungs, liver, bones and brain, although the heart, adrenal glands, peritoneal cavity and ovaries may also be affected (Fig. 13.2). Various studies put the average survival time with metastases from 18 months to 3 years (Efficace and Biganzoli, 2008; Leonard *et al.*, 2000; McEvilly and Dow, 1998). This does, of course, depend on where the metastases occur. For example, a woman with a single metastasis in her femur may live for many years, whilst a woman with multiple metastases affecting her liver may live for a much shorter time.

COMMON SITES OF METASTASES IN BREAST CANCER

Bone metastases

At any one time in the United Kingdom, it is estimated that approximately 25 000 women are living with bone metastases, which originate from primary breast cancer (Rees *et al.*, 1994). Metastases can arise in any bone in the body. However, metastases most commonly occur in the vertebrae, pelvis, ribs and long bones such as the femur or humerus. The incidence of bone metastases among women with advanced disease is thought to be as high as 73%, making the skeletal system the most common site of recurrence.

The prognosis for people with bone metastases is still relatively poor as, although bone metastases are not life threatening in themselves, they suggest blood-borne metastatic spread from the original tumour and therefore are often indicative of other soft-tissue metastases. If the metastases are confined predominately to the bones, life expectancy can be anywhere from 2–5 years (Chow and Yee, 2008). Often, even when there is no evidence of other metastatic disease, the complications associated with bone metastases, such as spinal cord compression, hypercalcaemia, pathological fractures and musculoskeletal pain, all contribute to a reduction in the patient's quality of life and often to their eventual decline (Heatley and Coleman, 1999; Hoskin and Makin, 1998).

Presentation

Some bone metastases are asymptomatic and may only show on X-rays or scans that are carried out for other reasons. Often, however, people will present with pain that may be described using the following characteristics:

- Dull;
- Deep aching;
- Persistent;
- Oppressive pain;
- Pain worse on movement or when weight bearing;
- Pain unrelieved by rest.

If bone metastases are suspected in a woman with breast cancer, initial investigations may include an X-ray of the affected area. The X-ray may show a lytic bony lesion. However, often a bone scan is required as pain can predate radiological changes and therefore a bone scan is more sensitive and can give more accurate information, often being able to detect bone metastases 2–18 months before changes are evident on plain radiographs (Waller and Caroline, 2000).

When bone metastases are discovered, treatment may be needed over a prolonged period of time. The aim of treatment should be to relieve pain, to strengthen bones, to try and control further spread and to improve the patient's quality of life. The relatively long prognosis should be taken into account when treatment decisions are being made.

Radiotherapy, hormone therapy, chemotherapy and, more recently, bisphosphonates (discussed later in this chapter) all have an important role to play in the control and palliation of bone metastases.

Lung metastases

The lung is the second most common site for metastases in women with advanced breast disease. Metastases can be solitary or multiple and, depending on the area of lung affected, can be asymptomatic or cause distressing symptoms.

Dyspnoea and cough are usually the most obvious symptoms that patients present with. Breathlessness is indicative of lung-tissue infiltration but may also be associated with infection or with infiltration of the lymphatic system, all of which cause reduced lung capacity. The presence of a malignant pleural effusion caused by metastases invading the pleura will also compound symptoms and may cause a degree of pain.

A chest X-ray or computerised tomography (CT) scan usually confirms lung metastases.

Treatment is very much based on controlling the disease and on symptom control. Systemic chemotherapy has been used, and Hoskin and Makin (1998) suggest that, in women with metastatic breast cancer, that its use can increase the median survival rate to 20 months, although this is very dependent on tumour response and other sites of disease.

Shortness of breath is probably one of the most anxiety-provoking symptoms a patient can experience, and therefore it is essential that any active treatment given must be used in conjunction with measures to ensure adequate symptom control.

Liver metastases

Liver metastases are found in approximately 5% of all patients with metastatic breast cancer (Hayes and Kaplan, 1991). The discovery of liver metastases carries with it serious consequences, as prognosis is often dramatically cut and, if the disease is symptomatic, a patient can deteriorate dramatically in a very short period of time.

How a person may present with liver metastases can vary; they may have one or more of the following signs.

- Enlarged liver on palpation;
- Tenderness in hepatic region caused by irritation of stretched liver capsule;
- Nausea;
- Reduced gastric emptying/feeling of being bloated;
- Oesophageal reflux;
- Jaundice (this is usually apparent in late stages of liver disease);
- Abnormal liver function test (LFTS) – although liver metastases are not the only reason why these may be elevated;
- Bruising or bleeding due to impaired production of clotting factors.

Liver metastases are usually confirmed by performing an ultrasound scan, and blood tests will normally be taken to assess the degree to which liver function is impaired.

The best course of treatment for patients with liver metastases must be carefully weighed up both by the doctors involved and by the patient, who should be given specialist support. Treatment, more often than not, will not extend a person's life but may reduce symptoms.

Systemic chemotherapy is one option that may be offered to some patients, but obviously if liver function is impaired, the drug type and dosage must be carefully considered. It is important to discuss the side effects that can be caused by chemotherapy, as this often proves influential in a patient's decision whether to go ahead with treatment. For some patients with liver metastases, a change in their hormone therapy is an option, especially if chemotherapy is too potent. Rarely, radiotherapy may be given, but this is mainly with the aim of reducing any soft-tissue swelling. Whether a patient chooses to have treatment or not, symptom control and psychological support are essential in maintaining their quality of life.

Brain metastases

Breast cancer is the second commonest source of brain metastases, and cerebral deposits have been found in approximately 25% of all patients when a series of post-mortems were carried out (Hoskin and Makin, 1998).

Patients may present with a variety of symptoms:

- Headache;
- Vomiting;
- Dizziness;
- Visual disturbance;
- Impaired intellectual function;
- Weakness;
- Mood swings;
- Fits.

When brain metastases are suspected, a CT or magnetic resonance imaging (MRI) scan of the brain will be carried out. Often, an MRI scan will prove more sensitive and may detect metastases, which do not show up on the CT scan.

Patients with brain metastases will often exhibit very distressing symptoms, and first-line treatment is to commence high-dose steroids (12–16 mg dexamethasone daily) even prior to metastases being confirmed by scan. The use of steroids aims to reduce the cerebral swelling, thus reducing symptoms and improving neurological function. Any significant improvement is usually apparent within 24–48 hours.

Steroid treatment is only really a short-term measure and, even if initially an improvement is noted, it is usually only for a limited period of time. Depending on the physical condition of the patient and depending on the patient's wishes, other treatment may be considered. For patients with multiple metastases, whole-brain radiation is an option. A short course of radiotherapy may be given and would be given with high-dose steroids to reduce excessive oedema. The success of the radiotherapy, however, is limited and it may only be effective for a short period of time. Occasionally, an isolated cerebral metastasis may be treated with stereotactic radiotherapy or, in some cases, surgery, but this is only in cases where there is no evidence of any other metastatic disease. Unfortunately, even if treated, the median survival rate for patients with brain metastases is 3–6 months (Broadbent and Hruby, 2008).

COMPLICATIONS OF METASTATIC BREAST CANCER

The following sections outline some of the more common complications encountered by women with advanced metastatic breast cancer.

Pathological fracture

A serious pathological fracture is thought to occur in approximately 9% of all patients with bone metastases. Of those patients, more than half have metastatic breast disease (Waller and Caroline, 2000). Bone affected by metastases is often very unstable and can fracture spontaneously or with relatively little trauma.

Pathological fractures can be prevented and are possible to predict in some cases. High-risk bony lesions can be spotted on bone scan and/or X-ray and may be considered for prophylactic internal fixation to prevent future pain and complications. A sharp increase in pain over days or weeks may be indicative of impending fracture, and again surgery may be required. Treatment will obviously depend on the bone involved and the overall condition of the patient.

If internal fixation is performed, the surgery will usually be followed by radiotherapy once the wound has healed. Patients who are too unwell to undergo surgery will be treated with palliative radiotherapy, immobilisation and effective pain relief.

For bones such as the ribs and pelvis that cannot be treated with surgery, local radiotherapy will be given to relieve pain and promote bone healing.

Spinal cord compression

Spinal cord compression is a palliative-care emergency and occurs in approximately 5% of all patients with advanced cancer (Waller and Caroline, 2000). It is caused by metastases travelling from the breast to the vertebrae, where they develop and thus exert pressure on the spinal canal. Cord compression can occur at any level in the spine. However, the majority of cases diagnosed (70%) will be found in the thoracic vertebrae (Twycross, 1997).

A patient with spinal cord compression may present with the following symptoms:

- Back pain – a constant nagging pain, local to site of lesion or a tight band of pain radiating from front to back;
- Limb weakness – a loss of power/strength in limbs, unsteady gait;
- Sensory loss – a feeling of numbness/tingling starting in lower limbs;
- Sphincter dysfunction – a loss of bowel/bladder control, retention.

It is essential that, if a patient complains of any of the above symptoms, they are investigated immediately. A detailed history should be taken and a neurological examination carried out. If there is any suspicion of spinal cord compression, an urgent MRI scan must be performed to ensure that the necessary information is available to make a quick and accurate diagnosis. X-rays may also be taken and, in the majority of cases, these will show the level of vertebral collapse.

Time is of the essence when treating spinal cord compression, and high-dose steroids (usually 16 mg dexamethasone daily) to reduce swelling around the spinal cord will often be prescribed prior to the MRI scan taking place. If spinal cord compression is confirmed, then urgent radiotherapy will be given to reduce tumour size. Very occasionally, there are cases whereby, if there is an isolated metastasis causing compression and the patient is deemed fit, surgical decompression may be used (Leonard et al., 2000).

Spinal cord compression, if left untreated, carries a very real threat of paralysis. Recovery is very much linked to performance status at presentation. The experience for patients is extremely traumatic, and they are often left with significant mobility problems and a poorer quality of life. It is important that physiotherapy, occupational therapy and specialist palliative care input are offered to support all patients and their families/carers dealing with spinal cord compression.

Malignant hypercalcaemia

Patients with advanced breast cancer are accountable for more than 20% of all reported cases of cancer-related hypercalcaemia (Waller and Caroline, 2000).

In the past, high calcium levels in the blood were thought to be linked to patients with bone metastases. However, this is no longer the case, and many patients with bone metastases have been found to have normal calcium readings. The cause of hypercalcaemia in the majority of patients is thought to be the release of parathyroid hormone–related protein excreted by the tumour in to the body's system. This prompts increased bone resorption, which consequently leads to more calcium entering into circulation.

The symptoms a patient may present with when hypercalcaemic are varied and range from mild to severe. Some symptoms may initially be overlooked as they are common in patients with advanced cancer. However, they may develop as the calcium level increases.

The symptoms of hypercalcaemia are:

- Fatigue;
- Weakness;
- Anorexia;
- Constipation;
- Thirst;
- Nausea and/or vomiting;
- Confusion;
- Drowsiness;
- In severe cases, coma.

A simple blood test is able to detect the corrected serum calcium level, which normally runs below 2.62 mmol/litre. When above 2.62 mmol/litre, patients may start exhibiting symptoms.

Hypercalcaemia is treatable; however, it does usually indicate a poor prognosis. Initial treatment involves rehydration, often with intravenous saline, followed by intravenous infusion of a bisphosphonate such pamidronate. Bisphosphonates work by binding themselves to the exposed surface of the bone and thus interrupting the process of bone resorption. The effect of bisphosphonates is usually significant in 1–2 days (Woodruff, 2004). However, it is common for patients with hypercalcaemia to require repeated treatment every 3–4 weeks.

Pamidronate is the bisphosphonate used most commonly to treat hypercalcaemia in cancer patients. A dose of 60–90 mg is given as an intravenous infusion, usually over a 2-h period. The most common side effects reported are mild nausea and fever.

More recently, zoledronic acid has started to be used, mainly treating those patients whose raised calcium levels have failed to respond to pamidronate.

In studies, zoledronic acid appears to be more potent than pamidronate, having a higher response rate, a more rapid onset and a longer duration of action (Woodruff, 2004). A dose of 4–8 mg is given via intravenous injection over a 5-minute period. The side effects are as for pamidronate.

Pleural effusion

A pleural effusion is an abnormal volume of fluid in the pleural space. It will occur in approximately 50% of all women with breast cancer (Leonard *et al.*, 2000) and is a sign of advanced, widespread disease.

Symptoms may include a dry, nonproductive cough, progressive shortness of breath and pain that may be pleuritic in nature. A simple chest X-ray will initially detect if there is an accumulation of fluid in the pleural cavity. However, an ultrasound scan can also be useful in differentiating between fluid and consolidation.

The treatment for a pleural effusion can vary slightly. Pleural aspiration may initially be tried, as drainage of as little as 250 ml of fluid can prove to relieve symptoms. However, the fluid soon re-accumulates, and therefore the insertion of a chest tube and drainage of fluid over a 24–48 hour period is far more effective in controlling malignant pleural effusions (Leonard *et al.*, 2000). Pleural effusions are likely to reoccur within a relatively short period of time and therefore, depending on the condition of the patient, a chemical pleuradhesis may be considered. This involves draining the effusion and then introducing a chemical irritant such as bleomycin tetracycline or talc into the pleural space, which causes the pleural lining to stick together thus preventing a re-accumulation of fluid. In a small majority of cases, surgery in the form of a pleurectomy may be considered, but this is a major procedure and the patient would need to be very fit for this to be entertained.

It is important to remember that a patient can be diagnosed with a pleural effusion and yet have no distressing symptoms. If this is the case, no treatment is required.

Often patients who are symptomatic with pleural effusions may chose not to have treatment and may prefer instead to have specialist palliative care input.

PALLIATIVE CARE IN ADVANCED BREAST CANCER

Although there have been many advances in the treatment of breast cancer, as yet there is still no cure for metastatic disease. Statistics show that approximately 11 000 women a year die from breast cancer and many more will be diagnosed with metastases. For those women, the main goals of treatment therefore must be to control disease and to palliate symptoms (Powles, 1997).

For years, there has been much mystery and misunderstanding surrounding palliative care. Recently, however, with documents being published by the National Institute for Health and Clinical Excellence (NICE) on *Improving Supportive and Palliative Care for Adults with Cancer* (2004) and the Department of Health's *End of Life Care Strategy* (2008), palliative care is evolving and becoming more widely understood by both health professionals and the public alike.

Palliative care involves so much more than symptom control or the care of patients in the last few weeks of life. The World Health Organization (WHO) (1990) has defined palliative care as 'the active total care of patients whose disease is not responsive to curative treatment'.

Within palliative care, there are underlying principles and aims as identified and listed by NICE (2004).

Palliative care aims to:

- Provide relief from pain and other distressing symptoms;
- Integrate the psychological and spiritual aspects of patient care;

- Offer a support system to help patients to live as actively as possible until death, and to help the family to cope during the patient's illness and in their own bereavement;
- Be applied early in the course of illness in conjunction with other therapies Aintended to prolong life (such as chemotherapy or radiation therapy), including investigations to better understand and manage distressing clinical complications.

    (National Council for Hospice and Specialist Palliative Care Services, 2002; WHO, 2002).

Palliative care is very much focused on how best to help people living with cancer, to live the life they have left to the best of their ability. As Twycross (1997) states: 'the primary aim of treatment is not to prolong life but to make the life which remains as comfortable and as meaningful as possible.'

Quality of life is a term that is often used within palliative care. It is a term that will mean many different things to different patients at different times. Ultimately, it is about setting realistic goals and standards that are achievable by the patients. It is about working with the patients to enable them to make informed choices about treatments and the care they wish to receive.

There is still some debate as to when cancer care becomes palliative care. However, the principles of palliative care are such that they can and often should be applied to a patient's care from the moment of diagnosis. The Department of Health in the NHS Cancer Plan (Department of Health, 2000) expresses the view that palliative care has a major role to play in a patient's care whatever stage of the illness they are at, and ideally palliative care should be offered alongside active treatment when appropriate.

SYMPTOM CONTROL IN ADVANCED BREAST CANCER

Poor symptom control can make a patient's life and that of their family miserable (Waller and Caroline, 2000). In women with breast cancer, there are a whole range of symptoms, which arise for different reasons and at different stages in a patient's life. These symptoms may be caused directly by metastases, indirectly from systemic effects of disease, from treatment being given and as a result of medication being taken. It is also important to remember that some patients will show symptoms that may be due to pre-existing conditions, such as arthritis, osteoporosis and heart disease.

WHO (1990) advocates that careful evaluation is the essential basis for symptom management, and that this is the responsibility of both doctors and nurses. Nurses at all levels are fundamental in achieving good symptom control for patients. Whether in hospital or in the community, nurses with the ability to assess patients, to identify the possible cause of symptoms and with the knowledge to implement appropriate care, will ensure that patients receive a much higher quality of care and thus a greater quality of life.

PAIN CONTROL

Pain is often the symptom feared most by patients when they learn they have cancer (Woodruff, 2004; Grond *et al.*, 1994). Many see pain as synonymous with cancer and yet, in reality, approximately 25% of patients do not experience pain (Twycross, 1997). Of the remainder, the pain experienced can, in the majority of cases, be controlled using effective analgesia and pain-management techniques.

Pain is rarely one dimensional. There are many different aspects of a person's life that will influence the pain they experience. The concept of 'total pain' recognises this fact and outlines key components that need to be looked at when assessing a patient's pain.

Components of 'total pain' (Saunders, 1996) comprise:

- Physical;
- Emotional;
- Social;
- Spiritual.

The intensity of emotions such as anxiety, depression, anger and hostility should always be noted when initially assessing a patient. Such features may often serve to lower a patient's' pain threshold and intensify their physical pain (Corcoran, 1991).

Classification of pain

Pain in cancer patients is usually divided into one of two categories, that of nociceptive pain and that of neuropathic pain (see Table 13.1). The physiology of pain is somewhat complex and is not always fully understood. However, it is important when making treatment choices to be able to classify pain.

Nociceptive pain

Receptors that respond to painful stimuli are called nociceptors. Nociceptive pain usually occurs as a result of tissue damage as nociceptors respond directly as a result of chemical, physical or thermal stimulation. The pain message travels from the nociceptors that are found in the skin, bone, organs and connective tissue, along intact neurons to the brain.

Neuropathic pain

Neuropathic pain is conveyed by pathways that are similar to those for nociceptive pain. However, it occurs as a direct result of injury or abnormal functioning of any nerve in the peripheral or central nervous system.

Assessment of pain

Many patients with advanced cancer will present with more than one pain. Up to 80% of patients will have at least two pains (Grady and Severn, 1999). 'Assessment of pain is an essential part of nursing care and a prerequisite of effective pain control' (Bird, 2003). Careful assessment of each individual pain, associated signs and symptoms and determination of the underlying cause, are essential if appropriate treatment is then to be initiated (Hoskin and Makin, 1998). Corcoran (1991) outlines four major components which nurses should consider when assessing a patient's pain.

1 A detailed history;
2 Accurate measurement;
3 Consideration of a patient's 'total pain';
4 Repeated review.

Table 13.1   The classification of pain.

	Category	Characteristics	Examples	Response to opiates
Nociceptive pain	Somatic pain	Dull, aching, throbbing, or gnawing. Well localised.	Bone pain, incisional pain, musculo-skeletal pain	Excellent
	Visceral pain	Results from injury to sympathetically inervated organs. Caused by infiltration, compression, distention or stretching of thoracic/abdominal viscera. Poorly localised, deep dragging, squeezing, or pressure like. When acute, colicky associated with autonomic symptoms (nausea, sweating etc). Often referred to cutaneous sites remote from lesion.	Bowel obstruction, stretching of the liver capsule, tumour invasion of parietal surfaces, perforation of a hollow organ	Good
Neuropathic pain		Results from injury to peripheral and/or central nervous system, by tumour compression or infiltration or damage from surgical radiation, or chemotherapy. Superficial burning, stinging sometimes with lancinating electric shock like pain. Often associated with sensory changes. There may also be associated muscle atrophy, autonomic changes and trophic changes in the skin.	Brachial lumbosacral plexopathies, postpherpatic neuralgia, vincristine or cisplatin neuropathy, diabetic neuropathy	May be inadequate

Reproduced with kind permission from Waller A and Caroline NL (2000) *Handbook of Palliative Care in Cancer*, 2nd edn. Boston/Oxford: Butterworth-Heinemann. Copyright © 2000 Elsevier.

A detailed history

The time spent with a patient, listening to her story is very valuable. It is time in which patients can open up and tell their version of what is happening. It is frequently the first real chance that patients have to express the true extent of the pain and the anxieties that go with it. Patients may try and protect their loved ones by covering up the severity of the pain, and therefore the relief at being able to share the burden is often evident. Spending time with the patient, listening to what is being said and being able to interpret what is being communicated is crucial to an accurate pain assessment being completed. In some cases, a patient may not be able to communicate her story, and therefore the nurse should seek to obtain as much information as is possible from someone who knows and is close to the patient.

A detailed history should include the following information:

- Sites of pain: How many? Where are they?
- Referral of pain: Does the pain radiate anywhere?

- Timing: Is the pain continual, intermittent or on movement? What makes it worse?
- Quality: What is the pain like? Burning, stabbing, dull or aching?
- Severity: How bad is the pain? Does it disturb sleep? Does it stop the patient doing normal activities?
- Medical disorders: Are there any conditions other than cancer that could cause pain?

Accurate measurement

It is important, when assessing pain, that the information received is as accurate as possible. Different methods may be used to measure the severity of a patient's pain. Rating scales such as the ones shown in Fig. 13.3 and Table 13.2 are commonly used and can prove very successful in determining whether pain relief is effective.

Some, although not all, patients may find it helpful to maintain a pain diary. This can be personalised to each individual's needs, but can record material such as increased need for breakthrough analgesia, effectiveness of analgesia, development of new pains and sleep disturbance due to pain. Many areas will have standardised pain diaries that can be given to the patient.

Whatever method is used to ensure accurate measurement of severity of pain, it must be one that is patient/carer friendly. A pain-intensity scale is worthless if the patient is unable to understand how to use it.

Consideration of 'total pain'

Pain, as has been noted earlier in this chapter, is far more than a physical phenomenon. It is important for the nurse to be able to see the patient as a whole, and this means identifying signs of psychological, spiritual and social distress. It also means recognising cultural differences, which can affect the way a patient copes with pain. Anxieties, fears and worries about how family/friends/carers will cope with death, finances and emotional issues are all commonplace and need to be addressed and dealt with if optimum pain relief is to be achieved. If the patient is anxious or depressed, satisfactory pain relief can be delayed by up to 2–4 weeks (Twycross, 1997).

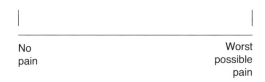

No pain | Worst possible pain

Fig. 13.3 Visual analogue scale.

Table 13.2 Numeric pain-intensity scale, 0–10.

1	2	3	4	5	6	7	8	9	10
No pain				Moderate pain			Worst possible pain		

Repeated review

It is more than likely that a patient with metastatic cancer will find that her situation changes regularly. Therefore, it is safe to say that new pains will occur and previously controlled pains may worsen. By repeatedly reviewing pain at regular intervals, problems can be identified and dealt with at the earliest possible time.

Complete pain relief may take time to achieve, and the patient needs to be reassured about this. Twycross (1997) advocates that it is best to aim for a programme of progressive pain relief. This starts with aiming for pain relief at night, followed by pain relief at rest during the day and, finally, aiming for pain relief on movement. In a small number of patients, the latter aim is not achievable.

PAIN MANAGEMENT AND INTERVENTION

Analgesia

WHO (1996) has outlined six principles which it hopes should be adopted internationally when managing pain in patients with cancer.

By mouth

Whenever possible, the oral route of administering analgesia is preferred.

By the clock

Analgesics should be given regularly to prevent pain recurring. The patient should not be allowed to feel pain before the next dose of analgesia is given. Analgesia given on an 'as needed' basis is not an effective means of pain relief.

By the analgesic ladder

WHO has developed a three-step analgesic ladder (Fig. 13.4). If analgesia in step one is not effective, move up to the next step.

For the Individual

Analgesia will affect everyone differently. Therefore, there is no correct dose of analgesia. The right dose of morphine is that which controls the pain.

Use of adjuvants

Adjuvants are a group of medications that enhance analgesic effects, control adverse side effects of opioids and manage symptoms that are contributing to a patient's pain.

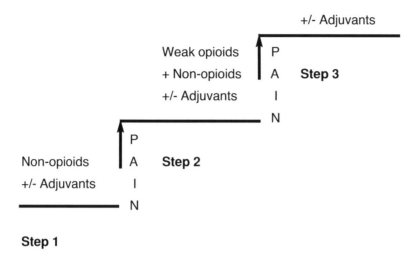

Fig. 13.4 World Health Organization analgesic ladder (1996).

Attention to detail

Do not assume anything. Take accurate precise history. Explore the patient's 'total pain'. Talk about the patient's fears and anxieties. Give the patient clear verbal and written instructions on how to take prescribed medication.

Non-opioid analgesia

Non-opioid analgesics are used in step one of the analgesic ladder and include aspirin, paracetamol and other non-steroidal anti-inflammatory drugs (NSAIDs).

Aspirin is not the drug of choice in patients with advanced cancer, owing to the increased risk of side effects such as gastric irritation and increased bleeding time. Paracetamol and NSAIDs should be used, especially in patients with metastatic bone disease (common in women with advanced breast disease) and for those with soft-tissue pain.

It is important to be aware that many NSAIDs, e.g. diclofenac, indomethacin and ketorolac, should be used with caution. They can cause severe gastric irritation and should never be used in patients with a past history of peptic ulcers. New selective COX-2 inhibitors such as ofecoxib are now available. They have reduced gastric toxicity, and therefore should be considered in patients with bone pain who have previously been unable to tolerate alternative NSAIDs.

Opioids for mild to moderate pain

Opioids for mild to moderate pain comprise step 2 analgesics in the WHO (1996) ladder and may also be known as weak opioids. Often analgesics in this group are combination drugs combining weak opioids with non-opioids. For example, some of the most common drugs prescribed are:

- Co-codamol 8/500 = 8 mg codeine + 500 mg paracetamol
- Co-codamol 30/500 = 30 mg codeine + 500 mg paracetamol
- Co-proxamol = dextropropoxyphene hydrochloride 32.5 mg + paracetamol 500 mg

Codeine phosphate, dihydrocodeine and tramadol are also prescribed at this level.

Tramadol has a role as an opioid in both the upper level of step 2 and the lower level, and may have some additional activity in neuropathic pain. Tramadol works within 1 hour of taking it and reaches peak plasma concentration within 2 hours.

Tramadol is thought to be less constipating than codeine or morphine. However, it has the potential to lower the seizure threshold, especially in patients taking tricyclic anti-depressants and therefore should be used with caution.

If pain is not controlled when opioids at this level are being given regularly and at maximum dosage, then the next step should be upwards not sideways.

Opioids for moderate to severe pain

Opioids for moderate to severe pain comprise step 3 analgesics and are often called strong opioids. Morphine is the drug recommended for use as a strong opioid in the management of moderate to severe cancer pain (European Association for Palliative Care, 1996).

Oral morphine

Before starting oral morphine, it is important that several issues are discussed in depth with the patient.

Firstly, there are many misconceptions and fears surrounding the use of morphine, and these need to be explored prior to commencing the drug. For many patients, morphine signifies 'the end', i.e. there is no further treatment and death is near. This is not the case. Morphine does not hasten death; it is often used whilst patients are still undergoing active treatment and generally is given to control pain and thus improve quality of life. Morphine will not cause patients to become dependent nor, if given correctly, will it turn them into 'zombies' or stop them breathing. These fears, however, are very real for many patients, and it is crucial that nurses acknowledge them and spend time reassuring and educating patients about the use of morphine.

Secondly, anticipated side effects should be talked through. Side effects such as nausea and sleepiness can cause a patient to stop taking morphine, believing that they are allergic to it. Yet it is often the case that, if they had persisted for 24–48 hours, the side effects may have worn off and effective pain relief achieved. Often anti-emetics are prescribed when a patient first commences morphine to counteract the possibility of nausea as a side effect.

Nurses need to educate themselves about the use of strong opioids. Unfortunately, studies have shown that some of the misconceptions and fears held by the patients are also held by some health professionals. Amongst nurses, lack of knowledge, personal beliefs and attitudes towards opiate use, fear of patient addiction and respiratory depression all contribute to ineffective pain management (McCaffrey et al., 1990; Clark et al., 1996; Warden et al., 1998).

Oral morphine: dosage

For patients who have never taken opiates before, or who have been on weak opioids, it is recommended that a starting dose of between 2.5–10 mg of immediate-release morphine, either in liquid or tablet form, be taken four times a day.

If changing onto oral morphine from an alternative strong opiate, this dose may need to be increased.

Additional doses of morphine should be available in between regular doses to allow for breakthrough pain.

The dose of morphine should be reassessed every 24 hours and titrated as necessary according to the pain. There is no ceiling dose on morphine and, in some cases, patients can tolerate 1000 mg or more daily to control pain.

Ultimately, when a morphine dose is reached that provides pain relief, the aim will be to convert patients onto sustained-release preparations that only need to be taken once or twice daily. An immediate-release medication should always be available in case of breakthrough pain.

Morphine sulphate may also be used in patients with syringe drivers or as a subcutaneous injection for breakthrough pain. Morphine sulphate in injectable form is twice as potent as oral morphine

Diamorphine

Diamorphine is three times more potent than morphine. It is used in palliative care in injection form because large amounts of the drug can effectively be given in small volumes. It is most frequently used in advanced cancer when a syringe driver is set up due to a patient being unconscious, unable to swallow or when a patient cannot take oral medication owing to uncontrolled vomiting.

Alternative opioids for moderate to severe pain

Transdermal fentanyl has proved increasingly useful in patients who are unable or reluctant to swallow tablets. It is also thought that fentanyl may be less constipating, nauseating and sedating than morphine.

Fentanyl comes in the form of a patch, of which there are varying strengths. The patch should be changed every 72 hours, and the site of application should be rotated.

Analgesia for breakthrough pain should be prescribed at the same time as the fentanyl patch. Until recently, the choice of breakthrough analgesia was fairly limited and, most commonly, immediate-release morphine was prescribed. More recently, there have been several fast-acting fentanyl preparations that have come onto the market. The fentanyl transmucosal 'lozenge on a stick' was the first preparation of its kind but, more recently, two further fast-acting fentanyl tablets have been developed, one of which can be used sub-buchally and one of which is used sub-lingually. Each come in varying doses which can be titrated up until the correct dose is reached to control the breakthrough pain.

When changing a patient from an alternative sustained-release opiate, the fentanyl patch should be applied at the same time as the last tablet is taken, because the fentanyl patch will take at least 12 hours to take effect.

Hydromorphone is relatively new in this country, but is becoming more widely used in controlling cancer pain. It comes in the form of controlled-release and immediate-release capsules, and 1 mg of hydromorphone is equivalent to 7.5 mg of morphine. The side effects of hydromorphone are similar to those of morphine; however, recent studies have shown it to be less sedating in some patients who are unable to tolerate morphine. It is a useful alternative in patients whose fears about morphine cannot be alleviated.

Oxycodone is an increasingly popular opiate that can be used as an alternative to morphine. Again, it comes in the form of an immediate-release and a sustained-release tablet. It also comes in an injectable form and can thus be used in syringe drivers.

Each 1 mg of oxycodone is equivalent to 2 mg of morphine. Oxycodone is now widely used in the UK as an alternative for those patients who have experienced side effects from morphine. Some doctors may choose to use it with patients who have renal impairment as they believe it to be less nephrotoxic than morphine.

Other opiates such as methadone may be used in patients with cancer, but generally this should only be done under the guidance of a palliative care or acute pain team.

Adjuvant analgesia

As discussed previously, adjuvants are a diverse groups of drugs in which the primary role is not as an analgesic. However, especially in cases of neuropathic pain, which is rarely sensitive to opioids, they have a successful analgesic effect.

Tricyclic anti-depressants

Tricyclic anti-depressants are often used to treat the burning and tingling sensations associated with neuropathic pain. Commonly used anti-depressants are:

- Amitriptyline 10–25 mg nocte;
- Lofepramine 70–210 mg nocte.

The role of newer anti-depressants (selective serotonin reuptake inhibitors) is still controversial, although work is being carried out to prove their effectiveness (Allen and Taylor, 1999).

Anti-convulsants

Anti-convulsants are again useful in treating neuropathic pain and are particularly useful when pain is shooting or stabbing. Commonly used drugs are:

- Carbamazepine – doses vary up to 200 mg, four times a day. Maximum 1200 mg/24 hours;
- Gabapentin – doses vary up to 900 mg, three times a day. Maximum 3600 mg/24 hours;
- Sodium valproate – 100–200 mg twice a day.

Doses can be titrated up depending on need and whether the patient can tolerate the medication.

Anti-arrhythmias

In neuropathy that does not respond to the above therapies, anti-arrhythmias such as flecainide 50–100 mg twice a day or mexiletine 50 mg twice a day may be used. This group of drugs should only be used under close supervision.

Steroids

Steroids, especially, when given in high doses (dexamethasone 8–16 mg) have an anti-inflammatory analgesic property. They work by reducing swelling and relieving pressure caused by the growth of tumours. They are particularly useful when used to treat symptomatic cerebral metastases, liver capsule pain and spinal cord/nerve compression. Attempts to avoid toxicity from prolonged use should be made, and alternative analgesics should be considered.

Bisphosphonates

Bisphosphonates were initially used to treat hypercalcaemia in malignant hypercalcaemia. However, they are now being used as key agents in the analgesic management of pain due to bone secondaries. They are also now evidence that bisphosphonates reduce skeletal complications such as pathological fractures in breast cancer when given to women with known metastatic bone disease (Lipton, 1997).

Bisphosphonates such as pamidronate 90 mg are usually given by intravenous infusion on an intermittent basis.

Oral preparations may be given but are poorly absorbed.

ALTERNATIVE PAIN MANAGEMENT IN ADVANCED BREAST DISEASE

Radiotherapy

A short course of palliative radiotherapy is often effective in relieving pain in both primary and metastatic cancer. Often, only one fraction of radiotherapy is required to achieve adequate pain relief. Although some patients may experience some pain relief within days, the maximum benefit will usually be seen 2–3 weeks after treatment. Because of this delayed effect, adequate alternative analgesia will need to be used initially. Radiotherapy is particularly effective in treating pain caused by bone metastases and gives partial or full pain relief in 80% of patients (Smith, 2001).

Radiotherapy may also be useful in treating pain due to fungating breast tumours, solid growths on the surface of the body and pain due to metastatic liver enlargement which is unresponsive to other medications.

Chemotherapy

Chemotherapy is worth mentioning in regard to pain control as some breast cancers are chemotherapy-sensitive. Chemotherapy, when given to women with metastatic disease, is very often palliative in intent – the hope being that it will reduce tumour size. Therefore, pain such as liver capsule pain may reduce as the liver metastases reduce in size. It is always important, however, to weigh up the benefits against the risks and side effects, and to allow patients to make an informed decision about treatment.

Hormone therapy

Hormone therapy is widely used in the treatment and control of breast cancer and, as such, has the potential to reduce tumour size in metastatic disease. Reduction in tumour size can lead to effective pain relief, and thus hormone manipulation is worth considering as a valid treatment of pain when used in conjunction with analgesic medication.

Anaesthetic procedures

Nerve blocks

Some difficult cases of cancer pain can be controlled by blocking the nerve pathways along which pain stimuli travel to the central nervous system. Nerve blocks can be short term (using injection of local anaesthetic) or more long term, lasting for several weeks(using chemical injection e.g. phenol) They should be carried out under specialist supervision and only after a full explanation has been given to the patient.

Spinal analgesia is becoming more widely used and can be given either epidurally or intrathecally. These methods are particularly effective in controlling chest wall pain or pain radiating through the lower half of the body. Not all patients will be suitable for this type of analgesia, and those that do partake will have to be fully informed and have a close support network.

Physical therapies in pain control

Many women with advanced breast disease will benefit from the use of non-pharmacological approaches to pain control. They are increasingly popular and are used well alongside drug therapy. Nurses need to be aware of these treatments and should be able to offer help and advice to patients.

Superficial heat or cold

The application of heat or cold to an area affected by localised pain can help bring relief.

Heat is particularly effective in alleviating pain caused by joint stiffness or muscle spasms, and pain can be relieved by a hot shower or bath. Heat acts by stimulating nerve fibres, increasing blood supply to the tissues and generally relaxing the patient. Heat pads are available for use in some hospitals, and wheat bags can be advocated as a safe alternative for patients to use at home. Care must always be taken to ensure the patient is protected from being burnt, and heat should not be applied to areas post-radiotherapy or to areas where bleeding is likely to occur. Warmth is a great comforter and, when used effectively, can produce significant pain relief.

The application of cold may often relieve burning pain or muscle spasm. Cold can be applied with ice packs or even with a bag of frozen peas. The cold packs should be wrapped in a soft cloth/towel to protect the patient from skin irritation. Cold packs should not be applied for longer than 15 minutes. Whilst cold has a more prolonged analgesic effect, many patients find it less comforting than heat and therefore it tends to be used less.

Transcutaneous electrical nerve stimulation

Transcutaneous electrical nerve stimulation (TENS) works by stimulating large-diameter nerves in the skin and subcutaneous tissues, using small electrodes which are placed on the body surface and connected to a compact battery-operated generator. TENS is thought to work because these nerve fibres relay the stimuli along the spinal cord, activating an agent called enkephalin which, in turn, inhibits painful stimuli being transmitted from the same area at a slower rate along smaller nerve fibres.

TENS can be useful in patients with moderate cancer pain, especially if pain is in the head and neck region, if it is due to nerve compression or if it is bone pain due to metastases.

TENS does not work in every patient. Its success relies on the correct positioning of the electrodes and on accurate adjustment of the electrical output which will both differ from person to person (Sykes *et al.*, 1997).

TENS has virtually no side effects and, if used correctly, can give the patient a sense of control over her pain. It should not be used in patients with pacemakers or on broken/irritated skin.

Massage

Massage is a technique that can be used by carers, nurses and trained therapists to provide patients with advanced cancer a pleasurable relief from both physical and mental tensions, thus decreasing pain.

The physical act of massage can relax muscles and increase skin circulation, whilst the gentle touch can prove to be of great comfort to patients. The intimacy of massage can often lead to a patient opening up and sharing their anxieties and fears.

Patients with advanced cancer usually only tolerate gentle massage, often only to one area of their body. Care should be taken if a patient is known to have clotting disorders or a history of deep vein thrombosis.

The therapies described in this chapter are just a few of the ones that may prove beneficial in the treatment of pain. More information on additional complementary therapies can be found in Chapter 14.

SYMPTOMS

Nausea and vomiting

Nausea and vomiting occurs in approximately 60% of patients with advanced cancer at some point in their illness. It is particularly prevalent in women with breast cancer (Waller and Caroline, 2000). Knowledge and understanding about the cause of the symptom can lead to effective management.

The physiological process involved in nausea and vomiting is complex and the causes are multiple. Two main areas within the brain are involved in the process – the chemoreceptor trigger zone (CTZ), which is able to detect blood-borne chemicals, and the integrated vomiting centre (IVC,) situated in the lateral medulla, which coordinates incoming impulses and results in the actual vomiting process. Impulses to the IVC can come from higher centres such as memories, sights and smells experienced when in a conscious state and from the balance organs of the inner ear.

The chemoreceptor trigger zone is activated when toxins within the circulatory system or cerebrospinal fluid stimulate receptor cells which send messages to the IVC. There are also chemoreceptors situated throughout the gut, in the liver and the brain. All are activated by toxins which cause stimuli to be transmitted via the vagus nerve to the IVC.

The common causes of nausea and vomiting are:

- Chemotherapy;
- Radiotherapy, particularly to the brain or GI tract;
- Medication: opiates, antibiotics, steroids, NSAIDs, oestrogens and iron;
- Electrolyte imbalance;
- Uraemia;
- Hypercalcaemia;
- Gastric hypomotility/stasis;
- Constipation;
- Brain metastases;
- Hepatomegaly;
- Pain;
- Anxiety/anticipation.

When treating nausea and sickness, it is important first of all to identify all possible causes and then correct any that may be reversible. Therefore, if sickness is being caused by constipation, a laxative should be given. If it is a sign of hypercalcaemia, intravenous bisphosphonates should be used.

Anti-emetics are commonly used to treat nausea and sickness in women with advanced breast cancer. Drugs will usually be given orally and should be taken regularly to achieve the best results. If a patient is vomiting excessively and is therefore unable to tolerate oral medications, anti-emetics can be given rectally, intra-muscularly or subcutaneously. Often, a subcutaneous infusion via a syringe driver is the most effective means of control in prolonged vomiting.

Different anti-emetics work at different points in the vomiting mechanism. It is therefore important that the prescription of anti-emetics is tailored to the potential causes. Often a combination of anti-emetics is required.

Cyclizine 50 mg is a good drug of choice when there are no obvious reasons for vomiting. It works on the histamine transmitters in the IVC and is better at controlling vomiting than it is at nausea.

For vomiting induced by opiates such as morphine, haloperidol 1.5–3 mg, a dopamine antagonist can prove very effective and should possibly be prescribed prophylactically when starting patients on morphine.

Metaclopramide 10 mg and domperidone 10–20 mg act on the gut wall. They are useful in the treatment of gastric stasis and in vomiting induced by chemotherapy/radiotherapy.

Explanation and reassurance when a patient is nauseated or vomiting is crucial. Nurses are often the professionals best placed to provide advice and reassurances. Many patients will find meal times traumatic if they are feeling nauseated or have recent experience of vomiting. Advice about eating small snacks or portions of food on a more frequent basis should be given to patients and their carers. Often carers may find this difficult to understand as the temptation is to try and 'feed their loved one up.' They may see it as the patient giving up. Carers need time to explore these issues and, with the nurse's help, need to be re-educated as to the revised needs of their loved ones. Tastes may change and, where as once a patient may have loved hot spicy food, the smell of curry may now make her vomit.

The comfort and dignity of the patient should always be at the forefront of any nursing intervention. Providing quick effective relief of nausea/sickness should be coupled with ensuring the patient's privacy, maintaining hygiene needs and providing a supportive controlled environment.

Weakness and fatigue

The problem of weakness is probably one of the most commonly reported symptoms in patients with advanced cancer. It is also one of the most difficult to treat. Studies show that up to 82% of patients may experience this symptom (Donnelly and Walsh, 1995).

Weakness is a term that is difficult to define, and many patients will use it synonymously with terms such as fatigue, exhaustion, lethargy and tiredness. Weakness and fatigue are often multifaceted and, when complained of, should be thoroughly investigated. Anaemia, steroids, biochemical abnormalities, anorexia and cachexia all contribute to the symptom of weakness. Problems such as anaemia and hypercalcaemia can be corrected but, for many patients, complaining of weakness and fatigue in advanced cancer there is no correctable cause.

The management of weakness and fatigue in most cancer patients is centred on the development of coping mechanisms. Nurses are often looked to for advice on these matters, and they should be able to talk on the subject of conserving energy through periods of rest and activity. They should also consider, with the patient's permission, referral to other members of the multidisciplinary team, such as the occupational therapist, physiotherapist and care managers, all of whom can offer services that will help maintain a patient's quality of life.

Shortness of breath (dyspnoea)

Breathlessness is greatly feared by many patients and is often one of the most distressing and debilitating symptoms experienced. Being unable to breathe will provoke anxiety and fear in both the patient and their family or carers.

The onset of dyspnoea should be carefully investigated. An accurate in-depth history should be taken, if not from the patient then from a carer or family member. The assessment should look at the initial onset, previous attacks, presence of cough, pleuritic pain, sputum colour/amounts and dyspnoea at rest or on exertion.

Possible causes of dyspnoea in patients with advanced cancer are:

- Lung metastases;
- Pleural effusion;
- Lymphangitis;
- Chemotherapy-induced damage;
- Radiation pneumonitis;
- Obstruction of bronchus by tumour;

- Chest infection;
- Heart failure;
- Pulmonary embolism;
- Anaemia.

Various measures are simple but will contribute to the effective management of breathlessness. Allowing the patient to assume a comfortable position is extremely important. Most breathless patients do not want to lie in bed; they prefer to be sitting semi-recumbent, upright, or sometimes leaning forward supporting themselves on a table. Reassurance should be given at all times, and the nurse should act with confidence, giving regular explanation to the patient. Some nurses are trained in basic relaxation techniques, and these can be beneficial in preventing a patient from panicking. The patient's room should be well ventilated either by opening a window or using an electric fan. In some cases, patients may find the use of oxygen helpful, but there is little proven benefit to this and, in most cases, it helps because that is what the patient perceives it will do.

Other interventions for breathlessness include the treatment of reversible causes such as the drainage of pleural effusions or the treatment of a chest infection. Various medications can be used to help control dyspnoea. Steroids can be used for their anti-inflammatory properties to treat lymphangitis and pneumonitis. Nebulisers and inhalers are sometimes worth trying as bronchodilators can be useful in the treatment of airway obstruction. One of the most useful drugs in the management of breathlessness is morphine. Morphine (5-mg starting dose) can reduce the respiratory drive and will ease the sensation of breathlessness in many patients (Boyd and Kelly, 1997). If a patient is very anxious and prone to panic, a small dose of a sedative such as lorazepam (0.5–2 mg) given sub-lingually can help with respiratory symptoms.

Many patients have to adapt to living with dyspnoea for what time they have left. This is often very difficult, affecting both the patients and their family/carers. Psychological, medical and practical support should be offered to ensure that the patients can achieve their optimum quality of life.

Constipation

Constipation is a common problem for many patients with advanced cancer. Constipation can be described as 'the evacuation of hard stools less frequently than is normal for the individual' (Twycross, 1997 p203). If allowed to go untreated, constipation can cause abdominal pain and swelling, retention of urine, incontinence and faecal overflow/diarrhoea (Fallon and Welsh, 1998).

Constipation can prove extremely uncomfortable for many patients, and its effect on quality of life should not be under-estimated. The main causes of constipation in patients with advanced cancer are as follows:

- Poor fluid and dietary intake;
- Low fibre intake;
- Medication – especially opioids, also chemotherapy, diuretics and anti-convulsants;
- Reduced mobility;
- Weakness;

- Immobility;
- Environmental factors, i.e. poor toilet facilities, lack of privacy.

(Maestri-Banks, 1998).

It is also important to remember that constipation can also be a symptom of hypercalcaemia, which is a serious condition needing urgent treatment.

The management of constipation can be very much nurse led. The nurse, on first meeting a patient, should be able to assess and identify certain factors that may lead to constipation. Simple advice given to the patients and their family/carers such as increasing fluid and food intake, adding bran to the diet and encouraging consumption of fruit juices may prove an easy solution to constipation. It is recognised, however, that the above measures may be difficult in a patient with far advanced cancer and, in fact if the constipation is drug induced, may not actually work. In these cases, laxative medication will be needed.

Laxatives are divided into several groups, the most common being:

Osmotic laxatives

Osmotic laxatives work by drawing fluid into the bowel lumen, thus softening stool.

Lactulose

Lactulose is the most frequently used in this group, but can cause abdominal cramps and flatulence. It is important to ensure an increased fluid intake, which is often difficult if patient is very unwell.

Movicol

Movicol is another increasingly popular osmotic laxative. It can be used for constipation and faecal impaction, is well tolerated and is often more effective than other osmotic laxatives.

Bulk-forming agents

Bulk-forming agents work by increasing faecal mass, which increases peristalsis. Fybogel is most commonly used in this group, and again an increased fluid intake is required. The full effect can take days to work. Bran can be used as a natural alternative.

Stimulant laxatives

Stimulant laxatives work by increasing intestinal motility.

Co-danthramer/co-danthrusate

Co-danthramer/co-danthrusate is the most commonly used stimulant laxative, and is often drug of choice in opioid-induced constipation.

Docusate sodium

Docusate sodium acts as both a stimulant and as a softening agent.

Senna

Senna is often used in combination with a softener such as lactulose. Senna can cause abdominal cramps and should not be used in patients with suspected bowel obstruction.

Rectal measures

Rectal measures includes suppositories and enemas. Approximately a third of patients will need rectal measures despite the use of oral laxatives (Twycross, 1997).

Dose of laxative

The dose of laxative given should be titrated slowly, depending on the patient's response to treatment. Regular assessment (looking at size, frequency and consistency) by a nurse should be carried out and it is often helpful to encourage the patient/ carer to keep a stool chart, especially when at home. The overall aim of laxative therapy is not to achieve a daily bowel action, but rather to achieve comfortable defecation (Maestri-Banks, 1998). It is important that the nurse conveys this to the patient.

Constipation in the majority of patients can, with time, be controlled effectively. A number of nursing interventions can ensure that it is dealt with efficiently and sympathetically. Information-giving and the education of patients and their carers is of primary importance in constipation management. Ensuring privacy and that appropriate toilet facilities are available both in hospital and at home is also crucial to the patient's comfort (Maestri-Banks and Burns, 1996). It should never be underestimated how much discomfort and upset constipation can cause to a patient. Its successful management can lead to the patient achieving comfort and therefore a better quality of life.

PSYCHOLOGICAL AND EMOTIONAL IMPACT OF METASTATIC BREAST CANCER

Many uncertainties are faced by women with breast cancer. Living with the knowledge that the cancer may reoccur has a huge emotional impact on the woman and her partner, family and friends. When metastatic disease is confirmed, the diagnosis is often more devastating that the original one and invokes all kinds of responses from the patient and those close to her.

Typical responses as outlined by Haber (1997) are:

- Personal responsibility – 'I did not do enough to stop the cancer, I have failed, why didn't I do something sooner?'
- Loss of hope – Many see recurrence as a sign of imminent death; they may become withdrawn and be seen to give up. As previously discussed, prognosis in metastatic breast cancer can be relatively long, depending on the extent of the recurrence.

- Denial – This response is similar to that witnessed at initial diagnosis. Women may put off going to the hospital for routine checks and may ignore new lumps developing. This type of response is associated with 'helplessness' (Levy *et al.*, 1985 cited in Haber, 1997). Denial is often a valid coping mechanism.
- Grief – This response may be centred around disappointment that all the efforts made to foster health have not worked. This grief can be worked through and may be short-lived if the woman can maintain the perspective that life is not over yet.

The patient with advanced breast cancer will have needs just as their families and friends will (Rutherford and Foxley, 1991). There is a need to be understood both on a practical and personal level. Patients with breast cancer may want explanations and they may need information. Studies have shown that the better informed the patient, the fewer cases of anxiety and depression there are (Fallowfield, 1991). Patients need to be able to make choices. They need, if they choose to, to hold on to some semblance of control in their lives and to feel that they have a role to play. Every patient will cope differently. Some patients will see the diagnosis as a challenge, using it to enhance their quality of life, to give a deeper meaning to their existence and relationships, and giving them a new sense of purpose (Ireland, 1987 p28). Some patients, as I have already said, may see it as the end, and will despair. Each individual patient will have different emotional needs, and therefore their psychological care should be tailored accordingly.

It is very important, especially when following the principles of palliative care, to recognise the emotional needs of the family. When a diagnosis of metastatic breast cancer is given, it can have a profound and far-reaching effect on the patient's partner, family and friends. The relationship between the patient and those closest to her can often change. Communication can be hindered between a patient and her loved ones. There is often a sense of wanting to protect one another, and this is especially true when looking at communication with children. Family members need to feel listened to. They need to be acknowledged as having emotions, as being involved. At a time when the majority of care centres on the patient, it is easy to forget that the family are equally anxious about what is happening and what the future might hold.

Specialist intervention is often helpful when dealing with problems such as isolation, withdrawal and depression. Often patients and their families will have very specialist needs, and this is being recognised by many cancer centres which employ psychologists, counsellors and social workers as part of the multidisciplinary team. Interventions will be discussed further in Chapter 15.

THE NURSE'S ROLE

Nurses have a huge role to play in not only delivering physical care but also in providing emotional support for women with breast cancer. Nurses at all levels, and whether they work in a hospital, in the community or in a hospice, will come into contact with patients who have metastatic breast cancer. Whilst many nurses are adept at providing the hands-on care, there is still much anxiety associated with providing emotional support for patients and their families. Many junior nurses express how ill equipped they feel in their role as comforter, supporter and bearer of 'bad news' in the care of the dying patient and her family (Costello, 1995).

The dying process, sexual issues, fears and anxieties are all subjects that women with breast cancer may want to address, and yet it is still often the case that these subjects are made light of, ignored or swiftly brushed aside. Nurses build up very close relationships with some patients and their families. They spend time with them, performing often intimate procedures, and it is therefore natural that a patient or family member will want to talk to that nurse. Allowing the patient and her family to express themselves is a very important support mechanism. Nurses are often worried about saying or doing the wrong thing, but often it is enough for the patient just to be able to talk. A combination of good communication skills and knowledge about cancer are required by the nurse (Tait, 1996). These are skills that will continually develop as the nurse becomes more experienced and more confident.

The NICE guidelines on *Improving Supportive and Palliative Care for Adults with Cancer* (2004) very much recognises the fact that, in reality, much of the professional support received by patients with advanced cancer is carried out by health professionals who are not palliative care specialists and who often have little training in this area.

Nurses need to know where to find support, not only for the patient and their families but also for themselves. 'If patients and their families are to be helped to cope with the traumas of a life-threatening illness in conjunction with unpleasant treatments and uncertain outcomes, support and supervision for nurses must be provided' (Craven, 2000).

ROLE OF THE PALLIATIVE CARE TEAM

Palliative care has continued to evolve on many levels. It is now expected that patients, families and staff will be able to access palliative care teams both in hospital and when at home in the community. Many specialist palliative care teams now offer a 7-day service, backed up by an out-of-hours advice line, which staff, patients and carers can all access.

The aims of palliative care teams are:

- To concentrate on quality of life;
- To provide effective symptom control;
- To provide psychological and spiritual care;
- To offer a source of support and understanding to the family, friends and carers involved with the patient both before and after death;
- To provide a high-quality, seamless service to patients, family, friends and carers;
- To provide support and education to other health professionals working with patients with palliative care needs;
- To give patients, if at all possible, a choice in where they want to die.

Palliative care teams vary in size, but are usually multidisciplinary. They may consist of consultants, specialist registrars, clinical nurse specialists, occupational therapists, physiotherapists, social workers, counsellors, dieticians and psychologists.

It can be argued that palliative care has a role to play right at the start of a cancer patient's journey. The truth is, however, that patients are often not referred to palliative care teams until the latter stages of their illness.

Hearn and Higginson (1998) carried out research within the area of specialist palliative care services and concluded that conventional care on its own is not enough for patients with advanced cancer and that a multi-professional approach in hospitals, hospices and the community is most beneficial to patients and their families.

Palliative care teams are happy to discuss referrals at any stage in a patient's illness. Patients do not have to have pain, or be in their last few days of life, before they can be referred. The team will carry out a thorough holistic assessment of the referred patient and will then offer continued advice and support to enable the patient and her family to maintain the optimum quality of life wherever they are. Palliative care teams do not take over from oncologists and GPs, but rather provide a complementary service working alongside other key health professionals. Liaison and communication are keys skills within a palliative care team, whether they are hospital or community based. Palliative care teams should be used as sources of information and support for staff of all levels dealing with patients with cancer.

The role of the palliative care team, as discussed, is complex and will vary from team to team. It is a role that is constantly evolving, and this is particularly so in the light of the publication of the Department of Health's, *End of Life Care Strategy* (2008). This document has placed a renewed emphasis on the importance of palliative care, both nationally and at local level. It calls for specialist palliative care teams to take the lead in helping to educate and train the many generalist nurses and health service personnel who constantly work with patients who have advanced cancer or other life-threatening illnesses.

Although the role of the palliative care team is likely to expand and change over the next few years, the overall principle of striving to provide the highest quality care for patients will remain the same.

CONCLUSION

In the UK alone, it is estimated that there are more than 100 000 women living with secondary breast cancer (Johnson and Swanton, 2006).The care and treatment of these women has evolved greatly over the past few years. Although there is still no cure for metastatic breast cancer, women are now able to live longer thanks to new treatments.

Caring for women with advanced breast cancer tests every aspect of holistic nursing care. Nurses are skilled professionals who can provide high-quality care, comfort and support to women with breast cancer and their family, as long as they themselves are well supported and given appropriate education.

Women with advanced breast cancer deserve the best possible care and that should include physical, psychological and spiritual care. Palliative care recognises all of these aspects and, as Julia Riley (2009), states: 'Palliative care is unique in that it is a patient-centred, multi-professional speciality that embraces a wide range of settings and disciplines.' (p 5)

Palliative care is a speciality that can adapt and complement a patient's care, whatever the stage of their illness.

Increasing importance is being placed on caring for those with advanced disease and end-of-life care issues. This can only be a good thing. Firstly, it will ensure that nurses and health professionals receive the training, education and support they need to become confident in providing supportive and palliative care. Secondly, it will improve and enhance the service provided for the patient and their family, which is ultimately what we as nurses are all striving to do.

REFERENCES

Allen M and Taylor R (1999) Pain control in palliative care. *The Pharmaceutical Journal* 262(7043): 620–624.

Bird C (2003) *Introduction to Breast Cancer*. London: Whurr Publishers.

Boyd K and Kelly M (1997) Oral morphine in symptomatic treatment of dyspnoea in patients with advanced cancer. *Palliative Medicine* 11: 277–281.

Broadbent A and Hruby G (2008) Brain secondaries. In: P Glare and N Christakis (eds) *Prognosis in Advanced Cancer*. Oxford: Oxford University Press.

Chow E and Yee A (2008) Bone secondaries. In: P Glare and N Christakis (eds) *Prognosis in Advanced Cancer*. Oxford: Oxford University Press.

Clark EB, French B, Bilodeau ML, Capasso VC, Edward A and Empoliti J (1996) Pain management knowledge attitudes and clinical practice. *Journal of Pain Symptom Management* 11: 18–31.

Corcoran R (1991) The management of pain. In: J Penson and R Fisher *Palliative Care for People with Cancer*. London: Edward Arnold.

Costello J (1995) Helping relatives cope with the grieving process. *Professional Nurse* 11(2): 89–94.

Craven O (2000) Palliative care provision and its impact on morbidity in cancer patients. *International Journal of Palliative Nursing* 6(10): 501–507.

Department of Health (2000) *The NHS Cancer Plan. A Plan for Investment, a Plan for Reform*. London: Department of Health.

Department of Health (2008) *End of Life Care Strategy. Promoting High Quality Care for All Adults at the End of Life*. London: Department of Health. Available: http://www.dh.gov.uk.

Dixon M and Sainsbury R (1998) *Handbook of Diseases of the Breast*, 2nd edn. London: Churchill Livingstone.

Donnelly S and Walsh D (1995) The symptoms of advanced cancer. *Seminars in Oncology* 22: 67–72.

Efficace F and Biganzoli L (2008) Breast cancer. In: P Glare and N Christakis *Prognosis in Advanced Cancer*. Oxford: Oxford University Press.

European Association of Palliative Care (Expert Working Group) (1996) Morphine in cancer pain. Modes of administration. *British Medical Journal* 12: 823–826.

Fallon M and Welsh J (1998) The management of gastrointestinal symptoms. In: C Faull, Y Carter and R Woof (eds). *Handbook of Palliative Care*. Oxford: Blackwell Science.

Fallowfield L (1991) *Breast Cancer*. London: Routledge.

Grady KM and Severn AM (1999) Key topics in chronic pain. Oxford: Bios Scientific Publishers Ltd.

Grond S, Zech D, Diefenbach C and Bischoff A, (1994) Prevalence and pattern of symptoms in patients with cancer pain: a prospective evaluation of 1635 patients referred to a pain clinic. *Journal of Pain Symptom Management* 9: 372–382.

Haber S (ed.) (1997) *Breast Cancer. A Psychological Treatment Manual*. London: Free Association Books Ltd.

Hayes D and Kaplan W (1991) Evaluation of patients following primary therapy. In: JR Harris, S Hellman, IC Henderson and DW Kinne (eds). *Breast Diseases*. 2nd edn. Philadelphia: Lippincott-Raven.

Hearn J and Higginson I (1998) Do specialist palliative care teams improve outcomes for cancer patients? A systematic literature review. *Palliative Medicine* 12: 317–332.

Heatley S and Coleman R (1999) The use of bisphosphonates in the palliative care setting. *International Journal of Palliative Nursing* 5(2): 74–80.

Hoskin P and Makin W (1998) *Oncology for Palliative Medicine*. Oxford: Oxford University Press.

Ireland J (1987) Life Wish. London: Century.

Johnson S and Swanton C (2006) *Metastatic Breast Cancer*. London: Informa Healthcare.

Leonard RCF, Rodger A and Dixon JM (2000) Metastatic breast cancer. In: M Dixon (ed.) *ABC of Breast Diseases*. 2nd edn. London: British Medical Journal Books.

Levy S, Herberman R, Maluish A, Schlien B and Lippman M (1985) Prognostic risk assessment in primary breast cancer by behavioural and immunological parameters. *Health Psychology* 4: 99–113.

Lipton A (1997) Bisphosphonates and breast cancer. *Cancer* 80 (Suppl.8): 1668–1673.

Maestri-Banks A (1998) An overview of constipation: causes and symptoms. *International Journal of Palliative Nursing* 4(6) 271–273.

Maestri-Banks A and Burns D (1996) Assessing constipation. *Nursing Times* 92(21): 28–31.

McCaffrey M, Ferrel B, O'Neil-Page E and Lester M (1990) Nurse's knowledge of opioid analgesic drugs and psychological dependence. *Cancer Nursing* 13: 21–27.

McEvilly JM and Dow KH (1998) Treating metastatic breast cancer. Principles and current practice. *American Journal of Nursing* 98 (Suppl. 4): 26–29.

McGinn K and Moore J (2001) Metastatic breast cancer: understanding current management options. *Oncology Nursing Forum* 28(3): 507–512.

National Council for Hospice and Specialist Palliative Care Services, (2002) *Definitions of Supportive and Palliative Care.* Briefing Paper 11. London: NCHSPC.

National Institute for Health and Clinical Excellence (2004) *Improving Supportive and Palliative Care for Adults with Cancer.* Available on: www.nice.org.uk.

National Institute for Health and Clinical Excellence (2006) *Advanced Breast Cancer Final Scope.* Available: www.nice.org.uk.

Office for National Statistics (2008) Cancer statistics registrations: registrations of cancer diagnosed in 2005, England. *Series MB1* 36: London: Office for National Statistics.

Overmoyer BA (1995) Chemotheraputic palliative approaches in the treatment of breast cancer. *Seminars in Oncology* 22 (suppl. 3): 2–9.

Powles TJ (1997) Efficacy of Tamoxifen as treatment of breast cancer. *Seminars in Oncology* 24 (Suppl.1) S1–48; S1–52.

Rees G, Coleman RE, Brennan JH, Mansel RE, O'Neill WM and Radstone DJ, (1994) Supportive care in breast cancer. *Journal of Cancer* 3: 188–196.

Riley J (2009) Palliative care is no longer the Cinderella speciality. *European Journal of Palliative Care* 16(1): 5.

Rutherford M and Foxley D (1991) Awareness of psychological need. In: J Penson and R Fisher, *Palliative Care for People with Cancer.* London: Edward Arnold.

Saunders C (1996) A personal therapeutic journey. *British Medical Journal* 313: 274–275.

Smith IE and de Boer RH (2000) Chapter 10: Role of systemic treatment for primary operable breast cancer. In: M Dixon (ed.) *ABC of Breast Diseases.* 2nd edn. London: British Medical Journal Books.

Smith J (2001) Recurrent breast cancer. In: K Burnet (ed.) (2001) Holistic breast care. London: Bailliere Tindall.

Souhami R and Tobias J (1995) *Cancer and its Management.* Oxford: Blackwell Scientific.

Sykes J, Johnson R and Hanks GW (1997) Difficult pain problems. *British Medical Journal* 315, 4th October, 867–869.

Tait A (1996) Psychological aspects of breast care. In: Denton S (ed) *Breast Cancer Nursing.* London: Chapman Hall.

Twycross R (1997) Symptom management in advanced cancer, 2nd edn. Oxford: Radcliffe Medical Press Ltd.

Waller A and Caroline NL (2000) *Handbook of Palliative Care in Cancer* 2nd edn. Boston and Oxford: Butterworth-Heinemann.

Warden S, Carpenter JS and Brockopp Y (1998) Nurses beliefs about suffering and their management of pain. *International Journal of Palliative Nursing* 4(1): 21–25.

Woodruff R (2004) *Palliative Medicine.* Oxford: Oxford University Press.

World Health Organization (1990) Cancer pain relief and palliative care. Report of WHO Expert Committee Vol 804, *WHO Technical Report Series.* Geneva: World Health Organization, pp. 1–75.

World Health Organization (1996) Cancer Pain Relief. Geneva: World Health Organization.

World Health Organization (2002) *National Cancer Control Programmes: policies and guidelines.* Geneva: World Health Organization.

14 Complementary and Alternative Therapies

Rosemary Lucey

INTRODUCTION

An important part of our role as health professionals is to provide good-quality and evidenced-based care and advice to those in our care, where our opinion and knowledge regarding all aspects of care has the potential to influence outcomes. This is especially true in the field of complementary and alternative medicine (CAM), where knowledge amongst fellow health professionals may be limited and patients and staff may be confused about the value of therapies.

Across Europe, about a third (35.9%) of people with cancer use some sort of complementary therapy. In the UK, that figure is 29%. The most common therapies used include herbal medicine (46.4%) and medicinal teas, relaxation techniques, spiritual therapies, homeopathy and vitamins/minerals.

The trend for the use of CAM is more prevalent in younger females, higher educated and with a higher annual income than those who do not use CAM (Molassiotis *et al.*, 2005). However, when looking at the data for use by those with breast cancer, the figure rises to 50% (Molassiotis *et al.*, 2006).

It is therefore vital that we have an understanding of these treatments so that we can give good-quality, evidenced-based advice where available. However, there is also a lack of evidence, which means that we must take a balanced approach. We need to understand why patients seek these therapies, the interactions and potential for good or harm and where to go for further information.

Which? reported in 2007, 'Overall, Britons will spend £191 million on the alternative treatments this year alone – up 32% in the past 5 years' and that nearly £120 million would be spent on herbal remedies, up 40% on 2002. It is predicted that sales will break the £250 million barrier by 2011. Almost half (49%) of the 1039 people aged 15 years and over questioned by Mintel said they had used complementary medicine and would do so again (Mintel, 2007).

It is estimated that 5.75 million people a year in the UK visit a complementary therapist (Thomas and Coleman, 2004). People with a long-term chronic illness are the most likely to use CAM, with the most common conditions being musculoskeletal problems, relief of stress, anxiety and depression and the desire to maintain a healthy body (Ong and Banks, 2003).

Breast Cancer Nursing Care and Management, Second Edition, Edited by Victoria Harmer
© 2011 by Blackwell Publishing Ltd.

THE RESPONSIBILITY AND ROLE OF NURSES

As nurses, we have a duty to be aware of the different types of therapies, to be knowledgeable about safety issues and to feel confident about discussing the subject with our patients. Nurses may practise complementary therapies if they have undergone the appropriate training and are within their competence.

The Nursing and Midwifery Council states in their guidance:

> It is the nurse or midwife's responsibility to judge whether the qualification awarded in a complementary therapy has brought them to a level of competence to use that skill for the people in their care. Where a nurse or midwife is working independently, self-evaluation of competence and accountability is particularly vital.
>
> It should be part of professional teamwork to discuss the use of complementary therapies with the doctor, pharmacist, and any other colleagues in the health-care team.
>
> Employers may wish to establish local policies to provide a framework for the use of complementary therapies by nurses and midwives in their employment. Employers are also advised to ensure they are aware of complementary alternative therapies and homeopathy. It is important to be aware that nurses and midwives remain accountable when practising complementary or alternative therapies (Nursing and Midwifery Council UK. Updated advice, April 2008).

It is important to find out what is available for your patients with regard to 'supportive care' generally, which should include the consideration of complementary therapies (National Institute of Clinical Excellence, 2004).

Patients and carers will be looking to health professionals for advice. There is increasing integration of care and recognition that caring for a patient with cancer does not just involve the administration of anti-cancer treatments (Young, 2007).

Alex Molassiotis, Professor of Cancer and Supportive care at Manchester University states with regard to complementary therapies and cancer patients, 'Oncology nursing is at the forefront of being a patient educator and a knowledgeable professional' (Molassiotis, 2007).

This chapter considers the following issues:

- What is CAM?
- What is the difference between complementary and alternative therapies?
- Regulation and standards;
- The evidence base and research;
- How to choose a therapist;
- Where to get more information;
- Descriptions of therapies commonly used by women with breast cancer;
- Brief descriptions of other complementary therapies;
- Supplements/herbs etc. sometimes used by women with breast cancer;
- Complementary therapies and menopausal symptoms;
  - Dietary and exercise advice;
- Further reading.

You cannot be expected to know everything about complementary therapies, but hopefully reading this chapter will enable you to ask appropriate questions and give safe, evidence-based advice.

WHAT IS CAM?

The term CAM covers a wide range of health-related therapies which are not part of orthodox medical care. Therapies may have statutory regulation (osteopathy and chiropractic), a voluntary code (acupuncture, homeopathy, aromatherapy etc.) or nothing in place. (Doctors, nurses and dentists who practise CAM are also subject to their own professional code). Some complementary therapies are available on the NHS. A therapy may be available at a hospital or GP's surgery alongside conventional therapies, or at a private health centre, sports club, at an individual therapist's house or the patient's own home.

In the UK, regulation was non-existent until the passing of the Medical Registration Act, so creating in fact, 'alternative medicine'.

In the early 20th Century, legislation limited the claims that non–medically qualified practitioners could make, which led to a decline in the numbers of alternative practitioners. In the 1960s, there was a renewed interest in the practice of alternative medicine, as people seemed to look for more control over their own wellbeing, although there was generally a negative response to this from the medical community. As late as 1986, a report from the British Medical Association (BMA) talked in terms of witchcraft and described alternative medicine as a 'passing fad' (British Medical Association, 1986). By 1993, a BMA report used the term 'complementary' and encouraged health professionals to learn about it (British Medical Association, 1993).

The 2000 National Cancer Plan (Department of Health, 2000) defined cancer treatment as a three-part system comprising diagnosis, treatment and 'supportive care'. Complementary therapies were one of 11 elements in the new supportive-care model. The *Cancer Reform Strategy* (Department of Health, 2007) further developed the role of complementary therapies in cancer care, aiming for provision of supportive care, regulation and guidance.

Following on from this, the *Manual for Cancer Services 2008: Complementary Measures* was published by the National Cancer Peer Review/National Cancer Action Team in 2008.

The Prince of Wales' Foundation for Integrated Health and the National Council for Hospice and Specialist Palliative Care Services collaborated to produce the *National Guidelines for the Use of Complementary Therapies in Supportive and Palliative Care* in 2004. These guidelines enable health-care providers to set up and maintain services and look at recruitment, working groups, supervision, ethics and accountability.

There is no one definition of CAM. The Cochrane Collaboration defines CAM as:

A broad domain of healing resources that encompasses all health systems, modalities, and practices and their accompanying theories and beliefs, other than those intrinsic to the politically dominant health systems of a particular society or culture in a given historical period (Zollman and Vickers, 1999).

Edzard Ernst, a professor of CAM at Exeter University, defines CAM as:

Complementary medicine is diagnosis, treatment and/or prevention which complements mainstream medicine by contributing to a common whole, by satisfying a demand not met by orthodoxy or by diversifying the conceptual frameworks of medicine (Ernst, 1995).

The British Medical Association (BMA) describes:

The practice of complementary and alternative medicine (CAM) involves any medical system based on a theory of disease or method of treatment other than the orthodox science of medicine as taught in medical schools' (British Medical Association, 2010).

Some countries run a dual system of medicine, e.g. Ayurvedic in India and traditional Chinese medicine in China, both alongside Western medicine. Definitions and explanations are as in the UK.

WHAT IS THE DIFFERENCE BETWEEN COMPLEMENTARY AND ALTERNATIVE THERAPIES?

There is a very important distinction to be made between 'complementary' and 'alternative' therapies in the way they are used. Complementary therapies are used alongside conventional medical treatment to help relieve symptoms, increase general wellbeing and ease side effects from treatment. Alternative therapies are used in place of conventional treatment, often in the hope of a cure. Some therapies can be either complementary or alternative depending on how they are used.

REGULATION AND STANDARDS FOR CAM

The status of most complementary therapies will change in the next few years due to work currently being undertaken at government and professional level. The report of the Science and Technology Committee of the House of Lords (2000) deliberated the future for regulation and standards. (Osteopathy and chiropractic are the only two complementary therapies currently regulated by Act of Parliament). The report divided the therapies into three levels, depending on evidence and organisation.

Group one

Group one encompasses acupuncture, chiropractic, herbal medicine, homeopathy and osteopathy. These are the 'big five' and incorporate diagnosis and treatment within an organised profession. The likelihood is that the other three will join chiropractic and osteopathy in statutory regulation in the next few years.

Group two

Group two therapies do not have a diagnostic feature, being those that complement conventional medicine, such as aromatherapy, Alexander technique, counselling, healing, hypnotherapy, massage, meditation and relaxation, reflexology and shiatsu.

Group three

Group three (a)

Group three (a) are therapies that may be long established and traditional with a philosophical approach such as Ayurvedic medicine, Chinese herbal medicine, traditional Chinese medicine and naturopathy.

Group three (b)

Group three (b) are therapies that 'lack any credible evidence' (Science and Technology Committee, House of Lords, 2000) and include crystal therapy, cranio-sacral therapy, dowsing, iridology, kinesiology and radionics.

Standards for CAM

There is evidence to suggest that therapies in groups one and two are valuable forms of treatment, and many have been subjected to scientific study including randomised controlled trials. There is also recognised training and standards, although not necessarily legally enforceable. It is likely that this will change in the next few years.

Although the therapies in Group three (a) are traditional and often linked to philosophies or religion, it can be difficult to find an established evidence base by Western standards, other than by accumulative observation. This does not mean that they are not effective, but rather that they have not been subjected to rigorous scientific research, so cannot be actively recommended.

As a nurse, be wary of recommending any of the therapies in group three (b) for their therapeutic value. It is difficult to find any scientific evidence of their efficacy at present.

We have moved in our national thinking since 2000, but still have a long way to go. Recently, the Health Professions Council was set up to regulate standards in many allied health professions, e.g. speech and language therapy, radiographers, etc. The aim is that this will eventually encompass all therapists engaged in clinical work. There is speculation that the NHS may insist on registration of any therapist working within the NHS with this body in the future. Although generally welcomed, there are cost implications for those many therapists who work voluntarily.

THE EVIDENCE BASE AND RESEARCH

Just because the evidence base for complementary therapies is small does not make them invalid as treatments. Resources are difficult to establish to fund research in an area where there is not a strong track record of research. Methodology is an important subject of debate as conventional research methods may not be suitable to measure the efficacy of CAM, due to the holistic approach. This can make it more difficult to run a randomised controlled trial, as standardisation of therapy could greatly reduce the effectiveness of that complementary therapy. Different research may require different methodologies with a more flexible design and alternative outcome measures. Research must embrace the holistic and individual approach whilst remaining scientifically robust.

Whilst traditional medical research uses more objective measurements, subjective outcome measurements are also widely used in most clinical trials, e.g. quality of life, severity of symptoms and structured interviews. The Government is encouraging more research into complementary therapies.

The National Cancer Research Institute (NCRI) was established to facilitate strategic planning relating to cancer research. NCRI is a collaborative body made up of the main funding supporters of cancer research, (Department of Health, the Medical Research Council, Cancer Research UK, industry leaders and several cancer charities). CAM research under the auspices of the NCRI fits into three main categories: (1) prevention, (2) treatment, (3) control, survival and outcomes.

A total of 558 patients were recruited to NCRI complementary therapies studies in 2008–2009.

The Complementary and Alternative Medicine Evidence Online (CAMEOL) database was set up by the Research Council for Complementary Medicine with the School of Integrated Health at the University of Westminster in London. The database reviews the evidence into the effectiveness of specific complementary therapies used within NHS priority areas, including cancer.

CAM research in the UK is currently 0.008% of total cancer research funding.

HOW TO CHOOSE A THERAPIST

Professional organisations exist to protect the public and set standards of education and practice. However, without statutory regulation, there is no protection of title (as with the title 'nurse') so, in theory, anyone can currently call themselves a therapist as there is no legal registration except for chiropractic and osteopathy. Professional organisations will tell you if a therapist is known to them – it is wise to check membership and qualifications. It is also important to consider the following issues before you recommend a therapist to anyone.

- What training have they undertaken and what qualifications do they hold?
- Are they a member of an organisation that has a code of practice and ethics?
- Do they have current insurance?
- What claims does the therapist make for the therapy? (As nurses, we should not be actively recommending alternative therapies, but must be able to support our patients if they decide to go down this route).
- Could this therapy interact with any conventional treatment the patient is having?
- Does the therapist have experience of treating patients with breast cancer?

Other factors that the patient may consider are:

- In what type of premises does the therapist work (e.g. hospital, health centre or private home)?
- Does the therapist make them feel comfortable and at ease?
- What is the cost?
- Can this therapy be provided on the NHS?
- Will the therapy involve buying books, videos or supplements etc?
- How many sessions are likely to be needed?

If it sounds too good to be true, then it probably is!

WHERE TO GET MORE INFORMATION

The Institute for Complementary and Natural Medicine
Can-Mezzanine

32–36 Loman Street, London SE1 0EH
Tel: 0207 922 7980

The Prince's Foundation for Integrated Health
33–41 Dallington Street, London EC1V 0BB
Tel: 020 3119 3100
Website: http://www.fih.org.uk

Note: Although this organisation is now closed, there is useful information on their website

Research Council for Complementary Medicine (RCCM)
The Royal London Homoeopathic Hospital, UCLH NHS Foundation Trust
60 Great Ormond Street, London WC1 3HR
Website: http://www.rccm.org.uk

Note: The website holds the most extensive collection of CAM research references in the UK.

Publications

Prince of Wales' Foundation for Integrated Health and National Council for Hospice and Specialist Palliative Care Services (2000) *The National Guidelines for the Use of Complementary Therapies in Supportive and Palliative Care* (Tavares, 2003). Available: http://www.fih.org.uk.

UK Cochrane Centre in Oxford has a limited number of reviews.
Magazines such as *Health Which?*

The Internet

The quality of information on the Internet is so variable and vast that it is important only to use good-quality sites such as those belonging to cancer information providers, for example:

* http://www.cancerhelp.org.uk
* http://www.macmillan.org.uk
* http://www.pennybrohncancercare.org
* http://www.nhsdirect.nhs.uk/
* http://www.library.nhs.uk (The National Electronic Library for Health)

Owing to the constantly changing organisation of CAM in the UK, it may be easier to obtain the most up-to-date information from websites.

ACUPUNCTURE

Yes, this is about needles – but not as we know them – the 'needles' used are very fine and mostly only inserted subcutaneously. Acupuncture is thought to be at least 2000 years old and comes from China, being brought to Europe in the 19th Century. Its modern revival in the West can be traced back to the 1930s when a French diplomat, Soulie de Morant, published a book describing the techniques used in China. There was a further revival of interest when President Nixon visited China in 1972 and saw acupuncture being used as an anaesthetic in surgery and the subsequent public interest in Chinese culture.

There are many types of acupuncture, of which two are most widely available in the UK. One is part of traditional Chinese medicine, where a practitioner would often also use herbs, acupressure, diet, moxibustion etc. The other type of acupuncture is medical acupuncture, (or Western acupuncture), practised by medical doctors who have undergone supplementary training in acupuncture. Medical acupuncturists use fewer points (20–30, compared with a traditional acupuncturist who has access to over 300) and tend to use it more for a symptom control, e.g. pain and nausea management or as an aid to smoking cessation etc.

A *Which?* survey conducted in 1995 found that 80% of respondents who had had acupuncture in the past 12 months were satisfied with the treatment that they had received. It is the fourth most popular therapy after osteopathy, chiropractic and homeopathy.

The body has Qi (or Chi), which flows along meridians. Chi is made up of Yin and Yang which should balance for good health. At times of illness, Yin and Yang are not in balance. Acupuncture needles are inserted at specific points along these meridians in order to restore the balance between Yin and Yang.

For what conditions is acupuncture useful for patients with breast cancer?

Acupuncture can be used for a wide range of symptoms and to promote energy levels and general wellbeing. Acupuncture is used to alleviate pain (e.g. bone or breast pain), to lessen side effects such as nausea and vomiting with chemotherapy treatment, to reduce or alleviate menopausal symptoms, e.g. for patients on hormone treatment or experiencing depression, headaches and much more. Acupuncture will help with menopausal-type side effects from hormone treatment for women with breast cancer.

What is the acupuncture experience like for the patient/practicalities?

At the first appointment, a full history is taken. Careful note is made of the appearance of the tongue for diagnostic purposes and pulses are taken. Some therapists will perform an abdominal examination. Other questions may involve asking about reaction to temperature, bowel function, emotion etc. Depending on which points are to be used, the patient may undress. Points can be anywhere on the body according to the condition being treated.

The sensation from the needles is often described as tingling or a dull ache. Needles can be stimulated by heat or electricity. Needle depth is usually less than a centimetre. (In the nail area, it would only be a millimetre and in the buttocks it could be deeper). Needles may be left in situ for an average of 20 minutes.

Note: A traditional Chinese acupuncturist may use other therapies in conjunction with acupuncture, e.g. moxibustion.

Sensations vary from no sensation at all to discomfort and occasionally pain. Sometimes a condition may become worse before it improves. Usually several sessions are needed, the acupuncturist being guided by how the patient feels. Patients describe a mixture of feelings following treatment such as drowsiness, relaxed or being full of energy.

Acupuncture contra-indications/points to note

Acupuncture is generally very safe with a qualified practitioner. Research published in 2001 showed that out of 34 407 acupuncture treatments, there were no serious adverse events (MacPherson *et al.*, 2001). A meta-analysis in 1995 showed that there were only 216 cases of serious complications worldwide (including such things as pneumothorax and tissue damage), over 20 years (Rampes and James, 1995).

A qualified therapist will always use sterile, disposable needles.

Care should be taken if patients have a low platelet count or other bleeding disorder. Electro acupuncture is not recommended for patients with a pacemaker.

Acupuncture qualifications and regulations

British Acupuncture Council

The British Acupuncture Council (BAcC) holds a register of members who follow a code of practice and ethics and have indemnity and insurance. BAcC are aiming for state registration and have set up the British Acupuncture Accreditation Board to determine standards of training. Members must have 3 years of full-time training or equivalent, which includes Western medical sciences, and will have MBAcC after their name.

British Medical Acupuncture Society

The British Medical Acupuncture Society (BMAS) is for members who are also doctors of medicine and is in addition to medical training. There are two levels of membership starting at basic competency gained over several weekends and presentation of case histories. Further training and case studies (100 of each) will gain a certificate of accreditation. Therapists will have BMAS after their name. Seventy per cent of doctors trained and registered with the British Medical Acupuncture Society are General Practitioners.

Acupuncture evidence and research

There is evidence that acupuncture is effective for treating chemotherapy-induced and post-operative nausea and vomiting, pain and menopausal symptoms (Vickers, 1996). It is used for wellbeing, to aid sleep and for a wide variety of conditions. There is much anecdotal and observational evidence for many other conditions, including menopausal type side effects during hormone treatment (de Valois, 2006; de Valois *et al.*, 2002, 2005, 2007).

Further reading about acupuncture

Birch SJ and Felt RL (1999) *Understanding Acupuncture*. London: Churchill Livingstone.
de Valois B (2007) Acupuncture. In: J Barraclough (ed.) *Enhancing Cancer Care: Complementary Therapy and Support*. Oxford: Oxford University Press, pp. 85–95.
Hicks A (1997) *Thorson's Principles of Acupuncture*. London: Thorsons.

AROMATHERAPY MASSAGE

Aromatherapy is the use of essential plant oils for therapeutic purposes. Aromatherapy massage is body massage using essential oils. Different oils have different properties, e.g. relaxing or stimulating. Usually oils are diluted with a base vegetable oil such as sunflower or sweet almond, (as undiluted they can damage the skin). A massage without essential oils can be enjoyable and beneficial, but not as effective. Oils can be massaged and absorbed via the skin, inhaled or used in a bath or in a cold compress.

Aromatherapy was used by the Ancient Egyptians, Greeks and Romans. In the sixteenth, seventeenth and eighteenth centuries, essential oils and perfumes were in great demand in Europe by doctors and herbalists. The term 'aromatherapy' was first used by the French biochemist Gattefosse in the 1930s, who discovered the healing effects of lavender after burning his hand. French army surgeon, Dr Valnet, used aromatherapy to treat wounds in the Second World War. In France, aromatherapy is practised by medical doctors who prescribe oils to be taken orally. Tisserand established training in Britain in the late 1960s.

The smelling of essential oils stimulates the limbic system, which is associated with emotion and affect (mood). Essential oils are absorbed through the skin and are thought to lead to the release of neurochemicals which affect various parts of the body.

Aromatherapy can also be used by associating a sense of smell with a physiological or psychological function, e.g. relaxing, and is sometimes used with cognitive behaviour therapy or hypnotic suggestion (as in Birmingham, where it has been used to treat epilepsy).

For what conditions might aromatherapy be useful for patients with breast cancer?

Aromatherapy is used to promote relaxation and increase general wellbeing. Other conditions it may help include anxiety, sleeplessness, menopausal symptoms, pain relief, respiratory congestion and nausea (e.g. anticipatory nausea and vomiting with chemotherapy). Some people describe a release of emotions. MIND (the mental health charity) includes massage and aromatherapy as being possible aids to relieve depression

What is the aromatherapy experience like for the patient/practicalities

An aromatherapy massage can be performed on any part of the body, e.g. hand, arm only (useful for patients with mobility problems), but is more commonly done on a wider area (e.g. back, neck). This will involve undressing to uncover the area to be treated.

The first session is usually longer, while the therapist takes a full history, but subsequent sessions would normally be 1 hour for a full massage. This would be adapted in different circumstances, e.g. in a ward setting, where there may be other constraints such as the condition or wishes of the patient.

The approach of aromatherapy is to ensure that the patient feels safe, comfortable and relaxed. After the massage, patients may experience a range of reactions such as feeling tired, energised, emotionally released or revitalised. The therapist usually discusses with the patient any negative or positive associations with a particular smell and the effect required.

For example, lavender or bergamot can be used for relaxation, while geranium or rosemary are used as stimulants.

The patient usually lies on a couch covered by towels or blankets to keep warm and will usually feel relaxed. Following treatment, patients are usually advised to drink extra fluid and to give themselves time before undertaking activity that requires concentration (e.g. driving).

Although most of the oil is absorbed by the skin, it is best not to wear clothes that may be spoiled by oil getting on to them.

Many therapists believe that full benefits are only felt after at least two or more sessions.

Aromatherapy contra-indications/points to note

Oils should not be used on broken or sensitive skin or in an undiluted form or taken internally. Cancer patients should go to a recognised practitioner with experience of treating patients with cancer. Oils may interact with sunlight (e.g. citrus oils) and can cause photosensitivity. Certain oils must be avoided if the patient is hypertensive or epileptic. During radiotherapy and until any skin reaction has gone, the area being treated should not be massaged or oils applied. As almond oil is often used, in theory care should be taken if the patient has a nut allergy, (although there is no evidence to support this). Aromatherapy massage is contra-indicated for someone with a deep vein thrombosis, and great care should be taken with osteoporosis so as not to damage the bones and cause fractures. Otherwise massage should be only carried out using gentle effleurage, especially if bone metastases are suspected.

Aromatherapy oils are widely available, but vary enormously from pure essential oils to synthetic ones or those already mixed with a carrier oil. Toiletry products labelled as 'aromatherapy' may have negligible amounts of essential oil. Price can be a good guide, so it is advisable to compare the same product from different manufacturers. Some oils are very expensive due to rarity and difficulty of extraction.

Because of the power of some of the oils, it is wise to advise your patients to visit a reputable aromatherapist who has experience of dealing with cancer.

Regulatory or professional body/qualifications

Fourteen aromatherapy organisations are represented by the Aromatherapy Organisations Council (AOC). It sets standards of training for schools of aromatherapy. If a therapist has trained at one of the approved schools, it indicates an acceptable level of qualification.

The Aromatherapy Trade Council was set up by the AOC and ensures the quality of the oils.

Evidence and research

Randomised controlled trials have shown a reduction in anxiety (Cooke, 2000). Anecdotal evidence is strong.

Further reading about aromatherapy

Jackson J (1993) *Aromatherapy*. London: Dorling Kindersley.
Stringer J (2007) Aromatherapy. In: J Barraclough (ed.) *Enhancing Cancer Care: Complementary Therapy and Support*. Oxford: Oxford University Press, pp. 97–106.
Tisserand, R (1988) *Aromatherapy for Everyone*. London: Penguin.

HOMEOPATHY

Homeopathy can be traced back as far as Hippocrates. The treatment is based on the premise of treating like with like, i.e. treating with a substance that causes the same symptoms that the disease it is trying to cure. However, the substances are administered in such a diluted form that the original substance is virtually undetectable. Traditionally, between each dilution stage, the remedy is shaken vigorously, a process known as 'succussion'. The dose of the substance is described as 'potency'. Most day-to-day remedies bought over the counter would be a 'sixth potency'.

The modern history of homeopathy started with Samuel Hahnemann, a German doctor who believed that he could help the body overcome its own health problems, instead of treating symptoms. He published 'The Law of Similars' in 1796 explaining his theories, maintaining that the greater the dilution, the greater the effectiveness of the substance. Therefore, he could use potentially fatal substances such as arsenic in such a dilute form as to be undetectable but get the effect that he wanted. The first homeopathic practitioner in the UK was Dr Quinn in 1827, who went on to establish the first homeopathic hospital in London in 1850. It gained added credence when the London Homeopathic Hospital had a much lower death rate than other London hospitals during the cholera epidemic of 1854 (16% compared to 60%).

Dr Fisher of St. Bartholomew's and the London Homeopathic Hospitals uses the analogy of a computer disc to explain how the dilutions work. A computer disc may contain a large amount of data, but in fact it is nothing more than metal. Likewise, homeopathic remedies may only contain water, the dilution medium and lactose for the tablets. This idea has also been termed as 'information medicine'.

Nobody really knows how homeopathy works. As previously explained, the remedies are so dilute by the time they are administered that it is not possible to identify the original substance. Homeopathic remedies come in a form of tablets, powder, liquid and also creams. They can be made from plant, mineral or animal. The fact that the original substance cannot be detected in what has been given has led some scientists to be sceptical about the effects of this treatment. Research is ongoing with differing results. The effects seem to lessen or disappear if the medicine is subjected to a strong magnetic force.

For what conditions might homeopathy be useful for patients with breast cancer?

Many women with menopausal symptoms (especially while taking hormone treatments), turn to over-the-counter homeopathic remedies or consult practising homeopaths. Remedies such as sepia and pulsatilla are thought to reduce the number and severity of hot flushes for some women and to help their general wellbeing. Anxiety, depression, sleeplessness, itchiness, allergies and promotion of healing may also be helped by homeopathy.

What is the homeopathy experience like for the patient/practicalities?

Patients can ask for referral to one of the five National Health Homeopathic Hospitals in the UK. There is one in London, Glasgow, Liverpool, Bristol and Tunbridge Wells in Kent. These hospitals are seeing increasing numbers of patients as outpatients while retaining very few inpatient beds. Patients can also visit a practising homeopath, who may be medically qualified, or buy remedies over the counter. Over-the-counter sales were worth £38 million in 2007 in the UK, with a 60% growth over the decade 1995–2005 (Mintel, 2007).

An initial consultation with a homeopath will take 1–2 hours. The patient would normally be asked questions about their medical history, what sort of person they are, their moods, their sleep pattern, did they feel worse in hot or cold weather etc. to build a picture before the treatment was decided. They would also look at body type and structure. There are nearly 3000 different homeopathic remedies, but usually less than 50 are used. A single homeopathic remedy or several may be prescribed combined into one remedy. Tablets are often placed under the tongue to be dissolved and are generally taken on an empty stomach.

Dosage in the acute stage can mean taking the remedy every hour, or more frequently. Remedies could be extracted from animal, plant or mineral substances. Initially symptoms may get worse before they get better. Homeopaths believe that 1 month of treatment is needed for every year that the person has had the imbalance. Patients are usually asked to return for monitoring before a new prescription is issued.

Many people buy their homeopathic medicines over the counter. This tends to be rather imprecise compared with a full consultation as a homeopathic diagnosis is not made before treatment. However, this probably will cause no harm (but see below), except in the case where conditions are treated that should require medical attention. Advice in pharmacies can vary enormously. Many remedies will need to be taken for at least 1 month to see if they are going to be effective. It is important that any remedies that are taken are reported to the medical team and recorded in the case notes.

Homeopathy contra-indications/points to note

In about 20% of cases, there is a worsening of symptoms before they get better, so careful monitoring may be needed, e.g. asthma or epilepsy. Patients need to be aware whether or not the homeopath is medically qualified. It is thought that some conventional drugs may have a possibility of blocking the therapeutic action of homeopathic treatments. However, in most cases, homeopathic remedies appear safe to take with conventional therapies.

Regulatory or professional body/qualifications

There is, at present, no statutory regulation so, in theory, anyone can call themselves a homeopath. This situation is likely to change in the next few years. Apart from homeopaths with no qualifications, the decision is between medically or non–medically qualified homeopaths. The professional body is the Society of Homeopaths (RSHom)

- Medically qualified homeopaths have completed a 6-month post-graduate course and will have MFHom (Member of the Faculty of Homeopathy) after their names.
- Non–medically qualified practitioners should belong to the Society of Homeopaths and will have RSHom (Registered with the Society of Homeopaths) or FSHom (Fellow of the Society of Homeopaths) after their name. This indicates an approved 3-year training period.
- A patient must feel confident that the homeopath she chooses understands breast cancer and will not miss signs of serious disease that may need urgent medical treatment.

Research/further reading about homeopathy

Ernst E and Hahn EG (eds) (1998) *Homeopathy. A Critical Appraisal*. Oxford: Butterworth Heinemann.

Kleijnen J, Knipschild P and Ter Riet G (1991) Clinical trial of homeopathy. *British Medical Journal* 302: 316–323.

Swayne J (2000) *International Dictionary of Homeopathy*. Edinburgh: Churchill Livingstone.

Thompson EA (2007) Homeopathy. In: J Barraclough (ed.) *Enhancing Cancer Care: Complementary Therapy and Support*. Oxford: Oxford University Press, pp. 193–202.

Which? (1992) Homeopathy off the shelf. *Which? Way to Health* (October) 158–160.

REFLEXOLOGY

Reflexology, or reflex zone therapy, was used in India and China over 5000 years ago, but its modern history started in the early part of the 20th Century when an American surgeon used it instead of an anaesthetic for minor ENT surgery. He proposed that the body was divided into vertical zones which could be accessed in the feet. It was further developed by a physiotherapist, Eunice Ingham, and a pupil of hers called Doreen Bayley who introduced reflexology to the UK, setting up the Bayley School of Reflexology in 1968 which is still a major influence on the practise of reflexology today.

Reflexology can be used to restore and maintain the body's natural equilibrium and encourage healing.

Therapists believe that the body's anatomy and physiology have a corresponding and connecting area on the foot called a reflex which when stimulated or 'worked' enables the body to promote healing. A reflex showing an area of imbalance is often described as feeling like grains of salt under the skin, thought by therapists to be crystal deposits. (The breast reflex is on the top of the foot). The theory is that working the reflexes will rebalance the corresponding area on the body. Similar reflexes are found on the hand. A reflexologist applies gentle pressure to the feet using hands only, encouraging the body to heal itself at its own pace.

Some therapists believe this is connected with meridians and acupressure points.

For what conditions might reflexology be used by patients with breast cancer?

Reflexology can be used to reduce anxiety and aid relaxation, sleeplessness, menopausal symptoms, pain relief, depression, general wellbeing, nausea and vomiting and headaches.

What is the reflexology experience like for the patient/practicalities?

At the initial consultation, the history would be taken with subsequent treatment sessions lasting for about 1 hour. The patient sits on a comfortable reclining chair exposing only below the ankles. The therapist would normally sit in front of them on a low stall with easy access to the feet. While working the feet, a therapist will often use aqueous cream or cornstarch, only using essential oils if they are also an aromatherapist, or had them prepared. (If a therapist uses oils, see also the section on aromatherapy). The pressure used on the feet will vary from therapist to therapist and the treatment required. For patients with active disease, a gentle touch is usually recommended. Reactions can vary widely. Some people feel relaxed after treatment or sleepy and some may feel energised, while others report an increase in bowel and bladder function for up to a few days afterwards. Initially treatment would be once a week, the frequency reducing as the condition improved. Some will people seek 'top up' sessions once a month or once every few months.

Treatment may also be on the reflex points on the hands. Other variations are possible.

Reflexology contra-indications/points to note

Anyone who does not like their feet being touched is not to be recommended to this treatment! Also contra-indicated are leg and foot ulcers, and other vascular disease such as deep vein thrombosis, and any infection such as athlete's foot. Therapists will usually avoid any area of active disease and will not give a full treatment to patients within a few days of them receiving chemotherapy, although there is little evidence to specifically exclude this.

Qualifications and regulations

There are two main organisations, which both set standards of training and practise and check that their members are insured. Members of the Association of Reflexologists will have MAR after their name, while members of the British Reflexology Association will have MBRA.

Evidence and research

Very little evidence exists to prove the efficacy of reflexology. Research has been inconclusive or weak, although there is some evidence to show benefit in pre-menstrual symptoms (Oleson, 1993). Anecdotal evidence is convincing, but more research is needed. There is as yet no evidence to prove the theory of reflex zones.

Further reading about reflexology

Ernst E and Koeder K (1997) An overview of reflexology. *European Journal of General Practice* 3: 52–57.

Hall NM (1991) *Thorson's Introductory Guide to Reflexology*. London: Thorsons.

Mackereth PA and O'Hara CS (2007) Reflexology. In: J Barraclough (ed.) *Enhancing Cancer Care: Complementary Therapy and Support*. Oxford: Oxford University Press, pp. 235–244.

OTHER COMPLEMENTARY THERAPIES – BRIEF OVERVIEW

Detailing other complementary therapies, Table 14.1 is not intended to be an exhaustive list of therapies but, rather, is intended to give guidance on the type of therapies about which you may be asked for advice. I have only given information where it relates to patients with breast cancer – therapies are used for a wide variety of other conditions.

Table 14.1 Other complementary therapies.

Name	What is it?	For what conditions do women with breast cancer seek it out?	Evidence of effect	Contra-indications	Professional body
Alexander Technique	Teaching of improved posture to reduce stress on body.	General wellbeing, stress, pain.	Yes		Yes
Art	Use of art for communication and emotional therapeutic use	Verbal communication problems		May be used with other psychological methods	Yes if Art Psycho-therapist
Bach Flower Remedies	Use of plant infusions for correction of emotional imbalances	Anxiety, general wellbeing	Inconclusive		Yes
Healing (faith healing, spiritual healers, therapeutic touch, psychic healing)	Therapists channel energy to heal people	Wellbeing; chronic conditions	Some anecdotal	Be aware if patient has mental instability	Yes, various
Herbal medicine	Use of plant remedies taken as tablets, teas, ointments, etc.	Numerous	Yes, but varies with plant, quantity, and condition	Quality control over products; interactions with drugs	Yes
Hypnotherapy	Altered level of consciousness induced by deep relaxation; suggestions are made to enable change	Stress; pain; cessation of smoking; panic attacks	Yes	Exacerbation of psychiatric disorders; abreaction	Yes
Kinesiology	Rebalancing of body's systems to better fight disease using touch	Wellbeing	No		Yes
Meditation (different types)	Various techniques for inducing relaxation and awareness of body	Wellbeing; reduce anxiety and stress; headaches; insomnia; menopausal symptoms; increase self-awareness and confidence	Yes – many studies done by meditation organisations show benefit	No – but be aware of support needed if patient has mental instability	Various

(Continued)

Table 14.1 (Continued)

Name	What is it?	For what conditions do women with breast cancer seek it out?	Evidence of effect	Contra-indications	Professional body
Music	Listening to music in a therapeutic way with a therapist	Relaxation; verbal communication problems	Inconclusive		Yes
Naturopathy	Rebalancing the body to better fight illness using methods such as diet, exercise and other CAMs	General wellbeing; prevent cancer recurrence	Depends on which therapy used	Depends on which therapy used	Yes
Osteopathy	System of manipulation of musculo-skeletal system	Pain, back problems	Yes for back pain	Osteoporosis; recent fractures; spinal disease; (back pain could be undiagnosed metastases)	Yes. Statutory regulation
Reiki	Type of healing	Pain; relaxation; boost energy	No	None found	Yes
Shiatsu	Massage of points along meridians, positioning and stretching. Done through clothes, often on floor	Musculo-skeletal problems etc. stiffness (e.g., arm mobility following axillary surgery)	Anecdotal, and some small studies	Osteoporosis; bone metastases	Yes
T'ai Chi and Qi Gong	Ancient Chinese forms of gentle rhythmic movements	General wellbeing; energising and relaxation	Possible reduction of blood pressure, etc.	None; exercises can be adapted to abilities and function	Yes, various
Yoga	Exercise for posture, stretching, breathing and stamina, and for keeping fit; may be spiritual and meditation	Relaxation; reduce anxiety; breathing problems	Possible reduction of blood pressure, etc.	None; exercise adapted to suit function	Yes, various

SOME SUPPLEMENTS/HERBS USED BY WOMEN WITH BREAST CANCER

Many women consider using supplements which can be bought over the counter (Table 14.2). These enquiries should be referred to a specialist as there can be interactions with active treatment. It is important that patients understand what they are taking by consulting a reputable therapist or their breast cancer treating team. Refer to the questions in the section on research and evidence in the introduction. It is important to note that those supplements that have an oestrogenic effect are not normally recommended for women with breast cancer, especially if there is a positive oestrogen receptor status.

With some products, it can be difficult to ascertain the strength of the active ingredient, e.g. '100% pure juice' could mean the entire contents or a description before it was added to the finished product. One can usually be guided by the cost.

The list in Table 14.2 is only a few of the products available which are used by breast cancer patients – many of the products have other uses. It is very important that the oncologist is informed of any supplements that the patient is taking, especially during the active treatment phase and that this is recorded in the case notes. Patients may also discuss this with their breast care nurse or information centre or with one of the specialist organisations offering cancer support.

COMPLEMENTARY THERAPIES AND MENOPAUSAL SYMPTOMS

One of the most common complaints about side effects from women who have had breast cancer is that of menopausal-type symptoms. Symptoms may include hot flushes and night sweats, mood swings, vaginal dryness, tiredness and difficulty with confidence and concentration.

These symptoms can be caused by treatments for breast cancer that suppress or stop oestrogen production such as chemotherapy, ovarian oblation or hormonal treatments such as tamoxifen (e.g. Nolvadex, Tamofen,) or an aromatase inhibitor (e.g. Arimidex, Aromasin). They can be further exacerbated if a woman has had to stop hormone replacement therapy (HRT) before receiving treatment for breast cancer. Unfortunately, it is not possible to predict which patients will get these symptoms, their severity or how long they will last. With many hormone treatments likely to last for at least 5 years, these side effects can have a major impact on quality of life.

Women turn to complementary therapies to treat their symptoms because of the lack of an acceptable effective conventional treatment. HRT is effective, but women with breast cancer are not generally offered it because of the potential risk of increasing the risk of recurrence. Drug treatments such as clonidine (Catapres), venlafaxine etc. may be effective, but the side effects may be unacceptable. With many women, there is also a reluctance to take yet more drugs, and the complementary approach is perceived as a more gentle and natural way to tackle the problem.

Recent studies using traditional Chinese acupuncture (de Valois et al., 2002) and ear acupuncture (de Valois et al., 2004) have demonstrated a considerable decrease in the number and intensity of menopausal symptoms, as well as improvements in physical and emotional wellbeing.

Table 14.2   Supplements/herbs available over the counter.

Name	Perceived benefit sought by women with breast cancer	Clinical evidence	Comments/safety
Aloe vera	Wound and skin healing; general wellbeing	Conflicting	Possible drug interactions; often asked about topical use during and after radiotherapy
Black cohosh*	Relief of menopausal symptoms.	Yes, some	
Calendula (marigold)	Anti-inflammatory, healing, (used for post-mastectomy lymphoedema)	None found	
Chamomile	Relaxation	None found	
Cranberry	Prevention of urinary tract infection	Yes, randomised controlled trials shows reduction in incidence	Sugar-free available for diabetics; not proved to treat infections
Echinacea	Prevention and shortening of duration of infection e.g. common cold; general wellbeing	Yes, although some inconclusive	Treatment not usually recommended for longer than 2 months
Evening primrose oil	Relief of menopausal symptoms	Conflicting results from radomised controlled trials; anecdotal evidence strong!	Possible drug interactions
Garlic	Promote general wellbeing	Yes, for reducing cholesterol	Interact with anti-coagulants; discontinue before surgery
Ginger	Nausea and vomiting e.g. with chemotherapy	Yes	Possible interaction with anticoagulants, cardiac and antidiabetic therapy
Ginseng (various types) *(some products)	Promote general wellbeing	Some but more needed	Quality varies; differences with types e.g. Asian, American, Siberian; may interact with MAO inhibitors, anticoagulants, sedatives, hypoglycaemics etc.

Green tea	Prevention and treatment of cancer	None found	May cause sleeplessness
Lavender	Relaxation	Inconclusive	Widely used
Linseed*	Relief of menopausal symptoms	Some, for use in diet with soy products – more information needed	
Mistletoe (Iscador)	Treatment for cancer and side effects	Small evidence for improved quality of life and survival	Drug interactions; local reactions
Phyto-oestrogens*	Relief of menopausal symptoms and osteoporosis	Yes, seems beneficial to increase in diet but more research needed	
Red Clover*	Relief of menopausal symptoms	Some evidence	Interactions with anticoagulants or hormone treatment possible
Royal jelly	Relief of menopausal symptoms; cancer prevention	No	
Shark cartilage	Cancer prevention	Inconclusive	Do not use with liver disease
St John's Wort	Depression	Yes	Drug interactions
Valerian	Sleeplessness	Yes	Note other sedatives
Vitamin E	Relief of menopausal symptoms	Inconclusive	

*Substances with an oestrogenic effect. These are inappropriate for most women with breast cancer, especially if oestrogen-dependent. Most supplements are contra-indicated for pregnant women.

General practical measures may include reducing stress, not being too overweight, keeping generally fit, not smoking, wearing several thin layers, having a fan handy and making up lost sleep where possible. It can be helpful for patients to know the triggers for them as individuals, such as hot drinks, caffeine, spicy food etc. Keeping a hot flush diary might highlight triggers for an individual if a pattern emerges. It is not necessarily just the obvious factors. One patient explained to me that every time she went down a certain aisle at the local supermarket, she had a hot flush!

There are many different types of complementary therapy approaches that women have found helpful. Unfortunately, in most cases, there is no conclusive evidence from clinical trials that they are effective. However, anecdotal evidence is plentiful from women about remedies that have helped them. A holistic practitioner may argue that it is not possible to assess the effectiveness of these therapies using the assessment methods of traditional conventional medicine. Whatever your views, many patients do feel considerably better and are able to continue with hormone treatment who would otherwise have stopped. It is important that your patient follows the advice given earlier in this chapter by asking the right questions, going to a reputable therapist who has experience in treating cancer patients and keeping her doctor informed.

Treatments for menopausal symptoms may include the following:

- Homeopathy: remedies may include sepia and pulsatilla, sage, rhubarb root extract, sulphur and graphites.
- Oriental medicine: Chinese herbs, acupuncture, shiatsu etc.
- Herbal treatments, such as dong quai, black cohosh, lavender, fennel, false unicorn root and wild yam, evening primrose oil etc. (but note that some may not be suitable if there is an oestrogen-dependent tumour).
- Other treatments, such as aromatherapy, reflexology or relaxation techniques etc.

DIETARY ADVICE AND EXERCISE

One of the most common questions we are asked in the Support and Information Centre concern diet and nutrition. At a time when patients are experiencing cancer treatments over which they feel they have no control and cannot influence, making a change in one's diet can feel like a positive step towards self-help.

Most of us are familiar with dieting fashions and media focus on food in general. Some women feel that they want to embark on a complete change of diet at a time of shock after a diagnosis of cancer. It is perhaps the one thing that they feel they have some control over, perhaps feeling, like most of us, that our diet could be healthier. It is when perhaps the body is under stress, e.g. receiving chemotherapy or other treatment, that people may make sudden changes that can be a shock to the system. Going down the DIY route of adding supplements or cutting out nutrients may give your patients additional problems.

There has been so much written about cancer and diet that it can be confusing and difficult for patients and health-care professionals to determine what patients should do, if anything. Great care must be taken not to give advice that could conflict with treatment, e.g. taking vitamin C supplements that interact with chemotherapy drugs. If you are not a cancer-trained nurse or specialist in the field, the best advice is NOT to give any dietary recommendations. Refer your patient to their oncologist or specialist nurse or to the hospital dietician trained in the care of cancer patients.

The following report serves as a reminder of the complexities of dietary information. We obtain vitamin A from fish, eggs, milk etc. and by converting beta carotene from fruit and vegetables. Beta carotene is an anti-oxidant and has long been thought to have a role in cancer prevention. We know from various studies conducted in the 1970s that cancer patients tend to have a lower blood level of beta carotene, and it was thought that raising this level would reduce the incidence of cancer. Two studies found the opposite result. In Finland, 29 000 male smokers took beta carotene supplements or placebo for an average of 6 years which resulted in an increase in cases of lung cancer by 18%. A similar trial in the USA showed an increase of 28% in all cancers (The ATBC Cancer Prevention Study Group, 1998).

Do not assume that a naturally occurring substance in food is as good when taking it in a supplement form. Just because a substance is good for you in your diet doesn't mean more of it in a supplement form is better!

The 5-year research released from Oxford University sounds a similar cautionary note. A total of 20 500 individuals were followed to ascertain whether vitamin and mineral supplements could protect patients who are unwell from developing serious illness such as heart disease and cancer. The conclusions were that there was no protection offered at all to people who were already unwell and that people would be better off eating a good diet which included plenty of fresh fruit and vegetables (The Lancet, 2002).

There is emerging evidence of the influence of diet and exercise in reducing the recurrence of breast cancer. Big studies are underway across Europe. More research needs to be done. The current long-term study DietCompLyf is looking at the diet and lifestyle of 3000 women with breast cancer to see if there is a link between phyto-oestrogens and breast cancer, and also to see how diet and dietary supplements may affect quality of life.

Breakthrough Breast Cancer compared a group of overweight or obese women restricted to 900 calories a day for 1 month with a group eating a normal intake. The women who had followed the diet had lowered expression of a gene called SCD within their breast tissue which has been shown to be linked to cancer growth.

It is thought that anti-oxidants can play a part in preventing cancer. These are especially found in fresh fruit and vegetables such as spinach, greens, sweet potato, broccoli, parsnips, swede and carrots and in tea and green tea (Macmillan Cancer Support, 2006).

WORLD CANCER RESEARCH FUND
UK – RECOMMENDATIONS FOR CANCER PREVENTION

1 Be as lean as possible without becoming underweight.
2 Be physically active for at least 30 minutes every day.
3 Avoid sugary drinks. Limit consumption of energy-dense foods (particularly processed foods high in added sugar, or low in fibre, or high in fat).
4 Eat more of a variety of vegetables, fruits, wholegrains and pulses such as beans.
5 Limit consumption of red meats (such as beef, pork and lamb) and avoid processed meats.
6 If consumed at all, limit alcoholic drinks to two for men and one for women a day.
7 Limit consumption of salty foods and foods processed with salt (sodium).
8 Do not use supplements to protect against cancer.

Special population recommendations

9   It is best for mothers to breastfeed exclusively for up to 6 months and then add other liquids and foods.

10   After treatment, cancer survivors should follow the Recommendations for Cancer Prevention.

11   Do not smoke or chew tobacco.

What is a healthy diet?

Remember you do not have to have all the answers! Don't be afraid to involve the dietician. The following is the standard advice that we should all heed, whether we have cancer or not. (Individuals may have special needs).

- Aim to eat five portions of fruit and vegetables a day.
- Try not to eat red or processed meats more than once a day.
- Avoid too many high-fat products, e.g. fried foods.
- Try to eat plenty of fibre-rich foods.
- Drink alcohol in moderation.

A healthy diet should include plenty of variety. Table 14.3 is suitable for giving to anyone without special dietary needs who asks for advice about healthy eating. Any change from this, or patients with special requirements, should be under the guidance of a dietician or doctor.

Alternative cancer diets

Many different types of diets are recommended to effect a 'cure' or modify side effects, and it is easy to understand the attraction. Here is a way of regaining control over one's life

Table 14.3   A guide to healthy eating.

Food group	Examples	How much to eat	Other comments
Cereal/starchy foods	Bread; rice/pasta; breakfast cereals; potatoes with skins	Plenty from this group; something from this group at each meal	Choose high-fibre cereals
Meat/protein foods	Chicken, beef, lamb etc; fish, eggs; peas, beans, lentils, nuts	Two choices from this group each day is sufficient	Not more than one serving a day of red or processed meat (e.g. sausages, meat pies, salami etc)
Dairy foods	Milk, cheese, yoghurt; fromage frais	Aim for 1 pint of milk or equivalent (e.g. 1/3 pint of milk = 1 carton of yoghurt or fromage frais = 1oz of cheese)	Try to opt for low-fat dairy foods such as semi-skimmed milk and low-fat cheese
Fruit and vegetables	Fresh, tinned or dried fruit; fruit juice; fresh and frozen vegetables	Choose five a day from this group; examples in next column	Banana with cereal; glass of fruit juice; salad in sandwich; vegetables with meal; fresh fruit as a snack

Remember that ready-made meals or tinned products may contain extra salt and sugar (Lynda Jackson Macmillan Centre, 2008).

that promises to make one feel better. The reverse can sometimes be true. Some therapists reject conventional treatment in favour of dietary 'cures'. Whilst it is of course the right of each patient to accept or reject treatment, it should be done in the full knowledge of all the facts. A diet may involve a new philosophy to life or a complete change of lifestyle. Diets may be time-consuming to follow, have little or no scientific evidence or may not include all the nutrients required. There are big profits to be made from selling supplements (one in five of the population takes a multivitamin supplement in the UK), and patients need to be aware of the potential risks.

We must support patients to make fully informed decisions.

Questions patients should ask before deciding on an alternative diet

- What trials have been carried out to prove the success of the diet? Is the evidence anecdotal or scientific? Who did the research? Was it independent?
- What does the medical team think about this treatment?
- What advantages are there to following this treatment?
- What disadvantages are there to following this treatment?
- What effect will following this diet have on the family, friends, social life etc?
- What nutrition does the diet provide?
- Is it compatible with the conventional treatment?
- How much will it cost in time and money?

Encourage patients to mention any change in diet to their doctor, especially if undergoing current cancer treatment. If patients decide to go against medical advice, it is important that the patient is able to continue to receive care from us as health-care professionals so we can support them in the best way we can.

Exercise after breast cancer

Following diagnosis and treatment for breast cancer, women can have problems such as depression, fatigue, weight gain and lack of self-esteem. Research is ongoing into what impact exercise may have, after a diagnosis of breast cancer, on quality of life and recurrence. Results from a Cancer Research UK trial (Daley *et al.*, 2004) seem to indicate that exercise can improve depression, aid weight loss and give a sense of wellbeing.

A study of 3000 women in the USA showed that those who were active were less likely to die of breast cancer than those who did less than 1 hour of physical activity each week.

Approximately 75% of patients gain weight during treatment and seek help to cope with this. An ongoing trial in the UK is looking at the most effective way to help women keep a healthy weight.

There is enough evidence so far for us to encourage women to take moderate exercise following a diagnosis of breast cancer. Watch out for the results of current trials which are likely to re-enforce this message.

Further reading about Dietary Advice and Exercise

Costain L (2001) *Super Nutrients Handbook* London: Dorling Kindersley.
Daniel R (1996) *Healing Foods*. London: Thorsons.
Elliot R (2001) *Take Five*. London: Cassell.

Stewart M (1998) *The Phyto Factor*. London: Vermilion.

Thiebaut AC *et al*. (2007) Dietary fat and postmenopausal invasive breast cancer in the National Institutes of Health-AARP Diet and Health Study cohort. *Journal of the National Cancer Institute*.

Thomas R (2008) *Lifestyle after Cancer*. London: Health Education Publications.

van Straten M and Griggs B (1990) *Superfoods*. London: Dorling Kindersley.

World Cancer Research Fund/American Institute for Cancer Research (2007) *Food, Nutrition, Physical Activity and the Prevention of Cancer: A Global Perspective*. Washington DC: AICR.

FURTHER READING ABOUT CAM

Barraclough J (ed.) (2007) *Integrated Cancer Care*. Oxford: Oxford University Press.

Ernst E (ed.) (2006) *The Desktop Guide to Complementary and Alternative Medicine*. London: Mosby.

Glenville M (2002) *New Natural Alternatives to HRT*. London: Kyle Cathie Ltd.

Lerner M (1994) *Choices in Healing: Integrating the Best of Conventional and Complementary Approaches to Cancer*. Cambridge, MA: MIT Press.

Lewith G (2004) *Understanding Complementary Medicine*. Family Doctor Publications Ltd (Poole) in association with British Medical Association (London).

Macmillan Cancer Support (2006) *Cancer and Complementary Therapies*. London: Macmillan Cancer Support.

Manning M (2001) *The Healing Journey: A Complete Guide to Healing Yourself and Others*. London: Piatkus Publishing.

Mills S and Budd S (1997) *Professional Organisation of Complementary and Alternative Medicine in the United Kingdom*. Exeter: The Centre for Complementary Health Studies, University of Exeter.

National Library for Health Complementary and Alternative Specialist Library (now available at http://www.library.nhs.uk/cam).

Prince of Wales' Foundation for Integrated Health and National Council for Hospice and Specialist Palliative Care Services (2004) *National Guidelines for the Use of Complementary Therapies in Supportive and Palliative Care*. Available: http://www.fih. org.uk.

Rowlands B (1997) *The 'Which?' Guide to Complementary Medicine*. Hertford: Which? Ltd.

Russo H (2000) Integrated Healthcare: A Guide to Good Practice. Prince's Foundation for Integrated Health.

Select Committee of Science and Technology, House of Lords (2000) *Complementary and Alternative Medicine*. London: HMSO.

Shealy CN (ed.) (2000) *The Directory of Complementary Therapies*. My Press Ltd.

Speechley V and Rosenfield M (2001) *Cancer at your Fingertips*, 3rd edn. London: Class Publishing.

Vincent C and Furnham A (1997) *Complementary Medicine: A Research Perspective*. Chichester: Wiley and Sons.

Zollman C and Vickers AJ (2000) *ABC of Complementary Medicine*. London: BMJ Books.

See also suggestions within each section.

Journals about complementary therapies

- *Complementary Therapies in Medicine*
- *Journal of Alternative and Complementary Medicine*
- *Integrative Cancer Therapies*

CONCLUSION

As nurses, we are always interested in the wider care of our patients. There is now more emphasis in the national cancer agenda about 'supportive care' which includes complementary therapy. Therefore we need to be more aware than ever of what is available, what is desirable and how we should advise those in our care. Ask yourself if the therapy will cause any harm such as interacting with conventional treatment. If the answer is no, then is there a benefit in terms of wellbeing alone? It is important to remember the guiding principle of empowering patients to take decisions about their treatment in the light of good evidenced-based advice from their treating team – however, it is vital to take an overview of possible benefits where no evidence is available.

It can be hard for us to step aside emotionally when patients decide on a completely alternative route – but we must be there to offer support.

After reading this chapter, I hope you are now aware of what a potential minefield CAMs and diet can be for breast cancer patients. The message must be 'beware!' As nurses we must practise within our competences, so must be careful about giving advice where we may not have all the facts. It is our duty to facilitate patients to make their own choices and support them, confident in the knowledge that they are making fully informed decisions.

REFERENCES

ATBC Cancer Prevention Study Group (1998) The effect of vitamin E and beta carotene on the incidence of lung cancer in male smokers. *New England Journal of Medicine* 330: 1029–1035.

British Medical Association (1986) *Alternative Therapy*. London: British Medical Association.

British Medical Association (1993) *Complementary Medicine: New Approaches to Good Practice*. Oxford: Oxford University Press.

British Medical Association (2008) *Alternative and Complementary Medicine*. London: British Medical Association.

Cooke B and Ernst E (2000) Aromatherapy: a systematic review. *British Journal of General Practice* 50: 493–496.

Daley A *et al.* (2004) Exercise therapy in women who have had breast cancer: design of the Sheffield women's exercise and well-being project. *Health Education Research* 19: 686–697.

de Valois B (2006) *Using Acupuncture to Manage Hot Flushes and Night Sweats in Women Taking Tamoxifen for Early Breast Cancer: Two Observational Studies*. London: Thames Valley University, unpublished PhD thesis. Available from the British Library.

de Valois B, Young T, Hunter M, Lucey R and Maher EJ (2002) Using traditional acupuncture to manage hot flushes in women taking tamoxifen. *Focus on Alternative and Complementary Therapies (FACT)* 8(1): 134–135.

de Valois B, Young T, Robinson N, McCourt C and Maher EJ (2005) Evaluating the effects of the NADA protocol on physical and emotional wellbeing in women undergoing adjuvant treatment for early breast cancer. *The 12th Annual Exeter Symposium on Complementary Health Care. Focus on Alternative and Complementary Therapies (FACT)* 10 (Supplement 1): 14.

de Valois B, Young T, Robinson N, McCourt C and Maher EJ (2007) Using acupuncture to manage menopausal symptoms in women taking adjuvant hormonal treatment for early breast cancer. *Psychooncology* 16: 262–274.

de Valois B, Young T, Robinson N, McCourt C, Ashford R and Maher EJ (2004) Using the NADA protocol to manage menopausal side-effects in women with early breast cancer. *Focus on Alternative and Complementary Therapies* 9 (Supplement 1): 9–10.

Department of Health (2000) *National Cancer Plan*. London: HMSO.

Department of Health (2007) *Cancer Reform Strategy*. London: HMSO

Ernst E, Resch Mills SKL, Hill R, Mitchell A, Willoughby M and White A (1995) Complementary medicine – a definition' (letter) in *The British Journal of General Practice* (5): 506.

Lynda Jackson Macmillan Centre (2008) *Helpful Hints on Healthy Eating*. Northwood: Lynda Jackson Macmillan Centre.

Macmillan Cancer Support (2006) *Cancer and Complementary Therapies*. London: Macmillan Cancer Support.

MacPherson H, Thomas K, Walters S, and Fitter M (2001) The York Acupuncture Safety Study: prospective survey of 34 000 treatments by traditional acupuncturists. *British Medical Journal* (323): 486–487.

Mintel (2007) *Complementary Medicines – UK*. London: Mintel.

Molassiotis A *et al.* (2005) Use of complementary and alternative medicine in cancer patients: a European survey. *Annals of Oncology* 16(4): 655–663.

Molassiotis A *et al.* (2006) Complementary and alternative medicine use in breast cancer patients across Europe. *Journal of Supportive Care in Cancer* 14(3): 260–267

Molassiotis A *et al.* (2007) Acupuncture pilot study for chemotherapy-related fatigue. *Complementary Therapies in Medicine*. 15: 228–237

National Cancer Peer Review/National Cancer Action Team (2008) *Manual for Cancer Services 2008: Complementary Measures*. London: National Cancer Peer Review/National Cancer Action Team.

National Institute of Clinical Excellence (2004) *NICE Guidance on Supportive Care for Adults with Cancer*. Available: http://nice.org.

Nursing and Midwifery Council UK (2008) *The Code – Standards of Conduct, Performance and Ethics for Nurses and Midwives*. London: Nursing and Midwifery Council.

Oleson T and Flocco W (1993) Randomised controlled study of premenstrual symptoms treated with ear, hand and foot reflexology. *Obstetrics and Gynaecology* 82: 906–911.

Ong C-K and Banks B (2003) *Complementary and Alternative Medicine; the Consumer Perspective*. London: The Prince of Wales' Foundation for Integrated Health.

Rampes H and James R (1995) Complications of acupuncture. *Acupuncture Medicine* 13: 26–33

Science and Technology Committee, House of Lords (2000) *House of Lords Science and Technology Committee Report*. London: HMSO.

Tavares M (2003) *The National Guidelines for the Use of Complementary Therapies in Supportive and Palliative Care*. Available: http://www.fih.org.uk.

Thomas K and Coleman P (2004) Use of complementary or alternative medicine in a general population in Great Britain. Results from the National Omnibus Survey. *Journal of Public Health* 26(2): 152–157.

University of Oxford Clinical Trials Unit (2002) MRC/BHF Heart Protection Study of antioxidant vitamin supplementation in 20536 high risk individuals: a randomised placebo controlled trial. *The Lancet* 360: 7–22.

Vickers A (1996) Can acupuncture have specific effects on health? A systematic review of acupuncture antiemesis trials. *Journal of the Royal Society of Medicine* 89: 303–311.

Which? (1995) Consumer Association survey regarding use of acupuncture. *Which?* November.

World Cancer Research Fund UK (2007) *Recommendations for Cancer Prevention*. Available: http://www.wcrf-uk.org.

Young TE (2007) The oncology setting. In: J Barraclough (ed.) *Enhancing Cancer Care: Complementary Therapy and Support*. Oxford: Oxford University Press, pp29–40.

Zollman C and Vickers A (1999) What is complementary medicine? *British Medical Journal* 319(7211): 693–696.

15 Psychological Issues for the Patient with Breast Cancer

Jane Rogers and Mary Turner

INTRODUCTION

There is no shortage of literature for nurses interested in psychological aspects of breast cancer. Breast cancer in all its facets is the most researched of all cancers, and the psychological ramifications of the disease, which affects almost one in nine women in England and Wales (National Institute for Clinical Excellence, 2002) have been extensively documented. However, this vast wealth of relevant and useful work can be somewhat daunting for a nurse new to this field. The purpose of this chapter, therefore, is to provide an accessible introduction to this subject, and to highlight some of the key psychological issues that a nurse is likely to encounter when caring for a patient with breast cancer. This chapter aims to:

- Discuss some of the common psychological reactions to diagnosis and subsequent treatments;
- Explore body image and sexuality;
- Consider partner and family reactions to breast cancer;
- Suggest therapeutic nursing interventions to reduce psychological morbidity.

Although psychological reactions can occur at any time, in order to provide some structure to this chapter, they will be presented in chronological order, starting with issues around diagnosis and progressing through different treatments to longer-term psychological effects. As the majority of breast cancer patients are women, the female gender will be used throughout this chapter when referring to patients. However, the particular issues facing men with breast cancer will also be considered.

PSYCHOLOGICAL REACTIONS TO DIAGNOSIS

Diagnosis and treatment of breast cancer are stressful events that can affect both short- and long-term functioning. Women often need assistance to cope with the stresses associated with diagnosis and treatment, both immediately after diagnosis and during and after treatment (Friedman *et al.*, 2006). When the diagnosis is given, there are as many ways for a woman to react as there are women diagnosed; in other words, everyone will react in an

Breast Cancer Nursing Care and Management, Second Edition, Edited by Victoria Harmer
© 2011 by Blackwell Publishing Ltd.

individual and unique way. There are, however, some common reactions, which will be explored, and some of the factors that impact on these will be considered.

Distress

It has long been recognised that a diagnosis of cancer creates a time of crisis for patients and their loved ones, and much has been written about how nurses and doctors can provide psychological support at this critical time (for example, Maguire and Faulkner, 1988a; Fallowfield *et al.*, 1990; Faulkner and Maguire, 1994). With women living longer following diagnosis and treatment of breast cancer, attention has turned in recent years to survivors' quality of life and the distress they experience because of their illness (Vachon, 2006). Helgeston *et al.* (2004), for example, found that there are distinct differences in women's adjustment to breast cancer. In particular, they found that, whilst the majority of women experience consistent and steady improvements in psychological wellbeing over time, a sub-group of women demonstrated significant deterioration in psychological wellbeing following breast cancer.

The National Comprehensive Cancer Network (2003) addressed the stigma attached to psychological problems, and chose to use the word 'distress' because it is more willingly accepted and less embarrassing than a psychological term. Feelings of distress range along a continuum from sadness and vulnerability to disabling depression. A new diagnostic tool called the Distress Thermometer (DT), along with an accompanying Problem List, has made it easier to screen patients to identify distress stemming from emotional, spiritual or religious concerns, practical or family issues or physical problems (Vachon, 2006).

Shock

For many women, their immediate reaction to the news that they have breast cancer is one of shock and disbelief. They may also be very fearful and anxious, and it can be some time before these feelings start to diminish. During this initial period of shock, however, the woman is likely to be given a large amount of medical information about treatment options. She is then asked to assimilate this information and make difficult decisions whilst in the midst of a complex psychological reaction to the diagnosis (Haber, 1997). This clearly places a great psychological strain on the woman, who is likely to require much emotional support.

Anxiety

For a significant number of patients, the shock of a cancer diagnosis will trigger an anxiety state. Faulkner and Maguire (1994) explain that:

> Anxious mood should be diagnosed when patients complain of a persistent inability to relax or stop worrying and are unable to distract themselves from these worries or be distracted by others, and this represents a significant change both quantitatively and qualitatively from the patient's normal mood. (p. 3)

Although it can be difficult to diagnose an anxiety state, there are certain symptoms that should alert the nurse. These include: sleep disturbance; irritability and being 'on edge'; sweating; tremor; nausea; palpitations; impaired concentration; indecisiveness; and spontaneous panic attacks (Tait, 1996; Faulkner and Maguire, 1994). Tait (1996) suggests that symptoms need to be present for about 4 weeks before a diagnosis can be made; however, many women experience acute anxiety on being given a diagnosis of breast cancer, and this may require immediate treatment.

Depression

Like anxiety, depression is another common psychological reaction to a diagnosis of breast cancer. It is known that up to one third of women develop severe anxiety or a depressive illness within a year of a diagnosis of breast cancer (Maguire, 2000); psychological support must therefore be an integral part of the management of the disease. Common symptoms of depression include: persistent lowering of mood; lack of interest and enjoyment in social activities; poor concentration; low self-esteem and confidence; pessimism and hopelessness; anxiety and irritability; sleep disturbance; loss of appetite; significant change in weight; loss of energy; and constant tiredness (Lovejoy et al., 2000). Symptoms need to persist for a period of 2 weeks before a diagnosis of depression can be made (Vachon, 2006).

Loss of control

In one of many texts written by women who have experienced breast cancer, McCarthy and Loren (1997) describe how important it is for them to be in control of their own lives. They explain that control to them means 'discipline, freedom, self-determination, independence, self-reliance, and choice'. They then add:

> The feeling of being in control deserted us in an instant when we received our diagnoses of breast cancer. (p. 2)

This is a powerful illustration of one of the devastating effects of diagnosis. Patients have to contend with the idea of the disease being in control, and then hand their lives over to health-care professionals, allowing them to take charge of the treatment. It is therefore not surprising that, for many women, the loss of control associated with a diagnosis of breast cancer is difficult to cope with.

Loss and grieving

Both the diagnosis of breast cancer and its treatment may represent loss to a woman, from the loss of a breast to the loss of confidence and sense of security. Many women may undergo a grieving process in order to come to terms with their losses (Kubler-Ross, 1978; Parkes and Weiss, 1983). This process can take many months or even years to complete, and can encompass many emotions, including guilt, denial, sadness and anger.

FACTORS AFFECTING PSYCHOLOGICAL REACTIONS

So far, some of the possible psychological reactions to a diagnosis of breast cancer have been described. However, there are several factors that may influence the extent to which these reactions are experienced. These include a woman's previous experience of breast cancer, the manner in which the diagnosis is given, and the manner and the speed of the diagnosis and first treatment.

Previous experience

A woman's previous life experience, and her experience of cancer in general and breast cancer in particular, may influence her psychological reaction to diagnosis and treatment. If she has, for example, lost a member of her family to the disease at an early age, she may be more frightened than if she witnessed a family member make a full recovery. Friedman *et al.* (2006) identify some important factors that may render a woman more vulnerable to psychological morbidity. These include a history of psychiatric illness; lack of social support; low expectations of the success of the treatment; pre-existing relationship difficulties and treatment with aggressive chemotherapy. If several of these factors are present, the woman may be even more vulnerable to psychological difficulties.

Breaking bad news

Dixon and Sainsbury (1998) state that:

> There is no easy way to break bad news. However it is important to do it in such a way that the patient can bear the news, receive the information that she needs to know and to enable her to express her feelings and concerns. (p. 207)

The way in which the diagnosis is made and the news broken to the patient can have an enormous impact on her psychological reaction (Faulkner and Maguire, 1994). Most experts agree that women who have the news broken to them in a sensitive manner, and are given the opportunity to ask questions, are likely to suffer less long-term psychological morbidity than those who are told abruptly or hurriedly (Maguire and Faulkner, 1988b; Fallowfield *et al.*, 1990).

For this reason, it is clearly stated in breast cancer guidelines (Department of Health, 1996) that protocols and procedures for the breaking of bad news must be in place, and that a specialist breast care nurse should be on hand to support the patient and family. The National Institute for Clinical Excellence (2002) has also produced guidance on the management of breast cancer which includes the recommendation that all members of the breast care team who provide clinical care should have special training in communication and counselling skills.

Screen-detected cancers

Whether a woman is diagnosed through the NHS Breast Screening Programme or through the symptomatic service may have an impact on her psychological response. The majority (approximately 80%) of women who go to breast clinics for investigation of suspected breast cancer are referred by their GP (National Institute for Clinical Excellence, 2002). These women are symptomatic; in other words, they have discovered a lump or other symptoms, and have been concerned enough to seek the opinion and advice of their GP.

On first discovering a change in their breast, many of these women immediately fear the worst, and so to some extent start to prepare themselves for a diagnosis of cancer. Women with suspected breast cancer are seen very quickly in a specialist breast clinic due to the Government's cancer 2-week wait guidelines (National Health Service Executive, 1998). This speed of referral may add to a woman's anxiety pre-diagnosis, as she may feel that she would not be seen so quickly if it were not serious; it may also paradoxically sound a warning note, rendering the actual diagnosis much less of a shock.

However, about 20% of women are referred to breast clinics from the NHS Breast Screening Programme (National Institute for Clinical Excellence, 2002). These women usually have no symptoms, and go for breast screening once every 3 years, expecting to be given a clean bill of health. They may therefore be totally unprepared for a diagnosis of cancer, and it can come as more of a shock to them, precipitating greater psychological morbidity.

One-stop clinics

The value of one-stop clinics, where a definite diagnosis is made and given to the patient at their first visit, remains controversial. A study by Harcourt *et al.* (1999), for example, showed that women with benign breast disease derived psychological benefit from having a speedy diagnosis, as they were spared the distress associated with waiting. However, women with breast cancer did not experience the same benefit. On the contrary, the study showed that women with cancer who had been through the one-stop system reported higher levels of depression 8 weeks following diagnosis than women who had experienced the two-stop system. These findings would appear to support Faulkner and Maguire's (1994) contention that bad news needs to be broken slowly, in order to avoid too abrupt a transition for the patient from the perception of being well to that of having a potentially life-threatening illness.

Waiting for treatment

Many women find that the time between being given the diagnosis and having the first treatment seems long, and this waiting can cause anxiety. Many women fear that the cancer might be growing while they are waiting for treatment. For this reason, a Government target is to cut down the waiting time to 4 weeks:

> No patient should have to wait more than four weeks for any form of treatment or supportive intervention. (National Institute for Clinical Excellence, 2002, p. 8)

For most women, the first treatment is surgical. The psychological implications of the different sorts of breast surgery will now be considered.

SURGICAL TREATMENTS

Mastectomy

It has already been suggested that women react in many different ways to a diagnosis of breast cancer, and similarly there are a myriad of reactions to mastectomy. Some women regard mastectomy as mutilating surgery, and some find the psychological consequences devastating (see the section on body image and sexuality below). However, many others are not primarily concerned with losing a breast; for example, Fallowfield *et al.* (1990) found that only 12% of women in their study cited breast loss as their primary concern. Some are far more concerned about the cancer, and see mastectomy as a means to improve their prognosis; it can also give them more peace of mind in the long term by helping to assuage the fear of recurrence.

Breast-conserving surgery

There is an understandable tendency in the literature to focus on mastectomy when considering the psychological effects of surgery. However, breast-conserving surgery also has psychological consequences. The surgery may be disfiguring, altering the shape and size of the breast. In addition, a woman may have fears that the cancer will return in the breast. Fallowfield (1986) found that women who had breast-conserving surgery experienced the same levels of anxiety and depression as those who had mastectomy.

Axillary node clearance

Until recently, it was common practice to remove all the axillary lymph nodes adjacent to the affected breast, in order to stage the disease accurately and treat it adequately. However, recent advances in breast cancer research have shown that the status of the sentinel node is an accurate predictor of the status of the axillary nodes in breast cancer (Veronesi *et al.*, 2003). The sentinel node is the first lymph node or nodes in the axilla to which breast cancer can spread. If cancer cells have invaded the sentinel node, patients will need further surgery to the axilla to remove the remaining nodes (please refer to Chapter 5 of this book for more details about surgical procedures).

Removal of these glands carries with it a significant risk of developing lymphoedema of the arm in the future. For some women, this means a reduction in the mobility of their arm, which may in turn lead to a loss of independence. Even those who do not develop lymphoedema can experience high levels of anxiety about their risk of doing so.

Immediate or delayed breast reconstruction

Some women are given the choice of immediate breast reconstruction following mastectomy. One study in the UK investigated the psychological advantages of immediate rather than delayed breast reconstruction (Al Ghazal *et al.*, 2000). This study found that most of the women who had delayed reconstruction said they would have preferred immediate reconstruction, whilst the women who underwent immediate reconstruction reported less anxiety and depression, and better body image and self-esteem.

However, immediate reconstruction is not available for every woman. Indeed, some surgeons are reluctant to offer it, because they have concerns that it may delay or compromise adjuvant therapy that they consider to be of paramount importance. A woman who wants this procedure may therefore need to be quite assertive, and be prepared to travel to a breast unit where it is available.

Making decisions about treatment

When a diagnosis of breast cancer is confirmed, treatment options need to be discussed and decisions have to be made before treatment can commence. In the past, decisions were made by the surgeon alone, and the woman was not consulted. However, there is now research evidence showing that women suffer less psychological morbidity if they are offered a choice of treatments and involved in the decision-making process (Fallowfield *et al.*, 1990; Kravitz and Melnikow, 2001). It is therefore now standard practice to involve women in making decisions about their treatment.

However, some women find it very difficult and stressful to make decisions about treatment, and do not want to carry such a heavy responsibility. The National Institute for Clinical Excellence guidelines (2002) point out that:

> There is fairly strong evidence that breast cancer patients benefit from involvement in treatment decisions, but women vary considerably in the amount of responsibility they wish to take and clinicians need to be sensitive to the degree to which individual patients want to become involved in decision making. (p. 29)

Surgeons and other members of the breast care team therefore need to spend enough time with each patient in order to assess her information needs and her willingness to take part in decision making.

BODY IMAGE AND SEXUALITY

Defining body image

The effect of breast surgery on body image has already been alluded to, but what exactly do we mean by this much-used term? Fobair *et al.* (2006) define body image as 'the mental picture of one's body, an attitude about the physical self, appearance, and state of health, wholeness, normal functioning, and sexuality' (p. 580). Faulkner and Maguire (1994) identify three components of body image: the loss of physical integrity (feeling no longer whole as a result of the removal of part of the body); a heightened sense of self-consciousness; and feeling less sexually attractive.

Society and the media

Every day, we are bombarded with images in the media that serve to underline the link between breasts and sexual desirability. Tait and Wing (1997) explain that:

> There has never been a time since Adam and Eve when a woman's breasts were not important. Through the ages, the ways in which they were portrayed have changed, but the message remains essentially the same. The female breast is regarded as the symbol of intrinsic femininity, sexual desirability and maternal comfort and succour. Whether breasts are alluded to in a subtle and evocative way or explicitly exhibited, they are central to many peoples' views about 'being a woman'. It is small wonder, therefore, that any real or potential threat to a woman's breast is stressful. (p. 151)

Given society's preoccupation with breasts, it is hardly surprising that both the surgical treatment and the disease itself can have a devastating impact on a woman's confidence and self-esteem, and make her feel less attractive than before.

Sexuality

Closely allied to body image is the issue of sexuality. Love (2000) contends that sexuality is one of the least discussed subjects with life after breast cancer. This is perhaps not surprising, since the personal and private nature of sex and sexuality can make it a particularly difficult subject to broach. Many health-care professionals, if they were honest, would probably admit that they find it much easier to focus on issues such as treatment rather than sexuality. Indeed, they may lack both the skills and the confidence to deal with this subject effectively.

However, it is imperative that these issues are addressed, as sexual problems and sexual functioning have been found to persist years after a diagnosis of breast cancer (Ganz et al., 2002). Many patients may want and need to discuss these issues, and they may well choose a nurse rather than a doctor to discuss them with, especially if a good nurse–patient relationship has been established. Nurses should therefore ask patients about their personal relationships as part of their assessment, and provide opportunities for patients to discuss their concerns about sexuality and body image. Although each patient will of course have her own individual concerns, it is worth briefly highlighting some common problems.

Fear of rejection

Many women fear that their partners will be put off by their appearance following surgery, and that they will no longer find them sexually attractive. Partners too may have concerns about the woman's appearance, and how it might impact on their sexual relationship. One study explored the reactions of husbands to their wives' diagnoses of breast cancer (Woloski-Wruble and Kadmon, 2002). This study revealed that, although the husbands described their relationships with their wives as 'excellent', the majority of them experienced a change in their sexual interest, function or satisfaction following their wives' diagnoses of breast cancer. Men may also have concerns about hurting their partners, which may deter them from resuming sexual activity. However, it is also worth pointing out that many couples find that the experience of breast cancer brings them closer, particularly if they can share their concerns and reassure one another.

Loss of libido

Many patients experience a loss of libido in the weeks and months following diagnosis, which may be related both to their psychological reactions and to the effects of treatment. A woman who is experiencing pain following surgery, for example, is perhaps less likely to feel like lovemaking. Many women also find that their sexual relationships are relegated to lower down their list of priorities as they are preoccupied with trying to make a psychological adjustment to their new situation.

Making new relationships

Of course, many patients are not in sexual relationships at the time of diagnosis and treatment, and this can bring a different raft of problems. Body-image concerns such as hair loss, weight gain and the loss of a breast can affect women at any age following a breast cancer diagnosis (Avis et al., 2004), and a woman on her own may find it harder to embark on a new relationship if she feels that the treatment has impaired her sexual attractiveness.

Nurses can be instrumental in helping patients to cope with all these concerns. As Salter (1997) rightly argues:

> Knowledge about actual and potential problems associated with sexuality and an alteration in body image enables the nurse to assess the meaning of this for the individual patient and family, provide counselling before and after the surgery, and intervene so that the individual will be able to adapt to an alteration in body image and return to his or her previous activities of daily living and lifestyle. (p. 33)

ADJUVANT THERAPIES

In the past, the only effective treatment for breast cancer was surgery. In recent years, however, there has been a dramatic rise in the number of women given adjuvant therapies for breast cancer, and these carry with them their own potential psychological morbidity. Psychological issues associated with chemotherapy, radiotherapy and hormonal therapies will now be briefly considered.

Chemotherapy

Chemotherapy can bring about many physical changes that can have a negative impact on a woman's body image. One of the most significant and common is hair loss which, for some women, is the most distressing part of their cancer treatment. It is relatively easy to disguise the loss of a breast by using a breast prosthesis but, although wigs, scarves and hats can be used, it is sometimes much more difficult to disguise hair loss. Many women are also distressed by the speed with which their hair can fall out. The journalist Ruth Picardie, who was diagnosed with breast cancer when she was 32, describes her experience of hair loss:

> Meanwhile, my hair is falling out with amazing rapidity – I estimate total baldness will be achieved by the weekend, so the whole thing will have happened in a week. [. . .] I'm now used to hoovering the bed every morning. . . (Picardie, 1998, p. 1)

Even the treatments used to counteract the side effects of chemotherapy can cause side effects of their own, contributing to altered body image. For instance, it is now common practice to give steroids as part of the anti-emetic regime; many women find that steroids increase their appetite, with the consequence that they gain weight, and feel less attractive.

Fertility

Although the majority of women are post-menopausal when diagnosed with breast cancer, a significant minority are still of childbearing age, and many of them are given chemotherapy that may affect their fertility. If patients have not had children at the time of diagnosis, infertility can be a major concern, which can increase their emotional distress (Partridge *et al.*, 2004). Some patients who already have children may have been planning more pregnancies, and the thought of infertility may cause them concern (Avis *et al.*, 2005). Furthermore, issues around the safety of subsequent pregnancies and the biological possibility of them are also often an anxiety (Beaumont, 2007). It is therefore very important that an assessment is made of the patient's feelings about future pregnancy so that, if necessary, fertility can be preserved whenever possible.

Fatigue

Fatigue can occur with all forms of cancer treatment, but there is now clear evidence that it is the most common side effect for patients receiving chemotherapy (Richardson, 1995a, 1995b). The exact physiological mechanisms that lead to fatigue are not fully established, but research shows that patients relate it to treatment, as well as to other symptoms, levels of activity and psychological concerns. There is little doubt that psychological reactions and physiological fatigue are closely linked, and it can be difficult to untangle them. For example, if a patient is depressed it may be hard to tell whether this is a cause or a consequence of fatigue. Fatigue can have a detrimental effect on all aspects of a woman's quality of life, including her interpersonal relationships, and as such can be very difficult to cope with.

Radiotherapy

Radiotherapy is another widely used treatment that can induce fatigue. It can also have other side effects. One of the most common side effects of radiotherapy to the breast is a sunburn-like skin reaction which, although temporary, can nevertheless result in significant psychological morbidity.

Women who have radiotherapy following breast-conserving surgery face two additional psychological challenges. First, the treatment can alter the shape, texture, sensation and appearance of the breast, therefore altering the woman's perception of herself; in other words, her body image. Second, the treatment sometimes brings about changes within the breast tissue that make radiological assessment of the breast difficult in the future. This means that each time the woman has follow-up mammography; there may be uncertainty and increased anxiety about whether or not the disease has returned.

Hormone therapy

Hormonal therapies have been used to treat breast cancer for many years now and are widely considered to be both effective and well tolerated. However, they can have side effects that can be very distressing for some women. For example, menopausal symptoms such as hot flushes, night sweats, mood changes, vaginal dryness, vaginal discharge, and weight gain can all have an adverse effect on a woman's psychological wellbeing, her body image and sexuality. Once again, the nurse needs to be able to assess the psychological effect of these therapies in order to provide supportive care. The charity Breast Cancer Care has produced a factsheet on menopausal symptoms and breast cancer (Breast Cancer Care, 2006) which offers practical suggestions of how to manage such symptoms.

BREAST CANCER IN MEN

Breast cancer in the male breast is a rare disease and accounts for less than 1% of all breast cancers (Anderson *et al.*, 2004). The clinical features, treatments and prognosis are all similar to those of female breast cancers. However, there is a tendency for them to present later, perhaps due to the common misconception that breast cancer can only occur in women.

Because the vast majority of people with breast cancer are women, there is still a tendency in the literature to ignore breast cancer found in the male breast, or at best to pay it scant regard. Even the National Institute for Clinical Excellence guidelines (2002) make no attempt to deal with breast cancer in men, merely making the statement: 'This manual update deals only with services for women with breast cancer'. Although it may of course be legitimate to deal with men with breast cancer separately, nevertheless its omission from a major Government document may only serve to further isolate and marginalise those affected by it.

As well as having to face many of the same issues as women, a man may experience specific psychological ramifications of having what is widely considered to be a female disease. The effect of mastectomy on body image can be every bit as traumatic for a man as for a woman, and just as a woman might struggle with her femininity, a man may feel his masculinity is compromised by both the disease and its treatment. For example, it might be difficult for him to explain to his friends in the pub that he is experiencing menopausal symptoms as a result of hormonal therapy. If radiotherapy is recommended as part of treatment, hair will fall out in the treatment area, which may result as a visible difference if the man is hirsute. Many issues need to be considered by the nurse caring for a man with breast cancer.

BREAST CANCER DURING PREGNANCY

A diagnosis of breast cancer associated with pregnancy raises a number of difficulties and psychological issues. A delayed diagnosis is not uncommon and may contribute to some women presenting with more advanced disease (Byrd *et al.*, 1962).

The focus of attention is not only on the woman, but securing the future of her unborn child. In one study, Bandyk and Gilmore (1995) found the major concerns of pregnant women treated with chemotherapy were: 'living to see my child grow up', the cancer treatments and their effects on the baby, and the risk of not being there for other children if the pregnancy continues. The unpredictability of cancer with all of its uncertainties, plus the additional stress of treatment effects on the unborn child can be very difficult. Prior and during chemotherapy, there may be fears of potential congenital abnormalities to the unborn child.

Important issues relevant for these women are childcare, if the woman needs to return to work, and financial concerns. Some women may require further therapy following delivery, which may require time off work, and consequently a drop in income. If their job carries no maternity rights or sickness pay, financial difficulties may be on the horizon.

Many of the issues relating to pregnant women diagnosed with breast cancer may be pertinent to those young women who are diagnosed in their twenties and thirties. If unmarried, a young woman may be concerned about the possible threat to future relationships, or revealing scars and a diagnosis to a new or old partner, coupled with concerns over future sexual function and fertility.

The breast care nurse specialist and multidisciplinary team need to be involved in the woman's psychological adjustment to her diagnosis and reaction to illness, and may be key players in exploring further concerns or difficulties.

LIVING WITH UNCERTAINTY

For many people, a diagnosis of cancer is a life-changing event. Life as it existed before the diagnosis can never be the same, and a process of psychological adaptation needs to take place. Many people, during the recovery phase, express the desire for life to 'get back to normal'. This is in fact not possible, because what was 'normal' has now changed. However, with the passage of time, psychological adaptation takes place which allows the new, at first very frightening, situation to feel gradually more familiar and less frightening, and a new sort of 'normal' develops.

Long-term adaptation

Carter (1993) studied the process of adaptation that long-term survivors of breast cancer undergo, and she offers some useful insights from this research. She identified a six-phase survival process that involves interpreting the diagnosis, confronting mortality, reprioritising, coming to terms, moving on and flashing back. To begin with, informants first interpreted the meaning of the cancer diagnosis for them. Many then experienced an 'existential realisation of being mortal', which caused them to experience high levels of anxiety. In the third phase, many women made changes in their priorities concerned with their lifestyles and life goals. The author then describes what happens in the fourth phase, coming to terms:

> Informants commonly recognized that they were reconstituted or changed in some way by their cancer experience. Some informants accepted the fact of having had cancer, accepted changes that resulted from cancer, and integrated the changes into their life-styles in healthy and productive ways. (p. 358)

In the next phase, moving on, the informants proceeded with life after cancer, having placed the cancer experience into the background and the past. However, many women also revisited and relived their previous experiences in the final phase, flashing back, as a way of 'tying the past, present and future together in a meaningful context'. This work offers a useful explanation of the process that many women undergo in the months and years following the diagnosis and treatment of breast cancer.

Recurrent disease

Although many women have to learn to live with the fear of breast cancer recurrence, most will never have to face the disease again. Unfortunately, however, for a proportion of women such fears will become reality, as at least one third of patients develop recurrent disease, sometimes many years after the initial treatment (National Institute for Clinical Excellence, 2002).

When breast cancer recurs, women may go through similar psychological reactions to those they experienced the first time around. However, there may be additional emotional challenges to be faced. Tait (1996) explains that:

> It can be a shattering blow to a patient to find that all the effort, skill and courage used to cope with the primary disease has not been effective in stopping the disease spreading. (p. 21)

As a consequence, some women experience feelings of failure when the cancer returns. However, Fallowfield (1991) contends that some women actually feel relieved to discover the cancer is back, because they had always been anxious that it would, and the diagnosis allows their uncertainty to end.

PARTNER AND FAMILY REACTIONS

A diagnosis of breast cancer affects not just the person diagnosed but also the people surrounding her – her partner, children, grandchildren, parents, siblings, friends and work colleagues. (For reasons of simplicity, the term 'relative' will be used to encompass all these relationships). It is therefore not uncommon for relatives to experience their own psychological reactions. Tait (1996) points out that breast cancer can jeopardise a patient's close personal relationships, because it can be difficult for patients and relatives to talk about both the disease and their psychological reactions to it. Some of the more common reactions will now be considered.

Fear

Fear is a very common response amongst relatives, and can be related to many different issues. The most obvious is the fear that the patient will die. Children in particular may harbour this fear, and may also be afraid that their mother will be too ill to look after them.

Depending on their age, children may have great difficulty in understanding what is happening to their mother, and therefore need to be given information and support in a manner appropriate to their age. Of course, a young person aged 15 years can understand a great deal more than a 5-year-old child, but even very young children need to have explanations they can understand. They also need to feel they can voice questions and concerns, and will be listened to and answered honestly.

Relatives may have fears about the effects of treatment, and be worried that the woman will change in some way and no longer be the person they knew. They may also be very apprehensive about how she will look, for example if she experiences hair loss during chemotherapy.

Guilt

Guilt is another common emotion amongst relatives, often arising from the fact that the disease has struck the woman rather than the relative. Parents of breast cancer patients may feel that, in the natural order of things, it should be them and not their child facing a potentially life-threatening disease. This guilt may be particularly intensified if the patient is a member of a 'breast cancer family' and has inherited a faulty gene from a parent.

Children sometimes feel guilty as they wrongly believe they caused the disease by misbehaving or upsetting their mother. Partners can also feel guilty, possibly because they believe the patient is a better person than they are, and therefore less deserving of cancer. It may be particularly difficult for same-sex partners, especially in the case of screen-detected cancers where one partner is given the all clear and the other is told she has cancer.

Feeling protective

Some relatives react by being protective – sometimes over-protective. It is, of course, a natural instinct to want to protect our loved ones from pain and suffering. However, this can seem suffocating for the patient, as many do not want to be handled with kid gloves or treated any differently from usual. Some relatives even try to prevent health professionals giving the patient full information about her diagnosis and prognosis in an effort to protect her, and this can require skilful handling by the breast care team.

Although the nurse's primary concern is the patient, if she is offering truly holistic care then she will need to take the relatives into account. Brewin (1996) believes that, by helping the relatives, we help the patient, and that therefore nurses need to pay more attention to how we communicate with and support relatives.

NURSING IMPLICATIONS

So far, this chapter has considered the psychological consequences of breast cancer and its treatment for the patient. It is clear that nurses have a crucial role in helping patients to deal with their psychological reactions, and some aspects of the nurse's role will now be considered.

Communication skills

In 1996, the United Kingdom Central Council (UKCC) for Nursing, Midwifery and Health Visiting (now the Nursing and Midwifery Council) published a document entitled Guide-lines for Professional Practice, in which it is stated that:

> Communication is an essential part of good practice. [...] Effective communication relies on all our skills. Building a trusting relationship will greatly improve care and help to reduce anxiety and stress for patients and clients, their families and their carers. (UKCC, 1996, p. 15)

It is hard to imagine a more stressful and anxiety-inducing experience than being given a diagnosis of cancer; therefore good communication from the point of diagnosis onwards is of paramount importance.

However, the ability of nurses to communicate effectively with cancer patients should not be taken for granted. Some research evidence suggests that nurses specialising in cancer nursing lack appropriate skills in communication (for example Wilkinson, 1991; Faulkner and Maguire, 1994). Indeed, many cancer nurses use communication strategies (such as closed questions) that actually block effective communication (Wilkinson, 1991). The reasons for this are complex, and may include lack of training, lack of confidence, inadequate support, lack of time and pressures of workload.

In order to address some of these issues, and in response to the recommendations of the National Institute for Clinical Excellence (2002), Advanced Communication Skills training is now being promoted throughout all 34 Cancer Networks in England. The model for this training has been developed in recent years for senior health professionals working in the field of cancer, and consists of a 3-day, learner-centred course, which focuses on specific issues identified by the learner as difficult or problematic. The training involves role play, with actors taking the part of patients, and video-recording, so that participants can observe their own performance. This model has been shown to be effective in improving the communication skills of doctors and nurses (Department of Health, 2008), and large numbers of facilitators across the country are now being trained to lead Advanced Communication Skills training. There is also growing recognition of the value of communication skills training for all staff, not just those in senior positions within the field of cancer; the Department of Health's End of Life Care Strategy, for example, recommends that all health and social care staff engaged in end-of-life care should have communication skills training appropriate to their role (Department of Health, 2008).

Non-verbal communication

Northouse and Northouse (1991) describe communication in oncology settings as 'a complex and multifaceted process', and make the important point that a large part of the communication that takes place between nurses and patients is non-verbal. Begley (1996) suggests that non-verbal communication is five times more effective than verbal. It is therefore essential that nurses learn to be aware of their own body language and what messages they are tacitly sending to patients, so they can use non-verbal communication in a therapeutic way to promote the nurse–patient relationship, rather than to block effective communication.

Assessment

Faulkner and Maguire (1994) contend that, although the diagnosis and treatment of cancer is associated with a significant psychological morbidity, this often remains unrecognised and unresolved:

> Patients and relatives are reluctant to disclose any problems, while health professionals are loath to enquire actively about them. (p. 1)

Faulkner and Maguire (1994) recommend that, when assessing patients, nurses should try and keep the discussion focused on the patient's feelings, and they suggest some skills which promote disclosure, such as open directive questioning, prompting, responding to cues, using silence, and encouraging the expression of emotions. It must be acknowledged, however, that such assessments require time and privacy and, for this reason, may not be practicable in, for example, a busy surgical ward. The breast care specialist nurse can therefore play a key role in assessing the patient, and this will be discussed further below.

Giving information

It is also important for health professionals to understand that, at the time of diagnosis, a patient who is in shock is unlikely to be able to absorb very much information. For this reason, many women need to go over the information several times, and some experts advocate the practice of tape-recording the initial consultation so that the patient can take the tape home and reconsider the information in the days following the diagnosis (Hogbin *et al.*, 1992).

The importance of written information is also widely acknowledged, and it is now viewed as an essential part of good practice to give the patient written information suited to her needs at each part of the treatment process. The National Institute for Clinical Excellence guidelines (2002) state that:

> At every stage, patients should be offered clear, objective, full and prompt information in both verbal and written form. Each patient should receive information relevant to her case about the disease, diagnostic procedures, treatment options and effectiveness. The amount and timing of the information should take each patient's preferences into account. (p. 26)

The nurse therefore needs to be skilful in assessing the patient in order to ascertain her information needs.

Common assumptions about psychological reactions

The literature abounds with assumptions about how women react to a diagnosis of breast cancer. For example, Love (2000) states that:

> The first thing a woman thinks of when diagnosed with breast cancer is: 'Will I die?' This is quickly followed by 'Will I have to lose my breast?' (p. 347)

Whilst not denying that many women may indeed experience such fears, it is dangerous to assume that all women will react this way. Not all patients will be distressed at losing their breast; some will be hugely relieved, as they will be much more concerned about having cancer (Fallowfield *et al.*, 1990).

Others may focus on what some might regard as more trivial concerns. For instance, a woman who wears dentures may be very concerned about having to remove them in order to undergo surgery, because of the alteration this makes to her facial appearance; this may be the body-image issue she focuses on at that time. It is therefore very important that nurses do not make assumptions about patients' psychological reactions to breast cancer.

It should also be pointed out that, despite the literature exhorting nurses to explore the feelings of cancer patients (Faulkner and Maguire 1994), not every patient will want to share her deepest feelings with relative strangers when diagnosed. Even if a patient does experience feelings of fear about dying or losing a breast, this may not be what she chooses to divulge. Not all patients will want to unburden themselves emotionally; some will want to cope privately, or within their own support network. The challenge for nurses is to assess each patient on an individual basis without prejudice, and then endeavour to meet her needs.

Other resources

It is important for nurses to be aware of other resources that are available both locally and nationally to support patients with breast cancer. Many patients derive benefit from the support of others who have been through the experience of breast cancer and, for this reason, many breast cancer support groups exist. Of course, some patients prefer not to participate in such groups; nevertheless, all patients should be informed about what is available to them and how to participate if they so wish.

In recent years, there has also been a huge increase in the number and variety of complementary therapies that are available (Barnett, 2002), many of which can play a part in the psychological support of people with breast cancer and their families. However, the array of complementary therapies can be quite bewildering for patients, and nurses can help by knowing what is available in their locality and how to access it.

Caring for the carers

Since the advent of primary nursing in the 1980s, nurses have been encouraged to develop relationships with patients in order to enhance care and reduce the patient's fear and anxiety (Pearson, 1988; Salvage, 1990; Wright, 1994). Indeed, there is a large body of literature on caring, which extols the virtues of interpersonal relationships between nurses and patients. Watson (1985), for example, believes that through interpersonal relationships nurses can help patients achieve a higher degree of harmony within the mind, body and soul.

Some writers, however, sound a note of caution. Van Hooft (1987) believes that it is not possible for nurses to sustain this level of caring:

> If the nurse is to be responsible for the growth in a holistic sense of the client as a total person, or if the nurse has to open with every client a depth of communication that allows for the sharing of the most intimate levels of existence, then the practical professional life of that nurse will become impossible. And this is not just because there will not be enough time; it's just not going to be psychologically possible either. (p. 33)

In other words, forming relationships with patients can have negative consequences for nurses. Caring can be stressful; indeed, Benner and Wrubel (1989), despite being strong advocates of caring, acknowledge that it is inevitably stressful. The National Institute for Clinical Excellence guidelines (2002) also warn that:

> Health care workers may come to treat patients in detached or even dehumanised ways as a way of reducing their own emotional stress. (p. 28)

Each nurse therefore needs to be aware of how she is affected psychologically by caring and forming relationships with patients. Turner (1999) suggests that nurses have to go through a process of learning how to manage their involvement if they are to become proficient at establishing and sustaining relationships with cancer patients. They also require both educational and emotional support if they are to learn how to manage their involvement in a positive and constructive way (Turner, 2001). It is therefore vitally important that adequate support is available to nurses, through education, guided reflection, mentorship and clinical supervision. The breast care nurse also has a part to play in the provision of support for less experienced staff.

Role of the specialist breast care nurse

The breast care nurse is now viewed as an essential member of the breast team, and therefore every woman with breast cancer should have access to a breast care nurse who has appropriate post-registration qualifications and is trained in counselling and communication (National Institute for Clinical Excellence, 2002).

Traditionally, the primary focus of the role has been to provide support and information to breast cancer patients and their families. Faulkner and Maguire (1994) describe the competencies they expect of specialist nurses. These include the ability to identify patients with anxiety states, depressive illness, body-image problems, sexual difficulties or interpersonal problems. They also suggest that breast care nurses:

> ... should be aware of signs of over-involvement or over-identification with patients, and be familiar with the concepts of transference and counter-transference. They should be comfortable with empowering patients rather than trying to act for them. They should be encouraged to continue their education, evolve their own working methods, and accept ongoing supervision, as well as to scrutinize their time-management. (p. 183)

The role is therefore multi-faceted and complex. In addition, in recent years, roles have started to expand and develop in diverse ways in different breast units across the UK, and are continuing to do so. For example, some breast care nurses now hold their own clinics for triple assessment, breast cancer follow-ups, or family history risk assessment; clinics which were once the domain of the medical staff.

At the same time as focusing on patients, breast care nurses also have a key role in educating and supporting other staff. In the past, specialist nurses have sometimes been accused of undermining other nurses, because they assume all the responsibility for psychological care of patients, leaving other nurses in both the hospital and the community feeling they are not allowed to contribute as much as they would like (Faulkner and Maguire, 1994). Alternatively, other nurses may choose to leave psychological care in the province of the specialist nurse, because it prevents them from having to take on this responsibility. However, it is more beneficial for both patients and staff if part of the specialist nurse's role is to support other staff in developing self-awareness, confidence and communication skills.

CONCLUSION

With the incidence of breast cancer rising to one in nine (National Institute for Clinical Excellence, 2002), it is safe to assume that most nurses will care for women with this disease at some point in their career. It is therefore incumbent upon all nurses to acquire sufficient knowledge of the psychological issues faced by these patients, together with the necessary skills of building therapeutic relationships, in order to improve the quality of the care they can offer.

REFERENCES

Al Ghazal S, Sully L, Fallowfield L and Blamey R (2000) The psychological impact of immediate rather than delayed breast reconstruction. *European Journal of Surgical Oncology* 26: 17–19.
Anderson WF, Althuis MD, Brinton LA and Devesa SS (2004) Is male breast cancer similar or different than female breast cancer? *Breast Cancer Research and Treatment* 83: 77–86.
Avis NE, Crawford S and Manuel J (2004) Psychosocial problems among younger women with breast cancer. *Psycho-Oncology* 13: 295–308.
Avis NE, Crawford S and Manuel J (2005) Quality of life among younger women with breast cancer. *Journal of Clinical Oncology* 23: 15, 3322–3330.
Bandyk EA and Gilmore MA (1995) Perceived concerns of pregnant women with breast cancer treated with chemotherapy. *Oncology Nursing Forum* 22: 975–977.
Barnett H (2002) *The Which? Guide to Complementary Therapies.* London: Which? Books.

Beaumont J (2007) Breast cancer: what are the issues for young women? *Cancer Nursing Practice* 6(9): 36–39.

Begley CM (1996) Triangulation of communication skills in qualitative research instruments. *Journal of Advanced Nursing* 24: 688–693.

Benner P and Wrubel J (1989) *The Primacy of Caring: Stress and Coping in Health and Illness.* California: Addison-Wesley Publishing Company.

Breast Cancer Care (2006) *Menopausal Symptoms and Breast Cancer.* Available: http://www.breastcancercare.org.uk/upload/pdf/Menopausal_symptoms_factsheet_BCC18.pdf

Brewin T (1996) *Relating to the Relatives: Breaking Bad News, Communication and Support.* Oxford: Radcliffe Medical Press Ltd.

Byrd BF, Bayer DS, Robertson JC and Stephens SE (1962) Treatment for breast tumors associated with pregnancy and lactation. *Annals of Surgery* 155: 940–947.

Carter BJ (1993) Long-term survivors of breast cancer. A qualitative descriptive study. *Cancer Nursing* 16(5): 354–361.

Department of Health (1996) *Guidance for Purchasers: Improving Outcomes in Breast Cancer: The Manual.* London: National Health Service Executive.

Department of Health (2008) *End of Life Care Strategy: Promoting High Quality Care for All Adults at the End of Life.* London: Department of Health.

Dixon M and Sainsbury R (1998) *Handbook of Diseases of the Breast,* 2nd edn. London: Churchill Livingstone.

Fallowfield L (1991) *Breast Cancer.* London: Routledge.

Fallowfield LJ (1986) Effects of breast conservation on psychological morbidity associated with diagnosis and treatment of early breast cancer. *British Medical Journal* 293: 1331–1334.

Fallowfield LJ, Hall A, Maguire GP and Baum M (1990) Psychological outcomes of different treatment policies in women with early breast cancer outside a clinical trial. *British Medical Journal* 301: 575–580.

Faulkner A and Maguire P (1994) *Talking to Cancer Patients and their Relatives.* Oxford: Oxford University Press.

Fobair P, Stewart SL, Chang S, D'Onofrio C, Banks PJ and Bloom JR (2006) Body image and sexual problems in young women with breast cancer. *Psycho-Oncology* 15: 579–594.

Friedman LC, Kalidas M, Elledge R *et al.* (2006) Optimism, social support and psychological functioning among women with breast cancer. *Psycho-Oncology* 15: 595–603.

Ganz PA, Desmond KA, Leedham B, Rowland JH, Meyerowitz BT and Belin TR (2002) Quality of life in long-term, disease-free survivors of breast cancer: A follow-up study. *Journal of the National Cancer Institute* 94: 39–49.

Haber S (Ed) (1997) *Breast Cancer. A Psychological Treatment Manual.* London: Free Association Books Ltd.

Harcourt D, Rumsey N and Ambler N (1999) Same-day diagnosis of symptomatic breast problems: psychological impact and coping strategies. *Psychology Health and Medicine* 143: 57–71.

Helgeston VS, Snyder P and Seltman H (2004) Psychological and physical adjustment to breast cancer over 4 years: identifying distinct trajectories of change. *Health Psychology* 23: 3–15.

Hogbin B, Jenkins VA and Parkin JA (1992) Remembering 'bad news' consultations. *Psycho-oncology* 1: 147–154.

Kravitz RL and Melnikow J (2001) Engaging patients in medical decision making. *British Medical Journal* 323(7313): 584–585.

Kubler-Ross E (1978) *On Death and Dying.* New York: Macmillan.

Love S (2000) *Dr. Susan Love's Breast Book.* Massachusetts: Perseus Publishing.

Lovejoy NC, Matteis M and Lillis P (2000) Cancer-related depression: part 1 – neurologic alterations and cognitive-behavioral therapy. *Oncology Nursing Forum,* 27(4): 667–678.

Maguire P (2000) Psychological aspects. In: M Dixon (ed) *ABC of Breast Diseases.* London: BMJ Books.

Maguire P and Faulkner A (1988a) How to do it: improve the counselling skills of doctors and nurses in cancer care. *British Medical Journal* 297: 847–849.

Maguire P and Faulkner A (1988b) How to do it: communicate with cancer patients: 1. Handling bad news and difficult questions. *British Medical Journal* 297: 907–909.

McCarthy P and Loren JA (eds) (1997) *Breast Cancer? Let Me Check My Schedule!* Oxford: Westview Press.

National Comprehensive Cancer Network (2003) Distress management clinical practice guidelines. *Journal of National Comprehensive Cancer Network* 1: 344–374.

National Health Service Executive (1998) *Health Service Circular. Breast Cancer Waiting Times – Achieving the Two Week Wait Target*. London: National Health Service Executive.

National Institute for Clinical Excellence (2002) *Guidance on Cancer Services: Improving Outcomes in Breast Cancer: Manual Update*. London: National Institute for Clinical Excellence.

Northouse LL and Northouse PG (1991) Interpersonal communication systems. In: SB Baird, R McCorkle and M Grant (eds) *Cancer Nursing: A Comprehensive Textbook*. Philadelphia: WB Saunders Company.

Parkes CM and Weiss RS (1983) *Recovery from Bereavement*. New York: Basic Books.

Partridge AH, Gelber S, Peppercorn J *et al.* (2004) Web based survey of fertility issues in young women with breast cancer. *Journal of Clinical Oncology* 22(20): 4174–4183.

Pearson A (ed) (1988) *Primary Nursing: Nursing in the Burford and Oxford Nursing Development Units*. London: Croom Helm Ltd.

Picardie R (1998) *Before I say Goodbye*. London: Penguin Books.

Richardson A (1995a) Fatigue in cancer patients: a review of the literature. *European Journal of Cancer Care* 4(1): 20–32.

Richardson A (1995b) The pattern of fatigue in patients receiving chemotherapy. In: A Richardson and J Wilson-Barnett (eds) *Nursing Research in Cancer Care*. London: Scutari Press.

Salter M (1997) *Altered Body Image: The Nurse's Role*, 2nd edn. London: Bailliere Tindall.

Salvage J (1990) The Theory and Practice of the 'New Nursing.' *Nursing Times* 86(4): 42–45.

Tait A (1996) Psychological aspects of breast cancer. In: S Denton (ed) *Breast Cancer Nursing*. London: Chapman and Hall.

Tait A and Wing M (1997) Whole or partial breast loss and body image. In: M Slater (ed) *Altered Body Image: The Nurse's Role*, 2nd edn. London: Bailliere Tindall.

Turner JM (2001) *Managing Involvement: A Grounded Theory of Nurses' Personal Involvement in Relationships with Cancer Patients*. Unpublished PhD thesis; University of London.

Turner M (1999) Involvement or over-involvement? Using grounded theory to explore the complexities of nurse–patient relationships. *European Journal of Oncology Nursing* 3(3): 153–160.

United Kingdom Central Council for Nursing, Midwifery and Health Visiting (1996) *Guidelines for Professional Practice*. London: UKCC.

Vachon M (2006) Psychological distress and coping after cancer treatment. *Advanced Journal of Nursing* 106(3): 26–31.

Van Hooft S (1987) Caring and professional commitment. *The Australian Journal of Advanced Nursing* 4(4): 29–38.

Veronesi U, Paganelli G, Viale G *et al.* (2003) A randomized comparison of sentinel-node biopsy with routine axillary dissection in breast cancer. *The New England Journal of Medicine* 349: 546–553.

Watson J (1985) *Nursing: Human Science and Human Care: A Theory of Nursing*. New York: National League of Nursing Press.

Wilkinson SM (1991) Factors which influence how nurses communicate with cancer patients. *Journal of Advanced Nursing* 16: 677–688.

Woloski-Wruble A and Kadmon I (2002) Breast cancer – reactions of Israeli men to their wives' diagnoses. *European Journal of Oncology Nursing* 6: 93–99.

Wright SG (1994) *My Patient – My Nurse: The Practice of Primary Nursing*, 2nd edn. London: Scutari Press.

16 Survivorship Issues

Carmel Sheppard

INTRODUCTION

Over the past 2 years, there has been a growing interest in what is meant by the term survivorship. This chapter explores the meaning of survivorship and the continued journey that many patients face despite the successful completion of their initial treatment. The psychological impact for both the patients and their family is discussed together with the long-term side effects of treatments. Anonymous case illustrations are used to provide the reader with a greater understanding of the long-term impact of the disease. The potential for screening and examples of patient enquiry to elicit difficulties relating to survivorship are considered.

BACKGROUND

Over the past 30 years, there have been significant improvements in relation to the diagnostic process of breast cancer and subsequent treatments. Whilst mortality rates from breast cancer within the UK remain high in comparison to other European countries, mortality rates have fallen dramatically since 1989 when 15 625 women died from the disease compared with 12 319 in 2006 (Cancer Research UK, 2008). A number have factors have contributed to this fall. The introduction of the breast screening programme has led to earlier diagnosis and a subsequent increase in breast awareness within the general population (NHSBSP, 2002). The development of endocrine therapy in the early 1970s, the introduction of tamoxifen and, more recently, the increased use of aromatase inhibitors, improvements in chemotherapy, improved access to radiotherapy and treatment per se have all contributed to increased survival. Rapid access to diagnostic services (Health Service Circular, 1999), clinical guidelines (NICE, 2002; BASO, 2005) and multidisciplinary teams have also contributed to minimising the risk of recurrence through improvements in care generally.

Whilst the biomedical agenda of breast cancer care has dominated the focus of research in improving disease-free survival, less attention has been paid to the impact of the continued journey that many patients face following completion of treatment. More recently, parallels have been drawn between cancer and chronic illness, with greater cognisance of

Breast Cancer Nursing Care and Management, Second Edition, Edited by Victoria Harmer
© 2011 by Blackwell Publishing Ltd.

the subsequent life difficulties that many women face as a result of their past diagnosis (Corner, 2008). It is encouraging to see that, although there remains a dearth of literature relating to survivorship, there now appears to be an emerging recognition and growing body of knowledge in this area. Indeed, the recent *Cancer Reform Strategy* (Department of Health, 2007) pays particular attention to the longitudinal pathway for cancer patients, highlighting the need for good continuity of care, access for patients at key points throughout their journey, ongoing psychological support, and the recognition of the wider impact such as follow-up needs, potential loss of income and financial impact and discrimination in the work place as well as the long-term impact of treatment.

The *Cancer Reform Strategy* also sets out a future plan to work in collaboration with Macmillan Cancer Relief and other cancer charities to develop cancer-survivorship initiatives working towards the development of future policies. The development of such policies will hopefully be inclusive of the diversity of needs for patients, given that each patient will have her own unique experience of what it is to be diagnosed with breast cancer, to undergo treatment and subsequently to begin a period of adjustment.

MEANING OF SURVIVORSHIP

Peck (2008) describes survivors as those who have 'faced their mortality and altered their future memories as well as their self-identities in response to a life-altering event' (p 100). Certainly, this does have some resonance in clinical practice. Many of us go through life with carefully crafted life plans or dreams for our future which may include planning for retirement, enjoying new hobbies, watching grandchildren grow etc. In reality, we know that there are no certainties in terms of life expectation, yet most of us tend to ignore the 'what ifs' and exist in blissful ignorance until faced with a threat to these plans. Hence life-threatening illness has the potential to create an enormous chasm when our personal life expectations and long-term horizons are suddenly threatened. In relation to Peck's definition (2008), it is not uncommon in practice to hear that patients are feeling confused regarding personal identify, which can be caused by a number of factors such as loss of role within the family, loss of job, earnings, as well the impact of altered body image and loss of femininity etc. Whilst Peck's (2008) definition appears to encapsulate a number of survival factors, the process of adaptation can be extremely painful emotionally. Whilst some women may adapt relatively easily and may derive positive outcomes, such as redefining life values and taking the opportunities to refocus their lives, others will find themselves either exhausted trying to fill their day to avoid thinking about the future (Case study 16.1), or feel completely stuck, unable to accept the need to re-define the future or feeling too scared to formulate new plans for fear of further loss if their cancer returns.

Survivors are sometimes described as having won the battle or having conquered the disease in some way. Leigh (2008) identifies the beginning of the 'war on cancer', whilst Kaiser (2008) suggests that there is a shift from the historical stigma, secrecy and shamefulness associated with breast cancer towards almost honoring those who are thought to have beaten or survived breast cancer; indeed activities such as the annual moonwalk, breast cancer awareness month and pink ribbons to name but a few appear to bear testimony to this. These fund-raising activities can also offer a new focus and challenge to women who have suffered breast cancer and also to those around them who have been affected by it in some way. Engagement may create feelings of general wellbeing in the knowledge that

> **Case study 16.1   Helen**
>
> Helen was diagnosed aged 28 years. She was married and had an 18-month-old son. Helen underwent a wide local excision, chemotherapy (completing only five cycles owing to side effects) and radiotherapy. During her chemotherapy, Helen continued to work on the days she could. Her son was cared for during the day whilst she worked, but she tried to keep normality through the maintenance of her role as mother and wife. Helen was the type of person who never showed emotion and was determined not to let her cancer affect her ability to care for her son. Seven years later, Helen suddenly became tearful and came for counselling. It became apparent that Helen had maintained an outer façade, had exhausted herself with work and had avoided ever thinking about the possibility of death. Triggered by the death of a well-known celebrity, Helen had begun to reflect on her prior experience and, in particular, the fact that she had not completed her sixth cycle of chemotherapy. Helen was convinced that it would not be long before her 'luck ran out' and her cancer returned, and her memories of chemotherapy and the possibility of recurrence became overwhelming, and she subsequently contacted her breast care nurse.

they are not only contributing to the future treatment of breast cancer, but that they are also helping others. Furthermore, engagement in external activities can offer a distraction from their own personal journey, and thus may be argued to have therapeutic benefits through the investment in new things (Worden, 1982). Nevertheless, for others, the constant media attention means that the reality of the disease and potential for recurrence is never too distant from their thoughts.

Although a small qualitative study, Breaden (1997) describes the experiences of six women. Themes such as the recurrent threat of cancer never being far from their mind, questioning the future, feeling lucky to be alive and not wanting to feel ungrateful were all described. One of the questions raised here is whether such feelings lead to sub-optimal life choices, e.g. less rewarding jobs or even the extreme of accepting a new partner that they otherwise would not have considered because they feel they should be grateful for what they have? In practice, may patients tell us that they feel less attractive, perceive themselves to have lower self-worth, feel a loss of self-confidence together with weakness and vulnerability. It is not uncommon, in practice, to hear the frustrations of some women finding it difficult to move on and to adopt a survivor's view, feeling guilty and sometimes angry that others can adapt so well, feeling pressure from friends and family to move on, and feeling a need to almost hide their own emotional labour to protect others (McKenzie and Crouch, 2004, cited Corner, 2008). Naturally, some people may cope through denial of their emotions, which can be used to protect us from painful thoughts and keep us from being too vulnerable and exposed. Equally, long-term suppression of feelings may lead to further disturbance, family disruption, a break down in communications and, ultimately, the patient feeling exhausted in an attempt to maintain this exterior coping façade and feeling isolated within her own personal inner conflicts (Freud, 1948).

Mullan (1985, cited Thewes *et al.*, 2004) identifies three distinct phases of survival. The first phase, the acute phase where the patient is newly diagnosed, focused on surviving aggressive treatments and dealing with the devastating knowledge of potential death. The second stage is characterised as the extended phase, where the patient reaches the end of formal treatment and goes into remission, but nevertheless continues to encounter the fears of recurrence. The final stage is identified as the permanent survival stage, which is when sufficient time has elapsed. Although we can perhaps all identify patients we have known clearly in these phases, and a number of authors (Kubler-Ross, 1973; Parkes, 1993) have tried to identify distinct phases of grief, we also need to remember that grief processes vary considerably. Individuals do not always follow a clear pathway towards recovery, but frequently fluctuate between these phases depending on a number of external factors (Mast 1998; Gil et al., 2004). The constant media attention paid to breast cancer is a steady reminder of the number of people who die from breast cancer. The death of close friends or colleagues may also create a wave of emotional instability with a reminder of their own mortality. Although the majority of us dismiss general aches and pains and treat coughs and colds as a mild interruption to our everyday lives, for those having experienced a cancer diagnosis, even minor ailments will naturally trigger emotions about their cancer, the potential for recurrence and threat to life.

PSYCHOLOGICAL RESPONSES

In relation to psychological morbidity, there are numerous studies suggesting a prevalence rate of anxiety and depression of between 25–50% within the first 2 years (Fallowfield et al., 1990; Fallowfield and Hall, 1991; Hall et al., 1996). However, many studies have demonstrated significant improvement in both physical and psychological morbidity within 2 years of diagnosis (Maguire, 1994; Ganz et al., 1996; Luker et al., 1995).

Ganz et al. (2002) studied the quality-of-life effects for 817 patients over a 10-year period and, overall, reported minimal changes over time in relation to physical, emotional and social wellbeing, although past chemotherapy was a statistically significant predictor of poorer quality of life many years after. Given that there is little change in psychological recovery beyond the first 2 years, many have questioned the need for ongoing clinical follow-up for women (NICE, 2002). Indeed, there is little evidence to show that follow-up makes a difference at all to overall survival (Schapira and Urban, 1991; Rosselli Dell Turco et al., 1994; Donnely et al., 2001). These studies, however, have mainly focused on benefits of follow-up in relation to disease-free survival, rather than the benefits in terms of survivorship and adaptation, and there remains a lack of evidence that it improves the quality of remaining life. Whilst some women will adapt well, there will inevitably be a number of women who do have difficulty in adjustment and who will need ongoing support. The question is how we identify these patients and ensure that support is available to those that need it and target psychological care resources?

In a 10-year cohort study examining the emotional response of 578 women, both helplessness and hopelessness at baseline was identified as a correlate to increased later risk of recurrence (Watson et al., 2005). Epping-Jordan et al. (1999) explored the different background and dispositional factors that may predict anxiety and depression post-diagnosis in a study of 80 women with breast cancer. Their findings suggest that more optimistic women experienced lower levels of distress, whilst women who were more pessimistic used more emotion-focused disengagement coping, which included self-criticism and social withdrawal leading to increased emotional distress at 3 and 6 months. These findings may be considered similar to those of Norsati et al. (2002) and Declerck et al. (2002) in that social relationships, external support and engagement in positive thoughts appear consistently important. A study by Gallagher *et al.* (2002) involving 195 women at 2 and 6 months post-diagnosis demonstrated lower anxiety and depression scores in women who were confident with family support. These women also had a lower appraisal of further threat and greater confidence in the ability to cope. Higher grade tumours, higher levels of worry about the cancer and a woman's judgement that she needed additional support from a counsellor, as well as a prior psychiatric history, were associated with poorer psychological function and higher 6-month General Health Questionnaire (GHQ) scores.

These studies suggest that the early identification and assessment of supportive needs are fundamental in the long-term care of breast cancer survivors, and thus should be seen as a major role for breast care nursing. One of the potential benefits of the breast care nursing role is the ability to develop and maintain a long-term relationship with the patient over time. Naturally, as with any relationship, the ability to form a meaningful relationship is dependent on good communication skills as well as on the opportunity to form this relationship through several contacts. Although much of the breast care nursing role typically appears to focus around the diagnostic phase of illness, subsequent contacts at significant milestones throughout treatment and recovery should be considered important. Understanding the patient's supportive network and role within the family is essential, as is the need for further assessment of this with a recognition that this may change over time. For some patients, it can be helpful to get the patient to draw diagrammatically the relationships and the flow of support within their family and social circle, so that this not only becomes visible to them (which in-itself might be helpful) but can form the basis of discussion and ways to identify other possibilities of support (Fig. 16.1).

Initial screening and assessment will help to form the basis of this relationship and to negotiate future needs for information, advice, and psychological support; however, other significant points throughout the patient journey may be just as important. For example, many patients find the transition from completion of treatment to routine follow-up care a difficult time. This is not surprising since, during active treatment such as radiotherapy or chemotherapy, patients have regular access to a number of health-care professionals. Some patients develop a sense of trust and are able to hand over responsibility for care. Consequently, when this stops, the patient may feel isolated and unsupported and may need to talk through her feelings to gain some reassurance. Similarly, when patients are finally discharged, although there may be some element of celebration, to the contrary some patients may feel a sense of panic facing an unknown future alone. Importantly, we also need to avoid creating the potential for dependency. Equally, continued follow-up for the patient may be interpreted as a need to monitor illness and may again serve as a constant reminder of the threat of recurrence.

Given that clinical follow-up makes no difference to overall survival, an alternative model of follow-up would be to change the ethos and focus of the follow-up review from clinical examination to a educational process of managing side effects and other consequences of the disease as well as introducing survival techniques, e.g. techniques to encourage positive thinking, managing emotion, moving from long-term to short-term horizon etc. Ganz and Hahn (2008) describe a handing over of care from oncologist to experts in health and wellness and survivorship and providing survivorship care plans. Providing greater access to written and video information regarding survivorship issues and coping may also help adaptation (Mandelblatt *et al.*, 2008). Greater use of help-lines and a move towards individualised patient response services rather than the traditional scheduled approach may also be both more efficient and cost effective (Sheppard, 2008).

Directional flow of support

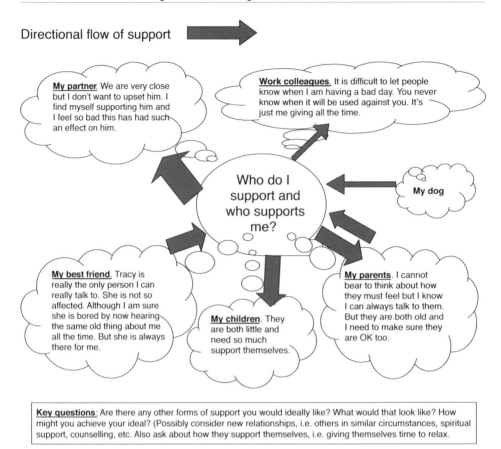

Fig. 16.1 The flow of support.

LONG-TERM TREATMENT EFFECTS

As well as the potential for ongoing fear, the physical effects of past treatment can equally have a long-lasting effect and subsequently can require ongoing support and advice from the breast care nurse over a protracted period of time. It is vital that the breast care nurse is not only aware of the side effects but can also, where possible, ameliorate the impact through information-giving, managing expectations, and intervention and adaptation advice. Ganz and Hahn (2008) provide an overview of such effects. Examples include effects of surgery such as body-image issues from both mastectomy and wide excision, difficulties with prosthesis and clothing, limitations of shoulder movements, chronic pain (Jung, 2003), lymphoedema, long-term issues relating to reconstruction from the donor site as well as actual reconstructed breast itself, and long-term potential problems with muscle transfer and implants etc.

Radiotherapy may have latent effects, such as swelling to the breast and arm due to fibrosis, potential damage to the ribs, chest wall, coronary arteries (Hooning *et al.*, 2007), myocardium, lung tissue and brachial plexus. Chemotherapy can result in infertility, neuropathy, menopausal symptoms, sexual dysfunction (Stead, 2003) and long-term decline in heart function (Abu-Khalaf *et al.*, 2007). Endocrine treatment typically extends over a 5-year period and continues to have ongoing side effects such as menopausal symptoms, particularly hot flushes, which can have the effect of sleepless nights, social embarrassment and weight gain, which may lead some patients to stop or not adhere to their medication (Atkins and Fallowfield, 2006). Further problems such as arthralgia and a potential increased risk of osteoporosis, endometrial cancers and thrombosis all add to the ongoing difficulties faced by patients trying to regain some normality (Sheppard, 2008).

FAMILY RESPONSE

As identified earlier, social support is of significant importance in psychological recovery, and therefore the breast care nurse should seek to understand the family context within the patient assessment. Exploration of the family structure and meaning of cancer and the experience within the family will provide the opportunity to help the patient understand her own family responses. In practice, we frequently hear the frustration of patients who believe that other family members just don't care any more, reporting that life has just gone back to normal within the family, leaving the patient to feel isolated in her grief.

Alternatively, for some patients, the family response can be completely the opposite, with the patients wanting to return to normal but feeling suffocated with family members still cosseting them. As breast care nurses, we must therefore also consider extending support to family members as well as the patients. Robinson *et al.* (2005) identify different types of family response.

- Families who focus on returning to life as it was before, with family members making frequent reference to wanting to get 'past it and put it all behind'. Frustration occurs when the patient or others want to go back over it and there is reluctance on the part of the patient to accept that life for the future is life with a past history of cancer.
- Families who allow the cancer to dominate their new world. This focus sometimes results in anticipatory loss, which subsequently causes families to pull apart in the anticipation of death (Case study 16.2).

Those families who did well appear to have a balanced view, whereby the possibility of death was not the sole focus. The authors capture the essence of the balanced world view in the following quote: *'prepare as if this is your last day on earth, live as if you are going to live forever'* (p 142). Encouraging openness within the family can help family members to develop an understanding of each other's response and to modify frustration when others within the family are not in the same phase or place in relation to their own grief.

Exploring the effects on children is also vitality important. Zahlis (2001) identified that as many as 81% of school-age children feared their mother was going to die from early-stage breast cancer. There is also some evidence that future parenting may also be affected, with some mothers distancing themselves in preparation for possible loss, or feeling that they are not as good a mother as those who are not ill (Lewis, 2006). Little work has been undertaken regarding education of children. and therefore this should be considered.

Case study 16.2   Rita

Rita is 54 years old, married and has an autistic child aged 16 years. Rita completed her chemotherapy treatment 4 months ago, having been diagnosed 1 year ago. She has found it increasingly difficult to cope and described herself as constantly emotional. She feels very angry with her husband, with the relationship between them becoming more strained. Exploring the process within the family and Rita's feelings about the future, it became apparent that, although Rita appeared superficially to have a balanced view of the future, her need to make plans for her daughter's future had become a constant anxiety. Rita had always assumed that she would be there for her daughter, knowing that her daughter would never be totally independent from the family home.

Rita had become acutely aware of the possibility that she may not be there in the future and had subsequently begun to disengage from her caring role, which subsequently led to her daughter to exhibit behavioural problems. Rita felt angry that her husband left it all up to her, and he was not helping, although naturally he had to work to maintain financial stability for the family. Her husband Jack was a senior manager and generally left the caring role to Rita. Jack was focused on getting family life back to normal and could not understand why Rita had suddenly become tearful, as things were just getting back to normal, as he saw it. The frustration between them had grown due to the fact that both of them had never been able to articulate their fears for the future of their daughter. Jack wanted to protect his wife and consequently avoided discussion regarding a less favourable outcome, and Rita equally wanted to protect Jack. Having the opportunity to explore her feelings with the breast care nurse enabled Rita to articulate these feelings in a safe environment and thus to understand what was happening in her relationship. Through this understanding, Rita was then able to explore the effects of a lack in communication and to seek ways to open these channels.

FINANCIAL AND WORK ISSUES

Further difficulties sometimes faced by women during rehabilitation are linked to issues relating in some way to actual or perceived discrimination. Difficulties in getting holiday insurance and increased loading of life-assurance policies not only increase the financial burden, but also pose as a constant reminder. Careers and future work may also be affected. To lose a job may further compound a feeling of loss of identity and role and result in a feeling of worthlessness and rejection. Whilst some patients may take the opportunity to change careers, retrain and invest in something new for the future to aid rehabilitation, others may feel forced financially to continue working despite ongoing struggles for fear of job loss or discrimination in terms of future career prospects. Although most patients return to work, approximately 20% report ongoing limitations in the ability to work up to 5 years post-diagnosis (Farley Short and Vargo, 2006).

In a survey of 378 women with breast cancer, 41% of women reported that their diagnosis had altered their priorities and ambitions at work, 25% reported a career change, 12% retired early, 5.2% felt afraid to change jobs in case of a recurrence, and 3% of women perceived discrimination at work (Steward et al., 2001). In the current climate of increasing unemployment and instability of jobs, this naturally puts further pressure on women to

> **Case study 16.3   Jane**
>
> Jane is 45 years old and is a single parent. She has two daughters aged 11 and 13 years. Jane struggles financially and, because of this, she continued to work throughout her chemotherapy. Her chemotherapy finished 4 months ago, but she still feels thoroughly exhausted. She feels a constant need to prove herself at work as she works in a highly competitive sales role, with a constant threat of redundancy and, because of this, Jane decided against considering breast reconstruction to minimise the time needed away from work. She gets home from work at 5 pm, begins to make dinner, encourages the children to do their homework and tries to help them, whilst at the same time clearing up. She feels desperately alone; she would love a new relationship but feels her diagnosis, mastectomy, and weight gain would prohibit any future relationship. She tries to convince others she is coping, but she is not sleeping owing to anxiety. She is frightened for her children and believes it will only be a short time before her cancer returns. She never has any time to just enjoy the children, but wants to try to build happy memories for them rather than memories of their mum being ill. She cannot afford any days out with them. The breast care nurse facilitated the opportunity for Jane to explore and consider other life opportunities, and also encouraged Jane to engage family members in offering help.
>
> A charitable grant enabled the family to have a holiday together to build some happy memories and to take some time out to rest and make plans for the future. A grant also helped to pay for some of the household bills. For the future, Jane decided to invest in something new and, having had some time away, she decided to complete her lifelong career plan. An educational bursary enabled her to undertake a teacher training course, with a placement in a local school.

attempt to return to work early and potentially to minimise the effects that are visible to others (Case study 16.3). Breast care nurses need to be aware of how to direct patients to seek advice. Information such as advice regarding statutory sick pay, incapacity benefit and disability allowance, as well as information for employers, is available from Macmillan Cancer Relief (http://www.macmillan.org.uk).

ASSESSING THE OVERALL IMPACT OF DISEASE

Understanding the needs of patients is the first step in being able to offer support and help. If we consider Maslow's theory (Fig. 16.2) (1943), he describes each of us as having a core pyramid of hierarchical needs in order to become fully functioning. Any interruption of this pyramid prevents us from achieving our full potential and thus leads to dysfunction. If we consider our patients in relation to the pyramid of needs, it is not surprising then that some patients do find it difficult to regain normality and to become fully functioning, as several layers of the pyramid become challenged. Physiological functioning may be affected due to treatment side effects. Understandably, some patients will also feel vulnerable and helpless, leading to potential loss of safety. Love, belonging and self-esteem may become threatened due to feelings of isolation and altered body image etc.

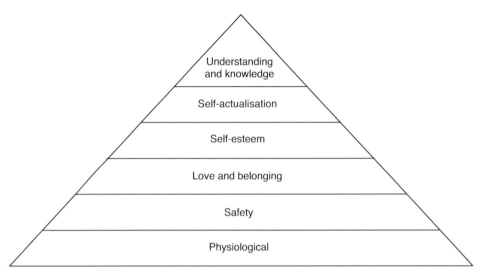

Fig. 16.2 Maslow's Hierarchy of Needs, originally published in *Psychological Review* (1943) 50 (4): 370–396.

Whilst a number of patients are capable of articulating their feelings, others may find this more difficult. Assessment tools to measure quality of life and psychiatric morbidity are particularly useful to identify those who otherwise would suffer in silence, and can be used to facilitate further exploration and discussion. Tools such as the Hospital Anxiety and Depression Scale (Zigmond and Snaith, 1983) and GHQ (Goldberg and Williams, 1988) can help the nurse to identify psychiatric morbidity, whilst quality-of-life tools such as the Functional Assessment of Cancer Therapy (Cella *et al.*, 1993), FACT-B (Brady *et al.*, 1997) and FACT endocrine subscale (Fallowfield *et al.*, 1999), or EORTC (Aaronson *et al.*, 1993) measures may help the nurse to identify specific difficulties such as body-image issues, functional, physical, sexual, social difficulties and endocrine problems etc.

More recently, tools to measure long-term survivorship have been developed (Zebrack *et al.*, 2006). Whilst formal measures can be extremely useful, they do not necessarily enable the individuals to present the full narrative of their individual experiences; simply encouraging the patients to tell their stories can be exceptionally powerful. Giving patients the time, the forum and the permission to do so is obviously important and signals to the patient that you want to hear them describe their thoughts and feelings and that you are interested in them as an individual. For those patients who find it difficult to articulate their feelings in a narrative or cogent way, encouraging them to describe their feelings in an abstract way through drawing, poetry or visualisation may provide a useful alternative approach.

Some patients may find it useful to draw a road map which identifies the road as they currently perceive it including road blocks, jams, road works and dangerous driving conditions analogous to their diagnosis and treatment. They may also wish to draw a road map to describe how they would like to see the future road as their journey continues. Writing down their feelings, fears and hopes may help to facilitate the patients in understanding what is happening to them emotionally and to recognise that this range of emotions is normal. Making priority lists (a combination of major and relatively 'trivial' items) for the future and introducing suitable timescales may help the patients to begin to map out their

---

Box 16.1   Examples of facilitative patient exercises

- To draw their family members, friends and other sources of support on a single piece of paper (could be stick people) and identify the relationship, the roles, the strength and direction of support.
- To draw a box on a piece of paper and then list all the things that concern them within the box. Where practical, it may be useful to assign a weighting to these concerns. They should then, metaphorically, take each concern out of the box, one at a time, to discuss so that it becomes less overwhelming.
- To draw a road map of their experiences since diagnosis, using traffic lights, bends, road blocks etc., to depict their perceived experience and consider how the future road could look.
- Identify priorities, hopes and ambitions and make a list for the future, together with suitable timescales.

---

hopes and ambitions and provide a means of engaging on the issue with their family and friends (Box 16.1).

CONCLUSION

The overall long-term effects of breast cancer are vast, but the uniqueness of individuals means that each of us will experience the impact of breast cancer in a different way; this in itself makes survivorship almost impossible to define. Through our longitudinal relationships with patients, we often find ourselves in a very privileged position when patients begin to trust us and to allow us to share in their continued journey. To observe and engage with patients on their emotional rollercoaster, with the celebration of completing treatment, yet sometimes struggling with adaptation, redefining their future, managing treatment side effects, family effects, and other aspects of their lives, often makes the experience as a nurse a very humbling one.

Given these experiences, it is essential that nurses contribute to the development of future policies in this area by engaging in debate, undertaking future research and seeking to better understand the long-term survivorship needs of patients. We need to build mechanisms for identifying patients who require ongoing support, so that we can target resources more effectively and ensure patients have access to the care and advice they need. We need to consider the points along the journey that are important to the patient and seek to provide some form of assessment at these points and to evaluate the benefits of interventional programmes to facilitate adaptation. Consideration of the effects on the family and children is also important.

In providing future care, we need to focus on enhancing services that are responsive to the long-term needs of patients. These should provide greater flexibility with more rapid access, and encompass the changing long-term needs of patients. As these needs become less medically orientated, we need to migrate the provision of service and support towards experts in the provision of survivorship education and rehabilitation. This may be supported by improved partnerships with relevant charities.

REFERENCES

Aaronson N, Ahmedzai S, Bergman B *et al.* (1993) The European Organisation for Research and Treatment of Cancer QLQ-C30: a quality of life instrument for use in international clinical trials in oncology. *Journal of the National Cancer Institute* 85(5): 365–376.

Abu-khalaf M, Juneja V, Chung G *et al.* (2007) Long term assessment of cardiac function after dose-dense and intense sequential doxorubicin, placlitaxel, cyclophosphamide as adjuvant therapy for high risk breast cancer. *Breast Cancer Research and Treatment* 104(3): 341–349.

Atkins L and Fallowfield L (2006) Intentional and non-intentional non-adherence to medication amongst breast cancer patients. *European Journal of Cancer* 42(14): 2271–2276.

BASO (2005) Guidelines for the management of symptomatic breast disease. *European Journal of Surgical Oncology* 31 S1–S2.

Brady M, Cella D, Mo F *et al.* (1997) Reliability and validity of the functional assessment of cancer therapy – breast quality of life instrument. *Journal of Clinical Oncology* 15(3): 974–986.

Breaden K (1997) Cancer and beyond; the question of survivorship. *Journal of Advanced Nursing* 26: 978.

Cancer Research UK (2008) *CancerStats Key Facts on Breast Cancer*. London: Cancer Research UK.

Cella D, Tulsky D, Gray G *et al.* (1993) The functional assessment of cancer therapy scale: development and validation of the general measure. *Journal of Clinical Oncology* 11(3): 570–579.

Corner J (2008) Addressing the needs of cancer survivors: issues and challenges. *Pharmacoecomics Outcomes Research* 8(5): 443–451.

Declerck C, Brabander B, Boone C and Geritis P (2002) Locus of control, marital status and predictors of early relapse in primary breast cancer patients. *Psychology and Health* 17(1): 63–76.

Department of Health (2007) *Cancer Reform Strategy*. London: Department of Health. Available: http://www.dh.gov.uk/en/Publicationsandstatistics/Publications/PublicationsPolicyAndGuidance/dh_081006.

Donnelly J, Mack P and Donaldson L (2001) Follow-up of breast cancer: time for a new approach. *International Journal of Clinical Practice* 55(7): 431–433.

Epping-Jordan J, Compas B, Osowiecki D *et al.* (1999) Psychological adjustment in breast cancer: Processes of emotional distress. *Health Psychology* 19(4): 315–326.

Fallowfield L and Hall A (1991) Psychosocial and sexual impact of diagnosis and treatment of breast cancer. *British Medical Bulletin* 47(2): 388–399.

Fallowfield L, Hall A, Maguire GP and Baum M (1990) Psychological outcomes in women with early breast cancer. *British Medical Journal* 301 6765.

Fallowfield L, Leaity S, Howell A, Benson S and Cella D (1999) Assessment of quality of life in women undergoing hormonal therapy for breast cancer: validation of an endocrine symptom subscale for the FACT-B. *Breast Cancer Research and Treatment* 55(2): 189–199.

Farley Short P and Vargo M (2006) Responding to employment concerns of cancer survivors. *Journal of Clinical Oncology* 24(32): 5138–5141.

Freud S (1948) The ego and the mechanisms of defence. London: Hogarth Press.

Gallagher J, Parle M and Cairn D (2002) Appraisal and psychological distress 6 months after diagnosis of breast cancer. *British Journal of Health Psychology* 7(3): 365–376.

Ganz P and Hahn E (2008) Implementing a survivorship care plan for patients with breast cancer. *Journal of Clinical Oncology* 26(5): 759–767.

Ganz P, Coscarelli A, Fred C, Kahn B, Polinski M and Pertersen L (1996) Breast cancer survivors: psychosocial concerns and quality of life. *Breast Cancer Research Treatment* 38 183–199.

Ganz PA, Desmond KA, Leedham B, Rowland JH, Meyerowitz BE and Belin TR (2002) Quality of life in long-term, disease-free survivors of breast cancer: a follow-up study. *Journal of the National Cancer Institute* 2; 94(1): 39–49.

Gil K, Mishel M, Belyea M *et al* (2004) Triggers of uncertainty about recurrence and long term treatment side effects in older African American and Caucasian breast cancer survivors. *Oncology Nursing Forum* 31(3): 633–639.

Goldberg D and Williams P (1988) *A User's Guide to the General Health Questionnaire*. Windsor: NFER-Nelson.

Hall A, Fallowfield L and A'Hern R (1996) When breast cancer recurs: a 3 year prospective study of psychological morbidity. *Breast Journal* 2(3): 197–203.

Health Service Circular (1998) *Breast Cancer* Waiting Times; Achieving the two Week Target. London: HMSO. Available: www.dh.gov.uk/PublicationsAndStatistics/LettersAndCirculars/HealthServiceCirculars/HealthServiceCircularsArticle/fs/en?CONTENT_ID=4004290&chk=Mvye/Y.

Hooning MJ, Botma A, Aleman BM *et al.* (2007) Long-term risk of cardiovascular disease in 10-year survivors of breast cancer. *Journal of the National Cancer Institute* 7; 99(5): 365–375.

Jung BF, Ahrendt GM, Oaklander AL and Dworkin RH (2003) Neuropathic pain following breast cancer surgery: proposed classification and research update. *Pain* 104: 1–13.

Kaiser K (2008) The meaning of the survivor identity for women with breast cancer. *Social Science & Medicine* 67: 79–87.

Kubler-Ross E (1973) *On Death and Dying.* Abingdon: Routledge.

Leigh S (2008) The changing legacy of cancer: issues of long-term survivorship. *Nursing Clinics of North America* 43(2): 243–258.

Lewis F (2006) The effects of cancer survivorship on families and caregivers. *American Journal of Nursing* 106(3): 20–24.

Luker K, Beaver K, Leinster S, Owens R, Degner L and Sloan J (1995) Information needs of women newly diagnosed with breast cancer. *Journal of Advanced Nursing* 22(1): 134–141.

Hooning M, Botma A, Aleman B *et al.* (2007) Long term risk of cardiovascular disease in 10-year survivors of breast cancer. *Journal of the National Cancer Institute* 99(5): 365–375.

Maguire P (1994) ABC breast disease; psychological aspects. *British Medical Journal* 309(6969): 1649–1652.

Mandelblatt J, Cullen J, Lawrence W *et al.* (2008) Ecomonic evaluation alongside a clinical trial of psychoeducation interventions to improve adjustment to survivorship among patients with breast cancer. *Journal of Clinical Oncology* 26(10): 1684–1690.

Maslow AH (1943) A theory of human motivation. *Psychological Review* 50: 370–396.

Mast M (1998) Survivors of breast cancer: Illness uncertainty, positive reappraisal and emotional distress. *Oncology Nursing Forum* 25(3): 555–562.

NHSBSP (2002) *Information and Advice for Health Professionals in Breast Screening.* Sheffield: NHS Cancer Screening Programme. Available: http://www.cancerscreening.nhs.uk/breastscreen/publications/nhsbsp53.pdf.

NICE (2002) *Improving Outcomes in Breast Cancer.* London: National Institute of Clinical Excellence.

Norsati C, Roberts J, Crayford T, McKenzie K and David A (2002) Early psychological adjustment in breast cancer patients. A prospective study. *Journal of Psychosomatic Research* 53: 1123–1130.

Parkes CM (1993) Bereavement as a psychosocial transition: Processes of adaptation to change In: M Stroebe, W Stroebe and R Hansson (eds) *Handbook of Bereavement: Theory, Research and Intervention.* Cambridge: Cambridge University Press.

Peck S (2008) Survivorship: a concept analysis. *Nursing Forum* 43(2): 91–102.

Robinson D, Carrol J and Watson W (2005) Experience building around the family crucible of cancer. *Families, Systems, & Health* 23(2): 131–147.

Rosselli Del Turco M, Palli D, Cariddi A, Ciatto S, Pacinic P and Distante V (1994) Intensive diagnostic follow-up after treatment of primary breast cancer. A randomised trial. *Journal of the American Medical Associate* 271(20): 1583–1597.

Schapira D and Urban N (1991) A minimalist policy for breast cancer surveillance. *Journal of the American Medical Association* 265(3): 380–382.

Sheppard C (2008) Aromatase inhibitors; helping patients choose. *Cancer Nursing Practice* 7(6): 18–20.

Stead M (2003) Sexual dysfunction after treatment for gynaecologic and breast malignancies. *Current Opinion in Obstetrics & Gynecology* 15(1): 57–61.

Steward D, Cheung A, Duff S *et al.* (2001) Long term breast cancer survivors: Confidentiality, disclosure, effects on work and insurance. *Psycho-Oncology* 10: 259–263.

Thewes B, Butow P, Girgis A and Pendlebury A (2004) The psychosocial needs of breast cancer survivors; a qualitative study of the shared and unique needs of younger versus older survivors. *Psycho-Oncology* 13: 177–189.

Watson M, Homewood J, Haviland J and Bliss J (2005) Influence of psychological response on breast cancer survival: 10 year follow up of a population based cohort. *European Journal of Cancer* 41: 1710–1714.

Worden W (1982) *Grief counseling and grief therapy.* New York: Springer.

Zahlis EH (2001) The child's worries about the mother's breast cancer: sources of distress in school-age children. *Oncology Nursing Forum* 28(6): 1019–1025.

Zebrack B, Ganz P, Bernaards C, Petersen L and Abraham L (2006) Assessing the impact of cancer: development of a new instrument for long term survivors. *Psycho-Oncology* 15: 407–421.

Zigmond A and Snaith R (1983) The hospital anxiety and depression scale. *Acta Psychiatrica Scandinavica* 67: 316–370.

17 Specialist Nursing Roles: What Are the Challenges?

Emma Pennery

INTRODUCTION

As the world around us changes, nursing practice is, of course, not immune to evolution and, within the specialty of breast care nursing, change has been inescapable over recent years. Inevitably, such change is both rewarding and challenging. The rewards include witnessing the emergence of new, improved breast cancer treatments, extended options for role development and the advancement of specialist breast care nurses as an influential professional group. However, challenges are also ongoing and involve significantly increased demands on individual post-holders, disappointment over pay grades and an increasing requirement to demonstrate one's worth (both in terms of economical value and in contributing to clinical and patient outcomes). Before considering these challenges in more depth, it is helpful to review the origins of various advanced nursing practice roles within the specialty.

CLINICAL NURSE SPECIALISTS

In the UK between the 1940s and 1970s, it became increasingly noticeable that nurses with ambition moved towards education or management because of the lack of career opportunities and remuneration in clinical care. Subsequent endorsement of Clinical Nurse Specialist (CNS) roles (a title adopted by the Royal College of Nursing in 1975) served as an attempt to retain and promote the value of clinical experts within practice whilst also raising the profile of nursing as a whole. Thus the evolution of CNS roles aimed at keeping successful and ambitious nurses in clinical care whilst also improving standards of specialist nursing input. Initially, application in the area of breast care was somewhat narrow in its focus, demonstrated by early references to post-holders as merely 'mastectomy nurses'. However, the past 15 years or so have witnessed an explosion, both in the numbers of CNSs in breast care and in their profile as a professional group. Broadly, conventional CNSs in breast care support people with benign breast disease, and those who are at high risk of, or already have breast cancer (as well as their families and friends). They provide information, monitor physical and psychological progress, provide emotional support and give practical advice at all points in the disease trajectory about all aspects of the diagnosis, management and impact of breast cancer (Royal College of Nursing, 1999), thus facilitating

Breast Cancer Nursing Care and Management, Second Edition, Edited by Victoria Harmer
© 2011 by Blackwell Publishing Ltd.

continuity and coordination (Armstrong, 2002). The clinical fields of practice associated with conventional CNS roles in breast cancer are as follows:

- Family history and genetics (includes prevention, screening and prophylactic surgery);
- Benign breast conditions;
- National Health Service breast screening;
- Patients newly diagnosed with breast cancer;
- Patients undergoing chemotherapy (and related side effects);
- Patients undergoing radiotherapy (and related side effects);
- Patients on endocrine therapy (and related side effects);
- Breast surgery;
- Breast reconstruction;
- Prosthesis fitting;
- Management of menopausal symptoms;
- Management of lymphoedema;
- Management of fungating wounds;
- Treatment-induced fertility issues;
- Metastatic disease;
- Social issues and finance;
- Recovery, rehabilitation and follow-up (including lifestyle changes).

Central to the development of CNS roles in all specialties was the notion that they would encompass more than just clinical work, and their multi-faceted nature has been repeatedly described in the literature, with core components including clinical practice expertise, education/teaching, management/consultation and research (Yates *et al.*, 2007; Royal College of Nursing, 1988). However, whilst clinical nurse specialism in theory offers an ideal opportunity to combine clinical and academic expertise (Hamric, 1989), the emerging reality is that CNSs struggle to fulfil the role in its entirety (specifically the research elements, which will be discussed later), and the clinical role predominates all others (Armstrong, 2002; McCreadie, 2001).

NURSE PRACTITIONERS

The UK in the 1970s and 1980s also witnessed an increasing number of Nurse Practitioner (NP) roles, which focused on expansion of nursing tasks especially in care traditionally regarded as medical, and existing nursing roles began to extend and expand (for example, undertaking cannulation). Even today, there is still no universally accepted definition of a NP, although the Royal College of Nursing has detailed domains of practice and core competencies required to ensure delivery of safe and effective practice (Royal College of Nursing, 2007a). Essentially, NPs should retain the capacity for advanced level practice but, whilst CNSs are more conventionally placed within a nursing model of care, NPs commonly undertake tasks more akin with medicine. Most NP models encompass assessment (seeing the patient and eliciting data); treatment (making decisions without a doctor and increasingly prescribing); carrying one's own caseload and receiving direct referrals. Within breast care, NP post-holders may also be engaged in nurse-led follow-up clinics but will also commonly run diagnostic clinics, having acquired skills in history taking, clinical examination, imaging and performing fine-needle aspiration and core biopsies (Chapman *et al.*, 2002; Garvican *et al.*, 1998).

CNS VERSUS NP

The above descriptions of two advanced nursing roles within breast care bring us onto one of the challenges post-holders face; that of potential competition between the roles and the pressure to take on extended clinical activity. In reality, CNS and NP roles probably both have legitimate places within breast care and, at least to some extent, will share a common core of knowledge and skills. Moreover, overlap of both roles is already apparent and considerable ambiguity regarding the roles remains, as it is sometimes difficult to clarify precisely the differences between CNSs and NPs within the specialty. This is not least because, as well as discrete NP post-holders, many conventional CNS roles have developed to include NP activity (such as nurse-led family history or follow-up clinics, seroma drainage and nipple tattooing). Thus, role boundaries are becoming more blurred, resulting in blended CNS and NP roles. This is epitomised by the recent publication of clinical standards for nurses working in breast care, which detail the essential knowledge and skills required for conventional and extended (nurse-led) care in 13 key clinical areas regardless of job title (Royal College of Nursing, 2007b).

Of course, NP and blended roles encompassing conventional CNS activity and nurse-led clinics, for example, are not without their potential challenges, and two key challenges relate to facing colleagues who publicly oppose such evolving roles and the time and resources they require to undertake.

With regards to the first of these, specialist breast care nurses have become embroiled in debates that controversially call into question their motivations for establishing NP, extended and nurse-led care, in terms of them representing legitimate areas for the advancement of nursing, versus nurses being utilised as the cheaper alternative. The literature reveals supporters of both camps; those who recognise the potential for NP and blended CNS roles to pioneer new aspects of nursing, versus those who suspect that anyone can be trained to perform mechanical tasks with a view to replacing the necessity for doctors to do them.

As the impetus for change has arisen as much from altered working practices in medicine as in purely nursing per se, tensions exist between those who recognise and welcome opportunities for practice and professional development and those who are concerned about the medicalisation of nursing and therefore the loss of its intrinsic value (Finlay, 2000). Certainly, if one performs only the medical and perhaps mechanical tasks of extended roles without integrating the substance and core of nursing care, there would be no difference between nurses and doctors, and no apparent qualitative improvement to the service offered to people with breast cancer. In fact, evidence suggests that such differences do exist and that the skills of NPs and CNSs adopting nurse-led care enable them to add strength and diversity to nursing practice. For example, a recently published meta-analysis reveals that patients are more satisfied if NPs rather than doctors provide care. It seems that NPs offer longer consultations, compile more complete records and are associated with offering more detailed and helpful advice to patients (Horrocks *et al.*, 2002). Such themes have also been demonstrated in studies on NP and extended CNS activity specifically in breast cancer care. Specialist nurses working in breast diagnostic clinics (taking histories, conducting examinations and giving patients test results) have been demonstrated to be safe, acceptable to patients and associated with more satisfaction, less anxiety, more information provision, equal decision-making skills and a lower percentage of inadequate cytology specimens when compared with doctors in a breast clinic (Hammond *et al.*, 1995; Garvican *et al.*, 1998).

Indeed, my own experience of providing nurse-led follow-up after treatment for breast cancer substantiates the above, with greater satisfaction reported in women seen in the nurse-led clinic when compared with traditional medical follow-up. A randomised controlled trial comparing follow-up by the two professional groups revealed that key advantages of the nurse-led clinic include improved continuity and greater attention paid to emotional needs and answering questions, thus attending to the issues that women perceive hinder rehabilitation and recovery. Although not always easy to articulate why, women noticed a shift of emphasis from the traditional medical model of physical examination of the breast, to a consultation that focused on the individual patient and the unique impact of breast cancer on their lives. According to the study, areas that specifically benefit from being attended to within the nurse-led clinic include management of menopausal symptoms, information regarding lifestyle changes and the opportunity to revisit prognosis and individual likelihood of disease recurrence (Pennery, 2005). Perhaps, therefore, any weaknesses in extending nursing roles in this way lie not in their underlying philosophy but in their execution.

The other key challenge, particularly for conventional CNSs extending their role activity, results from the increased pressures on the post-holder, specifically in terms of time. With traditional posts already evolving to reflect breast cancer treatment advances, an obvious concern is that further expansion of duties to incorporate even some extended-role activities, may result in compromised standards of care or individual burn out of the post-holder! Even without more widespread adoption of nurse-led activity, demands on time have already been mounting as recent years have heralded numerous changes in the management of breast cancer. For example, a greater understanding of cancer genetics has resulted in more women having prophylactic mastectomy; more sophisticated breast-reconstruction techniques require lengthy consultations to facilitate choice; and novel endocrine and targeted therapies necessitate complex explanations of treatment options.

Amid all of the above, the incidence of breast cancer is increasing worldwide every year, whilst mortality rates are beginning to fall (Cancer Research UK, 2008), resulting in greater numbers of patients undergoing routine follow-up after their treatment is over. Specialist nurses face the challenge of maintaining up-to-date knowledge in a fast-moving and complex clinical area, as well as developing the skills to deliver extended-role activity safely and effectively. An arguably counterproductive outcome of role extension, at least for some teams, is the sacrificing of other invaluable areas of care. This is illustrated by one study in which 20% of almost 300 breast care nurse specialists reported having insufficient time to spend with patients to be able to provide basic psychological support (Breast Cancer Care and Royal College of Nursing, 2004).

Thus, it may be prudent for all post-holders to consider the needs of their local area when planning implementation of extended nursing practice posts. CNSs with a predominant focus on surgery rather than chemotherapy and radiotherapy, for example, may consider surgically-related role extensions, such as seroma drainage, to achieve legitimate improvements in patient care. Selection of CNS, NP and blended skill-mix according to post-holders, local service needs and delivery gives further support to the concept of both posts existing in harmony rather than in opposition. However, an important consideration of extended-role practice, by a CNS or an NP, is whether it will result in a standard of service that is, at the very least, comparable (ideally superior) to the one that it replaces. Some years ago, the Royal College of Nursing (1999) suggested a checklist of relevant considerations to help individuals and teams considering adopting advanced nursing practice roles in breast care. This checklist for extended roles in breast cancer care is still in use today, and the following is adapted from the 1999 document.

- Is this new skill/role consistent with nursing practice?
- Is it consistent with my current job description?
- Does it fit current priorities – nursing and organisational?
- What changes will it entail?
- Will I need to stop some parts of my current role/care?
- Do I need accreditation?
- How will I get it?
- Do I need additional skills/training?
- How will I get them?
- How will I document them?
- Do I need a training period before I take on new responsibility?
- Do I have a mentor for this change?
- How will I evaluate my performance in this new role?
- Have I got clinical supervision?
- How will it improve patient care?
  (Reproduced with permission from the Royal College of Nursing)

Of course in the future CNS, NP and blended roles may be increasingly superseded by the introduction of Nurse Consultant posts. This newer advanced nursing practice role was introduced because of perceived ongoing limitations with the existing clinical career structure in nursing, which had resulted in expert nurses leaving due to the lack of practice-based promotional posts and to improve their earnings. Sub-roles of nurse consultants are expert practice; professional leadership and consultancy; education, training and development; and practice and service development. Nurse consultants aim to possess skills and competencies similar to those of CNSs, but with greater breadth and complexity (National Health Service Executive, 1999). However, with fewer overall numbers of nurse consultants in post than predicted (Department of Health, 2004) and limited application to breast care (at the time of writing, only six nurse consultant posts specifically in breast care have been appointed), the success, impact and proliferation of these roles have yet to be robustly appraised.

PROVING OUR WORTH

Changes in provision of health care generally have had an irreversible effect on how the management of breast cancer is organised. For example, patients experience shorter stays in hospital after operations, increasingly returning home on the day of surgery, and rapid access to services is to be the norm rather than the exception. In an attempt to mandate safe and effective care, the Government imposed standards that relate to expeditious management of patients with breast cancer, including a maximum 2-week wait for a hospital appointment following urgent referral by the general practitioner and a maximum 1-month wait from diagnosis to commencement of treatment (Department of Health, 2000). Strategies are ongoing to ensure that these standards are met (Department of Health, 2006), and the performance of individual hospitals is now available for scrutiny as summaries of cancer waiting times are published every quarter (Department of Health, 2008). Whilst such targets are undeniably virtuous, they inevitably place pressure on resources and this pressure, coupled with more stringent complaints procedures, ensures that there are penalties to getting it wrong. Interestingly, breast cancer is the most common diagnosis in medical malpractice claims in the USA (Anderson and Troxel, 2005). All this means that specialist breast care nurses are increasingly under pressure to detail their contribution to the key targets on which performance is measured and income is reliant. They have, in turn, become much more accountable for their contribution to the multidisciplinary approach to the management of breast disease.

In spite of this, documents that detail mandatory aspects of service delivery specifically related to breast cancer encouragingly always make reference to the pivotal role of specialist nurses. For example, the Association of Breast Surgery at the British Association of Surgical Oncology produces regularly updated guidelines on the management of breast disease that encompass primary care and diagnostic services, quality assurance and multidisciplinary working, medical therapies, recurrent and metastatic disease and workload and training issues. They reiterate the consensus opinion that all patients diagnosed with breast cancer should be offered the opportunity to access a breast care nurse specialist throughout the disease trajectory (Association of Breast Surgery, 2005). Similarly, the *Guidelines on Improving Outcomes in Breast Cancer* (National Institute of Clinical Effectiveness, 2002) detail recommendations for improving the process and consequence of numerous aspects of breast cancer management and care. Again, the suggestion that nurses invaluably contribute to team-working and inter-professional communication is decisive. Most recently, the *Cancer Reform Strategy* is very clear that 'commissioners ... should give particular consideration to the role of the clinical nurse specialists, who play a critical role in cancer care' (Department of Health, 2007 p 10).

This endorsement of specialist nursing roles comes in part from the increased recognition that high-quality cancer care encompasses far more than just survival rates from the disease. In addition to improving mortality figures, the unique impact of breast cancer and its treatment, and hence the importance of individualised care, is crucially acknowledged. Recent years have seen an upsurge in research studies which demonstrate the very real psychosocial, emotional and informational needs of people with breast cancer at all stages of their treatment and subsequent recovery (for example, Reich *et al.*, 2008; Parker *et al.*, 2007; Fobair *et al.*, 2006; Burgess *et al.*, 2005; Vivar and McQueen, 2005; Engel *et al.*, 2004; Oh *et al.*, 2004; National Institute of Clinical Effectiveness, 2004; Burstein and Winer, 2000; Maguire, 2000). Specialist nurses are particularly well placed to deliver high-quality psychosocial care, not only at diagnosis but also in response to the patient's complex needs arising during and after treatments (such as making treatment decisions, coping with menopausal symptoms and potentially impaired fertility and learning to live with the fear of recurrence).

BUILDING AN EVIDENCE BASE

Thus the imperative for psychosocial support for people with breast cancer (men and women) is widely accepted and few (health professionals or patients) would question the crucial contribution that specialist breast care nurses make. However, despite this public and professional endorsement, they have struggled as a professional group to produce meaningful, robust evidence to underpin their value and to demonstrate the improved outcomes they bring to their patients. This might be for several reasons.

First and foremost, nurses have not traditionally been skilled in research methodology (conducting or evaluating research) and have been relatively slow as a professional group in embracing the necessity for devising an evidence base of their own. However, this is changing, and the profession is noticeably moving from a reliance on tasks and procedures to interventions that are based on rigorous appraisal of evidence (Crinson, 1999). Secondly, even with this new knowledge, as alluded to earlier, nurses do not often have the time or resources to conduct evaluation activity. Thirdly, successful evaluation of nurse-led care is sometimes inhibited because it is notoriously difficult to articulate the art of caring, in other words to explicitly (and scientifically) describe and demonstrate how nurses actually make a qualitative and quantitative difference to care.

Bearing in mind these obstacles to specialist nurses conducting research, it was perhaps not unsurprising that a recent Cochrane review, designed to assess the effectiveness of interventions carried out by specialist breast care nurses, revealed a paucity of randomised, high-quality trials in this area (Cruickshank *et al.*, 2008). Only five studies met the criteria for the review, of which only three found some improvements in quality of life arising from specialist nursing interventions. The review authors conclude 'there is limited evidence at this time to support the contention that interventions by specialist breast care nurses assist . . . with the recognition and management of psychological distress for women with breast cancer' (Cruickshank *et al.*, 2008 p 2).

Yet, in spite of well-documented problems with methodology and comparability highlighted in this systematic review, as well as in other studies and previous reviews, specialist nursing input undoubtedly makes a unique contribution to improved patient outcomes. Benefits that specialist nurses bring to their patients, as described in the literature by both patients and other health professionals, include recognising and reducing psychological distress, anxiety, depression and insomnia; inspiring confidence with decision making and enhancing understanding of their disease and treatments; more efficient and effective multidisciplinary team performance including more appropriate referrals and prolonging continuity throughout the whole disease trajectory (Campbell *et al.*, 2006; Eicher *et al.*, 2006; Halkett *et al.*, 2006; Amir *et al.*, 2004; Haward *et al.*, 2003; Liebert *et al.*, 2003; National Breast Cancer Centre's Specialist Breast Nurse Project Team, 2003).

For example, in one study, 277 women having surgery were randomised to receive current routine care, routine care plus support from a voluntary counselling organisation, routine care plus input from a specialist nurse or all three. The researchers found that support from the specialist nurses alone was of more benefit in reducing psychological distress than any other combination of services (McArdle *et al.*, 1996). Similar findings are reported more recently by Ritz *et al.* (2000) in whose randomised study evaluating quality of life in more than 100 women seen by advanced nurse practitioners, specialist nursing interventions were found to contribute significantly to reducing anxiety compared to medical care alone, at 6 months following a breast cancer diagnosis. The strongest effects were recorded in the sub-scales of inconsistency and unpredictability, with nurses significantly reducing the effects of these and improving mood states and wellbeing overall (Ritz *et al.*, 2000).

THE IMPLICATIONS OF FAILING TO PROVE OUR WORTH

It seems, therefore, that specialist breast care nurses face a paradox in that their input is mandated in policy documents and highly valued by patients and health professionals alike, whilst failing (at least in part) to be underpinned by a robust evidence base. Some might question whether this matters. Arguably it does in a world in which hospitals are forced to focus on costs more than ever before (Snow, 2006), and CNS roles are being placed under ever-increasing scrutiny (Leary, 2007). This is evident in the results of two unpublished surveys of specialist breast care nurses, one carried out by the Association of Breast Surgery (at the British Association of Surgical Oncology, 2006), and the other jointly between Breakthrough Breast Cancer, Breast Cancer Care and the Royal College of Nursing (2006). The prevalent findings from both surveys revealed that CNSs in breast care felt at risk of redundancy or being down-graded; were unhappy with their Agenda for Change job banding; had been asked to return to ward duties; were under resourced because of vacant posts not being filled or frozen and being asked to take on extra (non-standard) CNS responsibilities; and felt enormously under-valued. A further Royal College of Nursing survey of 330 specialist nurses from a variety of clinical specialties (not all cancer) (Royal College of Nursing, 2008) echoed these exact themes, with a fifth reporting being at risk of redundancy (Royal College of Nursing, 2008).

The above has probably been compounded by the aforementioned gaps in the evidence base underpinning specialist nurses and by them finding it difficult to meaningfully describe what they do, thus rendering demands to produce business cases demonstrating their economic worth a real challenge. This might be relieved a little in the future by an innovative attempt to help CNSs articulate elements of their activity which are notoriously difficult to describe in a more sophisticated way using a mathematical model called Pandora (Leary, 2007). The absolute benefits of this approach are eagerly awaited.

EDUCATION AND TRAINING

Another key challenge and a major difficulty with standardisation of both CNS and NP roles relates to training and qualifications. Unfortunately, specific courses, especially for extended roles, may not be readily available and, certainly within breast care, there are very few accredited courses that prepare one for extended-role activities such as breast palpation. General programmes of study for NPs have begun to emerge (usually at Master's level) and largely include a greater focus on anatomy and physiology, comprehensive physical assessment, diagnostics, pharmacology, pathophysiology and disease management. Professional bodies suggest that recognised NP qualifications should be undertaken if extended-role tasks are a major focus of the individual job description. However, it is arguable as to what extent possession of core physical assessment skills, such as percussion and auscultation, will be relevant to specialist nurses in very specific clinical areas such as breast care.

As a result, new nursing roles akin with medicine are commonly undertaken only after informal training and without a record of competence or measurement of ongoing development. Learning 'on the job' does not automatically result in explicit documentation, not only of initial training but equally as important, maintenance of the skill through ongoing practice. Therefore, training and proficiency in extended-role tasks must be clearly documented, and such tasks should be practised continuously to maintain competence. It is essential that if specialist breast care nurses are to be accountable and to make professionally autonomous decisions for which they have sole responsibility, documentation of practical experience and training in order to demonstrate competence to perform extended-role tasks is essential. The recent implementation of one or two advanced clinical practice courses aimed specifically at nurses working in breast care practitioner roles should certainly help with this in the future.

Standardising minimum education and training for all specialist nurses will help to mitigate against the problem of substantial variations in the grades associated with such posts (from band 5 to 8C) and thus lessen the potential for unjust remuneration for work undertaken (both over- and under-payment of post-holders relative to experience and qualifications). In recognition of this, the Royal College of Nursing Breast Care Nurses Forum declared that consensus and clarity are vital to ensure optimum standards of specialist nursing care for individuals with breast cancer. Thus they propose definitions of advanced nursing practice roles and minimum educational and practice requirements for those aspiring to them (Royal College of Nursing, 2002). Of course, some diversity in role function will always be apparent because of several influencing factors.

The type of work-setting will determine overall numbers of referrals and treatment modalities offered. For example, not all centres offer specialist services such as cancer genetics or breast reconstruction. Some CNSs will not be involved with chemotherapy or radiotherapy on site and some have no input into palliative care. Also there is diversity in nursing practice according to the availability and extent of the local multidisciplinary team. For example, some CNSs will be actively involved in lymphoedema management and prosthesis fitting, whilst others will benefit from physiotherapists, lymphoedema nurse specialists and appliance officers who undertake the majority of such tasks. Finally, different practice settings will require the CNS to have different levels of input in outpatients versus inpatients, private versus National Health Service and on-site versus home visits.

CONCLUDING THOUGHTS

Amidst such daunting challenges, it is perhaps important to remind ourselves why specialist breast care nursing roles (NPs, CNSs or Nurse Consultants) exist and how. The *why*, of course, should always have patient care at its core. Opportunities for improving patient care and developing the professional value of nursing should always remain a priority over politics and power struggles, but this can be difficult in the face of increasing challenges and decreasing morale. Extended roles integrating medical tasks are welcomed if they do not compromise conventional specialist nursing care. Complementing rather than competing with existing medical or nursing models can only serve to enhance both patients and all professional groups. Indeed complementing is essential if we are to avoid the temptation of becoming all things to all people.

The requirement to demonstrate explicitly the value of specialist roles to patients with breast cancer is ongoing, yet crucial research into the impact of such roles on patient outcomes remains problematical and somewhat elusive. A unique feature of specialist breast care nurses is their close and prolonged interaction with their patients, and it may be worthwhile to direct future efforts towards evaluating this as well as the outcomes it produces. In other words, demonstrating what it is specifically about specialist nursing that enhances care (the process) in order to verify its continued investment. All health professionals have an obligation to measure in some way their impact in relation to the needs of the people they care for. If specialist breast care nurses were to succeed in producing comprehensive and high-quality evidence of the ways in which they benefit the delivery and outcomes of care, the future for them and their patients will be bright. However, as the

Cochrane review authors acknowledge, even without this they remain 'an integrated and respected part of the multidisciplinary team' (Cruickshank *et al.*, 2008, p. 16).

The *how* relates to appropriate selection, training and implementation of specialist nursing roles. CNS and NP roles (both separately and blended) are arguably invaluable in our increasingly complex specialist area, but such roles are not for everyone and any role changes must be voluntary and not coerced. Extended nursing roles should never be implemented without lengthy consideration of the prerequisite issues common to all:

- Time (to adequately conduct role);
- Training (formal and informal, by whom and level);
- Qualifications (and background);
- Litigation – an appreciation of the legal implications of extended roles (inexperience is not considered a defence);
- Accountability – approval and sanction of employer;
- Documentation (explicit and meaningful);
- Resources;
- Evaluation (rigorous outcome measures);
- Sound motivation.

An intriguing outstanding dilemma is to what extent NPs need a background in breast cancer care prior to undertaking the role. Some existing post-holders fulfil the NP role with backgrounds such as practice nursing and receive what is often comprehensive training in the extended-role *tasks*. However, my experience from the nurse-led follow-up clinic is that patients may ask numerous questions about all aspects of their disease and management other than those relevant to that consultation or task. It is my extensive knowledge of breast cancer that allows me to address rather than defer such concerns. I am unable to say how my effectiveness would have been appraised without this knowledge. Perhaps this further supports the notion of a working model that blends the two roles, rather than pitting them against one another.

Of course, unresolved issues pertaining to specialist nursing roles in breast care remain, not least regarding pay. Insisting on consistency in role titles might go some way to resolving this. Currently, such roles in breast cancer use a misleading variety of titles (including breast care nurse, breast care sister, clinical nurse specialist, nurse practitioner, specialist nurse practitioner, breast nurse clinician, consultant nurse and nurse consultant), hold different grades and are qualified to various different levels. This lack of consistency renders them somewhat meaningless with regards to expectations of colleagues, managers and patients and is undoubtedly an obstacle to instigation of new posts.

I would urge post-holders to contribute to professional debate and to ensure in the future that posts revolve around evidence-based discovery of the differences various health-care professionals offer and identification of the best professional to enhance patient care at that time. Salvage and Smith (2000) wisely advise letting go of resentments and boundary disputes and instead directing efforts towards capitalising on the wealth of skills that all professionals can bring to bear on solving health problems and improving services for patients.

Interestingly, similar conclusions were drawn by White (2001) some years ago, who suggested it is time for specialist breast care nurses to concentrate on precise role modelling and definitions, establishing core educational requirements and providing the evidence which proves effectiveness. However, whilst White perceived that the pioneering days for specialist breast care nurse were over, I assert that they still coming into their own. Breast cancer is a dynamic and exciting area in which to work, and I hope that you will share my confidence that we can look forward to seeing nurses (in various roles) very much at the forefront of this care in the future.

REFERENCES

Amir Z, Scully J and Borrill C (2004) The professional role of breast cancer nurses in multi-disciplinary breast cancer care teams. *European Oncology Nursing Society* 8: 306–314.

Anderson R and Troxel B (2005) Breast cancer litigation. In: R Anderson (ed.) *Medical Malpractice: A Physician's Handbook*. NJ: Humana Press, Chapter 12, p 153.

Armstrong S, Tolson D and West B (2002) Role development in acute nursing in Scotland. *Nursing Standard* 16(17): 33–38.

Association of Breast Surgery, at the British Association of Surgical Oncology (2005) Guidelines for the Management of Symptomatic Breast Disease. *European Journal of Surgical Oncology* 31: 51–521.

Association of Breast Surgery, at the British Association of Surgical Oncology. (2006) *Email Survey of Breast Care Nurses*. (Unpublished survey).

Breakthrough Breast Cancer, Breast Cancer Care and the Royal College of Nursing. (2006) *Breast Care Nurse Survey: Summary of Results*. (Unpublished survey).

Breast Cancer Care, Royal College of Nursing (2004) *Time to Care: Maintaining Access to Breast Care Nurses*. London: Alpine Press.

Burgess C, Cornelius V, Love S, Graham J, Richards M and Ramirez A (2005) Depression and anxiety in women with early breast cancer: five year observational cohort study. *British Medical Journal* 330: 702.

Burstein H and Winer E (2000) Primary care of survivors of breast cancer. *New England Journal of Medicine* 343(15): 1086–1094.

Campbell D, Khan A, Rankin N, Williams P and Redman S (2006) Are specialist nurses available to Australian women with breast cancer? *Cancer Nursing* 29(1): 43–48.

Cancer Research UK (2008) *Breast Cancer Key Facts*. Available: http://info.cancerresearchuk.org/cancerstats/types/breast.

Chapman D, Purushotham A and Wishart G (2002) Nurse practitioner training in breast examination. *Nursing Standard* 17(2): 33–36.

Crinson I (1999) Clinical governance: the new NHS, new responsibilities? *British Journal of Nursing* 8(7): 449–453.

Cruickshank S, Kennedy C, Lockhart K, Dosser I and Dallas L (2008) Specialist breast care nurses for supportive care of women with breast cancer. *Cochrane Database of Systematic Reviews* Issue 1, Art. No.: CD005634. DOI: 10.1002/14651858.CD005634.pub2.

Department of Health (2000) *The National Health Service Cancer Plan*. London: HMSO.

Department of Health (2004) *NHS Hospital and Community Health Service Non-Medical Workforce Census, England 2004: Detailed Results*. London: HMSO.

Department of Health (2006) *Waiting Times for Cancer: Progress, Lessons Learned and Next Steps*. London: HMSO.

Department of Health (2007) *Cancer Reform Strategy*. London: HMSO, p. 10.

Department of Health (2008) http://www.performance.doh.gov.uk/cancerwaits/2008/q1/part4.html.

Eicher M, Marquard S and Aebi S (2006) A nurse is a nurse? A systematic review of the effectiveness of specialised nursing in breast cancer. *European Journal of Cancer*, 42(18): 3117–3126.

Engel J, Kerr J, Schlesinger-Raab A, Sauer H and Hölzel D (2004) Quality of life following breast-conserving therapy or mastectomy: results of a 5-year prospective study. *The Breast Journal* 10(3): 223–231.

Finlay T (2000) The scope of professional practice: a literature review to determine the document's impact on nurses' role. *Nursing Times Research* 5(2): 115–125.

Fobair P, Stewart SL, Chang S *et al.* (2006) Body image and sexual problems in young women with breast cancer. *Psycho-Oncology* 5(7): 579–594.

Garvican l, Grimsey E, Littlejohns P, Lowndes S and Sacks N (1998) Satisfaction with clinical nurse specialists in a breast care clinic; questionnaire survey. *British Medical Journal* 316: 976–977.

Halkett G, Arbon P, Scutter S and Borg M (2006) The role of the breast care nurse during treatment for early breast cancer: the patient's perspective. *Contemporary Nurse* 23(1): 46–57.

Hammond C, Chase J and Hogbin B (1995) A unique service? *Nursing Times* 91(30): 28–29.

Hamric A (1989) History and overview of the CNS role. In: A Hamric and J Sproß (eds) *The Clinical Nurse Specialist in Theory and Practice*, 2nd edn. Philadelphia: WB Saunders.

Haward R, Amir Z, Borrill C *et al.* (2003) Breast cancer teams: the impact of constitution, new cancer workload and methods of operation on their effectiveness. *British Journal of Cancer* 89: 15–22.

Horrocks S, Anderson E and Salisbury C (2002) Systematic review of whether nurse practitioners working in primary care can provide equivalent care to doctors. *British Medical Journal* 324: 819–823.

Leary A (2007) Vital statistics. *Nursing Standard* 21(17): 18–19.

Liebert B, Parle M, Roberts C *et al.* (2003) An evidence based specialist breast nurse role in practice: a multicentre implementation study. *European Journal of Cancer Care* 12(1): 91–97.

Maguire P (2000) Psychological aspects. In: J Dixon (ed.) *ABC of Breast Diseases*, 2nd edn). London: BMJ Publishing Group.

McArdle J, George W, McArdle C, Smith D, Moodie A, Hughson A and Murray G (1996) Psychological support for patients undergoing breast cancer surgery: a randomised study. *British Medical Journal* 312: 813–816.

McCreadie M (2001) The role of the clinical nurse specialist. *Nursing Standard* 16(10): 33–38.

National Breast Cancer Centre's Specialist Breast Nurse Project Team (2003) An evidence-based specialist breast nurse role in practice: a multi-centre implementation study. *European Journal of Cancer Care* 12: 91–97.

National Health Service Executive (1999) *Health Service Circular: Nurses, Midwives and Health Visitor Consultants: Establishing Posts and Making Appointments*. Department of Health. London: HMSO.

National Institute of Clinical Effectiveness (2002) *Guidance on Cancer Services: Improving Outcomes in Breast Cancer – Manual Update*. London: National Institute of Clinical Effectiveness.

National Institute of Clinical Effectiveness (2004) *Guidance on Cancer Services – Improving Supportive and Palliative Care for Adults with Cancer: The Manual*. London: National Institute of Clinical Effectiveness.

Oh S, Heflin L, Meyerowitz B *et al.* (2004) Quality of life of breast cancer survivors after a recurrence: a follow-up study. *Breast Cancer Research and Treatment* 87(1): 45–57.

Parker PA, Youssef A, Walker S, Basen-Engquist K, Cohen L, Gritz ER, Wei QX and Robb GL (2007) Short-term and long-term psychosocial adjustment and quality of life in women undergoing different surgical procedures for breast cancer. *Annals of Surgical Oncology* 14(11): 3078–3089.

Pennery E (2005) *Providers and Recipients of Breast Cancer Follow-up: Addressing Needs and Optimising Service Delivery*. D. Phil thesis, University of Southampton.

Reich M, Lesur A and Perdrizet-Chevallier C (2008) Depression, quality of life and breast cancer: a review of the literature. *Breast Cancer Research and Treatment* 110(1): 9–17.

Ritz L, Nissen M, Swenson K *et al.* (2000) Effects of advanced nursing care on quality of life and cost outcomes of women diagnosed with breast cancer. *Oncology Nursing Forum* 27(6): 923–932.

Royal College of Nursing (1975) *New Horizons in Clinical Nursing*. London: Royal College of Nursing.

Royal College of Nursing (1988) *A Report of the Working Party Investigating the Development of Specialties within the Nursing Profession*. London: Royal College of Nursing.

Royal College of Nursing (1999) *Developing Roles: Nurses Working In Breast Care*. London: Royal College of Nursing.

Royal College of Nursing (2002) *Advanced Nursing Practice in Breast Cancer Care* London: RCN Direct.

Royal College of Nursing (2007a) Advanced Nursing Practitioner Competencies. http://www.rcn.org.uk/_data/assets/pdf_file/0014/114503/RCN_ANP_competencies_for_July_07_AU_Board.pdf

Royal College of Nursing (2007b) *Clinical Standards for Working in a Breast Specialty. RCN Guidance for Nursing Staff*. London: RCN Direct.

Royal College of Nursing (2008) *Briefing Paper: Final Results of Specialist Nurse Survey*. Available: http://www.rcn.org.uk/newsevents/news/article/uk/specialist_nurses_targeted_to_cut_nhs_costs.

Salvage J and Smith R (2000) Doctors and Nurses: Doing it Differently. *British Medical Journal* 320: 1019–1020.

Snow T (2006) Prove your worth. *Nursing Standard* 20(48): 12–14.

Vivar C and McQueen A (2005) Informational and emotional needs of long term survivors of breast cancer. *Journal of Advanced Nursing* 51(5): 520–528.

White S (2001) A dual role ... breast care nurse specialist. *Nursing Standard* 15(42): 59.

Yates P, Evans A, Moore A *et al.* (2007) Competency standards and educational requirements for specialist breast nurses in Australia. *Collegian* 14(1): 11–15.

Index

Page numbers in italics represent figures, those in bold represent tables.

Printed and bound by CPI Group (UK) Ltd, Croydon, CR0 4YY